ECGs MADE EASY

Barbara Aehlert, MSEd, BSPA, RN

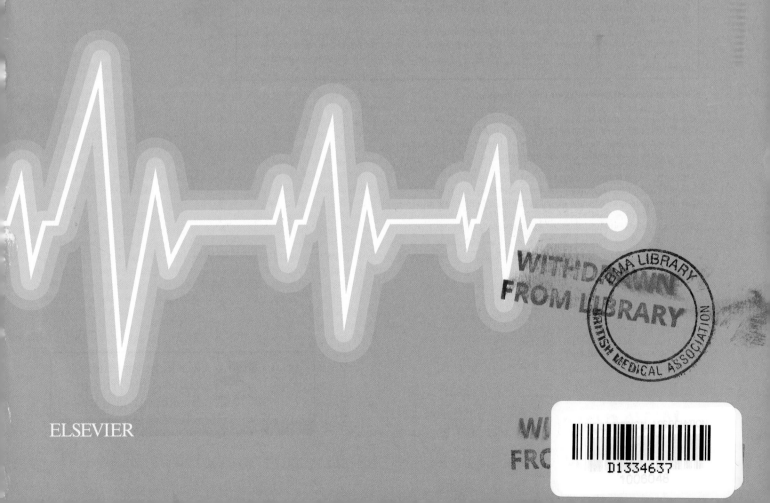

ELSEVIER

ELSEVIER

3251 Riverport Lane
St. Louis, Missouri 63043

Library of Congress Cataloging-in-Publication Data

Names: Aehlert, Barbara, author.
Title: ECGs made easy / Barbara Aehlert, MSEd, BSPA, RN.
Description: Sixth edition. | Phoenix, Arizona : Southwest EMS Education,
   Inc., [2018] | Includes bibliographical references and index. |
   Identifiers: LCCN 2017015081 (print) | LCCN 2017026543 (ebook) | ISBN
   9780323479059 () | ISBN 9780323401302 (pbk. : alk. paper)
Subjects: LCSH: Electrocardiography--Handbooks, manuals, etc.
Classification: LCC RC683.5.E5 (ebook) | LCC RC683.5.E5 A39 2018 (print) |
   DDC 616.1/207547--dc23
LC record available at https://lccn.loc.gov/2017015081

Executive Content Strategist: Sandra Clark
Content Development Specialists: Laura Selkirk/Melissa Kinsey
Publishing Services Manager: Deepthi Unni
Senior Project Manager: Umarani Natarajan
Design Direction: Brian Salisbury

Printed in Canada

Last digit is the print number: 9 8 7 6 5 4 3 2

Working together
to grow libraries in
developing countries

www.elsevier.com • www.bookaid.org

Preface to the Sixth Edition

Many years ago, as a green but enthusiastic nurse preparing to shift from medical-surgical nursing to critical care, I signed up for a course in basic ECG recognition. It was an intimidating experience. My instructor was extremely knowledgeable and kind, and I studied diligently throughout the course, yet I struggled to crack the code of heart rhythm interpretation. To make matters worse, I couldn't find any resources in which these complex concepts were presented in a practical, useful way. Although I passed the course, I decided to repeat it a few months later because I simply couldn't recall and apply the information I needed to help my patients.

After successfully completing the second course, I promised myself that I would someday present these concepts in a simpler way. That promise became my life's work. Ever since then, I have been looking for better ways in which to present the skill of basic ECG recognition to those who will apply that knowledge every working day:

- Paramedics
- Nursing and medical students
- ECG monitor technicians
- Nurses and other allied health personnel working in emergency departments, critical care units, postanesthesia care units, operating rooms, and telemetry units

This book can be used alone or as part of a formal course of instruction in basic dysrhythmia recognition. The book's content focuses on the essentials of ECG interpretation. Each ECG rhythm is described and accompanied by a sample rhythm strip. Then the discussion turns to possible signs and symptoms related to each rhythm and, where appropriate, current recommended treatment. At the end of each chapter, additional rhythm strips and their descriptions are provided for practice. (All rhythm strips shown in this text were recorded in lead II unless otherwise noted.) The Stop & Review exercises at the end of each chapter are self-assessment activities that allow you to check your learning.

In addition, resources to aid the instructor in teaching this content can be found on Evolve at http://evolve.elsevier.com/Aehlert/ecg/. These resources include:

- Image Collection
- PPT Slides
- PPT Practice Slides
- TEACH 2.4
- Test Bank

I have made every attempt to supply content consistent with current literature, including current resuscitation guidelines. However, medicine is a dynamic field. Recommendations change as medical research evolves, technology improves, and new medications, procedures, and devices are developed. As a result, be sure to learn and follow local protocols as defined by your medical advisors. Neither I nor the publisher can assume responsibility or liability for loss or damage resulting from the use of information contained within.

I genuinely hope this book is helpful to you, and I wish you success in your studies and clinical practice.

Best regards,
Barbara Aehlert

Acknowledgments

I would like to thank the manuscript reviewers for their comments and suggestions. Areas of this text were rewritten, reorganized, and clarified because of your efforts.

I would also like to thank the following health care professionals, who provided many of the rhythm strips used in this book: Andrew Baird, CEP; James Bratcher; Joanna Burgan, CEP; Holly Button, CEP; Gretchen Chalmers, CEP; Thomas Cole, CEP; Brent Haines, CEP; Paul Honeywell, CEP; Timothy Klatt, RN; Bill Loughran, RN; Andrea Lowrey, RN; Joe Martinez, CEP; Stephanos Orphanidis, CEP; Jason Payne, CEP; Steve Ruehs, CEP; Patty Seneski, RN; David Stockton, CEP; Jason Stodghill, CEP; Dionne Socie, CEP; Kristina Tellez, CEP; and Fran Wojculewicz, RN.

A special thanks to Melissa Kinsey for her humor, guidance, advice, and impeccable attention to detail throughout this project.

To

Deepak C. Patel, MD

whose knowledge, humor, and genuine compassion for his
patients are unparalleled.

Reviewers for the Sixth Edition

Kristen Borchelt, RN, MSN, FNP, NR-P, CPN
Care Coordinator
Cincinnati Children's Hospital Medical Center
Cincinnati, Ohio

Joshua Borkosky, BS, FP-C
EMS Education Manager
University of Cincinnati College of Medicine
Cincinnati, Ohio

Angela McConachie, DNP, MSN-FNP, RN
Assistant Professor
Goldfarb School of Nursing at Barnes-Jewish College
St. Louis, Missouri

Bill Miller
Paramedic Crew Chief
St. Louis Fire Department–BEMS
St. Louis, Missouri

Mark Nootens, MD, FACC
Cardiologist, Private Practice
Munster, Indiana

Ruth C. Tamulonis, MS, RN
Nursing Professor
Yuba College
Marysville, California

About the Author

Barbara Aehlert, MSEd, BSPA, RN, has been a registered nurse for more than 40 years, with clinical experience in medical/surgical nursing, critical care nursing, prehospital education, and nursing education. Barbara is an active CPR and Advanced Cardiovascular Life Support (ACLS) instructor with a special interest in teaching basic dysrhythmia recognition and ACLS to nurses and paramedics.

Contents

9 INTRODUCTION TO THE 12-LEAD ECG, 241

10 POSTTEST, 278

INDEX, 321

Anatomy and Physiology

LEARNING OBJECTIVES

After reading this chapter, you should be able to:

1. Describe the location of the heart.
2. Identify the surfaces of the heart.
3. Describe the structure and function of the coverings of the heart.
4. Identify the three cardiac muscle layers.
5. Identify and describe the chambers of the heart and the vessels that enter or leave each.
6. Identify and describe the location of the atrioventricular and semilunar valves.
7. Explain atrial kick.
8. Name the primary branches and areas of the heart supplied by the right and left coronary arteries.
9. Define and explain acute coronary syndromes.
10. Discuss myocardial ischemia, injury, and infarction, indicating which conditions are reversible and which are not.
11. Compare and contrast the effects of sympathetic and parasympathetic stimulation of the heart.
12. Identify and discuss each phase of the cardiac cycle.
13. Beginning with the right atrium, describe blood flow through the normal heart and lungs to the systemic circulation.
14. Identify and explain the components of blood pressure and cardiac output.

KEY TERMS

acute coronary syndrome (ACS): A term used to refer to distinct conditions caused by a similar sequence of pathologic events— a temporary or permanent blockage of a coronary artery. These conditions are characterized by an excessive demand or inadequate supply of oxygen and nutrients to the heart muscle associated with plaque disruption, thrombus formation, and vasoconstriction. ACSs consist of three major syndromes: unstable angina, non–ST-elevation myocardial infarction, and ST elevation myocardial infarction.

afterload: The pressure or resistance against which the ventricles must pump to eject blood.

angina pectoris: Chest discomfort or other related symptoms of sudden onset that may occur because the increased oxygen demand of the heart temporarily exceeds the blood supply.

apex of the heart: Lower portion of the heart that is formed by the tip of the left ventricle.

atria: Two upper chambers of the heart (singular, atrium).

atrial kick: Blood pushed into the ventricles because of atrial contraction.

atrioventricular (AV) valve: The valve located between each atrium and ventricle; the tricuspid separates the right atrium from the right ventricle, and the mitral (bicuspid) separates the left atrium from the left ventricle.

atypical presentation: Uncharacteristic signs and symptoms perceived by some patients experiencing a medical condition, such as an ACS.

base of the heart: Posterior surface of the heart.

blood pressure: Force exerted by the blood against the walls of the arteries as the ventricles of the heart contract and relax.

cardiac output (CO): The amount of blood pumped into the aorta each minute by the heart; defined as the stroke volume multiplied by the heart rate.

chordae tendineae (tendinous cords): Thin strands of fibrous connective tissue that extend from the AV valves to the papillary muscles that prevent the AV valves from bulging back into the atria during ventricular systole (contraction).

chronotropy: A change in (heart) rate.

diastole: Phase of the cardiac cycle in which the atria and ventricles relax between contractions and blood enters these chambers. When the term is used without reference to a specific chamber of the heart, ventricular diastole is implied.

dromotropy: Refers to the speed of conduction through the AV junction.

dysrhythmia: Any disturbance or abnormality in a normal rhythmic pattern; any cardiac rhythm other than a sinus rhythm.

ejection fraction: The percentage of blood pumped out of a heart chamber with each contraction.

endocardium: Innermost layer of the heart that lines the inside of the myocardium and covers the heart valves.

epicardium: Also known as the visceral pericardium; the external layer of the heart wall that covers the heart muscle.

heart failure: A condition in which the heart is unable to pump enough blood to meet the metabolic needs of the body; it may result from any condition that impairs preload, afterload, cardiac contractility, or heart rate.

inotropy: Refers to a change in myocardial contractility.

ischemia: Decreased supply of oxygenated blood to a body part or organ.

mediastinum: Middle area of the thoracic cavity; contains the heart, great vessels, trachea, and esophagus, among other structures; extends from the sternum to the vertebral column.

mitochondria: The energy-producing parts of a cell.

myocardial infarction (MI): Death of some mass of the heart muscle caused by an inadequate blood supply.

myocardium: Middle and thickest layer of the heart; contains the cardiac muscle fibers that cause contraction of the heart and contains the conduction system and blood supply.

myofibril: Slender striated strand of muscle tissue.

papillary muscles: Muscles attached to the chordae tendineae of the AV valves and the ventricular muscle of the heart that help prevent the AV valves from bulging too far into the atria.

pericardium: A double-walled sac that encloses the heart and helps protect it from trauma and infection.

peripheral resistance: Resistance to the flow of blood determined by blood vessel diameter and the tone of the vascular musculature.

preload: Force exerted by the blood on the walls of the ventricles at the end of diastole.

proximal: Location nearer to the midline of the body or the point of attachment than something else is.

sarcolemma: Membrane that covers smooth, striated, and cardiac muscle fibers.

sarcomere: Smallest functional unit of a myofibril.

sarcoplasm: Semifluid cytoplasm of muscle cells.

sarcoplasmic reticulum: Network of tubules and sacs that plays an important role in muscle contraction and relaxation by releasing and storing calcium ions.

semilunar (SL) valves: Valves shaped like half-moons that separate the ventricles from the aorta and pulmonary artery.

septum: An internal wall of connective tissue.

stroke volume (SV): The amount of blood ejected from a ventricle with each heartbeat.

sulcus: Groove.

systole: Contraction of the heart (usually referring to ventricular contraction), during which blood is propelled into the pulmonary artery and aorta; when the term is used without reference to a specific chamber of the heart, ventricular systole is implied.

tone: A term that may be used when referring to the normal state of balanced tension in body tissues.

venous return: Amount of blood flowing into the right atrium each minute from the systemic circulation.

ventricles: The two lower chambers of the heart

LOCATION, SIZE, AND SHAPE OF THE HEART

[Objective 1]

The heart is a hollow muscular organ that lies in the space between the lungs (i.e., the **mediastinum**) in the middle of the chest (Fig. 1.1). It sits behind the sternum and just above the diaphragm. About two thirds of the heart lies to the left of the midline of the sternum. The remaining third lies to the right of the sternum.

The adult heart is about 5 inches (12 cm) long, 3.5 inches (9 cm) wide, and 2.5 inches (6 cm) thick (Fig. 1.2). It typically weighs between 250 and 350 g (about 11 oz) and is about the size of its owner's fist. The weight of the heart is about 0.45% of a man's body weight and about 0.40% of a woman's. A person's heart size and weight are influenced by his or her age, body weight and build, frequency of physical exercise, and heart disease.

SURFACES OF THE HEART

[Objective 2]

The **base**, or posterior surface, **of the heart** is formed by the left atrium, a small portion of the right atrium, and **proximal** portions of the superior and inferior venae cavae and the pulmonary veins (Fig. 1.3). The front (anterior) surface of the heart lies behind the sternum and costal cartilages. It is formed by portions of the right atrium and the left and right **ventricles** (Fig. 1.4). However, because the heart is tilted slightly toward the left in the chest, the right ventricle is the area of the heart that lies most directly behind the sternum. The **apex**, or lower portion, **of the heart** is formed by the tip of the left ventricle. The apex lies just above the diaphragm at about the level of the fifth intercostal space in the midclavicular line.

The heart's left side (i.e., left lateral surface) faces the left lung and is made up mostly of the left ventricle and a portion of the left atrium. The right lateral surface faces the right lung and consists of the right atrium. The heart's bottom (i.e., inferior) surface is formed primarily by the left ventricle, with small portions of the right ventricle and right atrium. The right and left ventricles are separated by a groove containing the posterior interventricular vessels. Because the inferior surface of the heart rests on the diaphragm, it is also called the *diaphragmatic surface* (Fig. 1.5).

COVERINGS OF THE HEART

[Objective 3]

The **pericardium** is a double-walled sac that encloses the heart and helps protect it from trauma and infection. The tough outer layer of the pericardial sac is called the *fibrous parietal pericardium* (Fig. 1.6). It anchors the heart to some

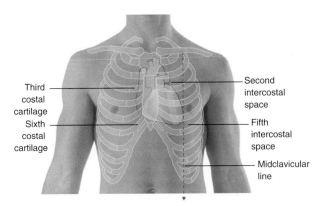

Fig. 1.1 Anterior view of the chest wall of a man showing skeletal structures and the surface projection of the heart. (From Drake R, Vogl AW, Mitchell AWM: *Gray's anatomy for students,* ed 3, New York, 2015, Churchill Livingstone.)

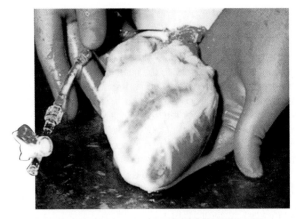

Fig. 1.2 Appearance of the heart. This photograph shows a living human heart prepared for transplantation into a patient. Note its size relative to the hands that are holding it. (From Patton KT, Thibodeau GA: *Anatomy & physiology,* ed 9, St. Louis, 2016, Mosby.)

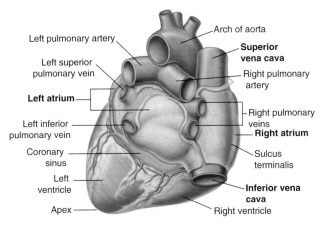

Fig. 1.3 The base of the heart. (From Drake R, Vogl AW, Mitchell AWM: *Gray's anatomy for students,* ed 3, New York, 2015, Churchill Livingstone.)

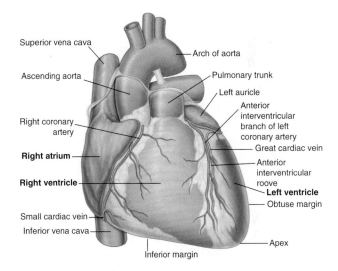

Fig. 1.4 The anterior surface of the heart. (From Drake R, Vogl AW, Mitchell AWM: *Gray's anatomy for students,* ed 3, New York, 2015, Churchill Livingstone.)

CLINICAL CORRELATIONS

The right and left phrenic nerves, which innervate the diaphragm, pass through the fibrous pericardium as they descend to the diaphragm. Because these nerves supply sensory fibers to the fibrous pericardium, the parietal serous pericardium, and the mediastinal pleura, discomfort related to conditions affecting the pericardium may be felt in the areas above the shoulders or lateral neck.

of the structures around it, such as the sternum and diaphragm, by means of ligaments. This helps prevent excessive movement of the heart in the chest with changes in body position.

The inner layer of the pericardium, the *serous pericardium,* consists of two layers: parietal and visceral (Fig. 1.7). The parietal layer lines the inside of the fibrous pericardium. The visceral layer attaches to the large vessels that enter and exit the heart and covers the outer surface of the heart muscle (i.e., the epicardium).

Between the visceral and parietal layers is a space (the pericardial space) that normally contains about 20 mL of serous (pale yellow and transparent) fluid. This fluid acts as a lubricant, preventing friction as the heart beats.

CLINICAL CORRELATIONS

If the pericardium becomes inflamed (pericarditis), excess pericardial fluid can be quickly generated in response to the inflammation. Pericarditis can result from a bacterial or viral infection, rheumatoid arthritis, tumors, destruction of the heart muscle in a heart attack, among other causes.

Heart surgery or trauma to the heart, such as a stab wound, can cause a rapid buildup of blood in the pericardial space. The buildup of excess blood or fluid in the pericardial space compresses the heart. This can affect the heart's ability to relax and fill with blood between heartbeats. If the heart cannot adequately

Continued

fill with blood, the amount of blood the ventricles can pump out to the body (cardiac output) will be decreased. As a result, the amount of blood returning to the heart is also decreased. These changes can result in a life-threatening condition called *cardiac tamponade*. The amount of blood or fluid in the pericardial space needed to impair the heart's ability to fill depends on the rate at which the buildup of blood or fluid occurs and the ability of the pericardium to stretch and accommodate the increased volume of fluid.

The rapid buildup of as little as 100 to 150 mL of fluid or blood can be enough to result in signs and symptoms of shock. Conversely, 1000 mL of fluid may build up over a longer period without any significant effect on the heart's ability to fill. This is because the pericardium accommodates the increased fluid by stretching over time.

The symptoms of cardiac tamponade can be relieved by removing the excess fluid from the pericardial sac. *Pericardiocentesis* is a procedure in which a needle is inserted into the pericardial space and the excess fluid is sucked out (aspirated) through the needle. If scarring is the cause of the tamponade, surgery may be necessary to remove the affected area of the pericardium.

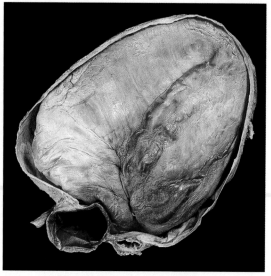
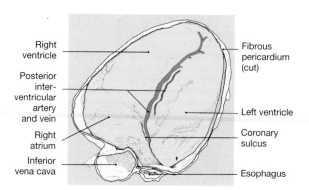

Fig. 1.5 The inferior surface of the heart. The inferior part of the fibrous pericardium has been removed with the diaphragm. (From Gosling JA: *Human anatomy: color atlas and text,* ed 4, London, 2002, Mosby.)

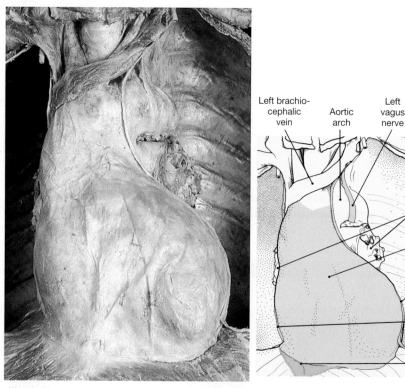

Fig. 1.6 The fibrous pericardium and phrenic nerves revealed after removal of the lungs. (From Gosling JA: *Human anatomy: color atlas and text,* ed 4, London, 2002, Mosby.)

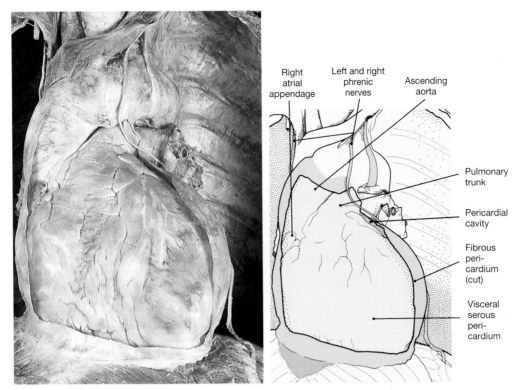

Fig. 1.7 The fibrous pericardium has been opened to expose the visceral pericardium covering the anterior surface of the heart. (From Gosling JA: *Human anatomy: color atlas and text,* ed 4, London, 2002, Mosby.)

STRUCTURE OF THE HEART

Layers of the Heart Wall

[Objective 4]

The walls of the heart are made up of three tissue layers: the endocardium, myocardium, and epicardium (Fig. 1.8 and Table 1.1). The heart's innermost layer, the **endocardium**, is made up of a thin, smooth layer of epithelium and connective tissue and lines the heart's inner chambers, valves, chordae tendineae (tendinous cords), and papillary muscles. The terminal components of the heart's specialized conduction system can be found within this layer (Anderson & Roden, 2010). The endocardium is continuous with the innermost layer of the arteries, veins, and capillaries of the body, thereby creating a continuous, closed circulatory system.

The **myocardium** (middle layer) is a thick, muscular layer that consists of cardiac muscle fibers (cells) responsible for the pumping action of the heart. The myocardium makes up about 30% of the total left ventricular mass (Anderson & Roden, 2010). The innermost half of the myocardium is called the *subendocardial area*. The outermost half is called the *subepicardial area*. The muscle fibers of the myocardium are separated by connective tissues that have a rich supply of capillaries and nerve fibers.

 Did You Know? _____

The thickness of a heart chamber is related to the amount of pressure or resistance that the muscle of the chamber must overcome to eject blood.

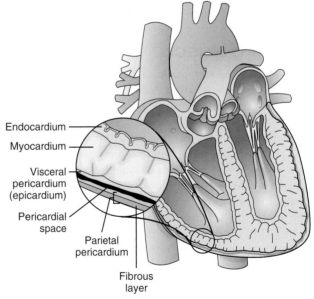

Fig. 1.8 The pericardial sac is composed of two layers separated by a narrow fluid-filled space. The visceral pericardium (epicardium) is attached directly to the heart's surface, and the parietal pericardium forms the outer layer of the sac. (From Copstead-Kirkhorn L, Banasik JL: *Pathophysiology,* ed 5, Philadelphia, 2013, Elsevier.)

The heart's outermost layer is called the **epicardium**. The epicardium is continuous with the inner lining of the pericardium at the heart's apex. The epicardium contains blood capillaries, lymph capillaries, nerve fibers, and fat. The main coronary arteries lie on the epicardial surface of the heart.

TABLE **1.1**	Layers of the Heart Wall
Heart Layer	**Description**
Epicardium	• External layer of the heart • Coronary arteries, blood capillaries, lymph capillaries, nerve fibers, and fat are found in this layer
Myocardium	• Middle and thickest layer of the heart • Muscular component of the heart; responsible for the heart's pumping action
Endocardium	• Innermost layer of the heart • Lines heart's inner chambers, valves, chordae tendineae, and papillary muscles • Continuous with the innermost layer of arteries, veins, and capillaries of the body

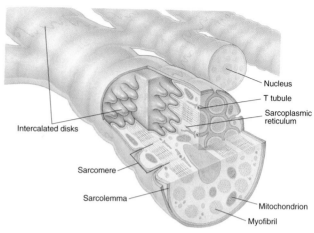

Fig. 1.9 Cardiac muscle fiber. Unlike other types of muscle fibers, the cardiac muscle fiber is typically branched and forms junctions, called intercalated disks, with adjacent cardiac muscle fibers. (From Patton KT, Thibodeau GA: *Anthony's textbook of anatomy & physiology*, ed 20, St. Louis, 2013, Mosby.)

They feed this area first before entering the myocardium and supplying the heart's inner layers with oxygenated blood. **Ischemia** is a decreased supply of oxygenated blood to a body part or organ. The heart's subendocardial area is at the greatest risk of ischemia because this area has a high demand for oxygen and it is fed by the most distal branches of the coronary arteries.

CARDIAC MUSCLE

Cardiac muscle fibers make up the walls of the heart. These fibers have striations, or stripes, similar to that of skeletal muscle. Each muscle fiber is made up of many muscle cells (Fig. 1.9). Each muscle cell is enclosed in a membrane called a **sarcolemma**. Within each cell (as with all cells) are **mitochondria**, the energy-producing parts of a cell, and hundreds of long, tube-like structures called **myofibrils**. Myofibrils are made up of many **sarcomeres**, the basic protein units responsible for contraction. The process of contraction requires adenosine triphosphate (ATP) for energy. The mitochondria that are interspersed between the myofibrils are important sites of ATP production.

The sarcolemma has holes in it that lead into tubes called *T (transverse) tubules*. T tubules are extensions of the cell membrane. Another system of tubules, the **sarcoplasmic reticulum** (SR), stores calcium. Muscle cells need calcium in order to contract. Calcium is moved from the sarcoplasm of the muscle cell into the SR by means of "pumps" in the SR.

There are certain places in the cell membrane where sodium (Na^+), potassium (K^+), and calcium (Ca^{++}) can pass. These openings are called *pores* or *channels*. There are specific channels for sodium (sodium channels),

potassium (potassium channels), and calcium (calcium channels). When the muscle is relaxed, the calcium channels are closed. As a result, calcium cannot pass through the membrane of the SR. This results in a high concentration of calcium in the SR and a low concentration in the **sarcoplasm**, where the muscle cells (sarcomeres) are found. If the muscle cells do not have calcium available to them, contraction is inhibited (the muscle stays relaxed). The force of cardiac muscle contraction depends largely on the concentration of calcium ions in the extracellular fluid.

 ECG Pearl

The heart consists of two syncytia: atrial and ventricular. The *atrial syncytium* consists of the walls of the right and left atria. The *ventricular syncytium* consists of the walls of the right and left ventricles. Normally, impulses can be conducted from the atrial syncytium into the ventricular syncytium only by means of the atrioventricular (AV) junction. The AV junction is a part of the heart's electrical system. This allows the atria to contract a short time before ventricular contraction.

Heart Chambers

The heart has four chambers, two atria and two ventricles. The outside surface of the heart has grooves called *sulci*. The coronary arteries and their major branches lie in these grooves. The coronary **sulcus** (groove) encircles the outside of the heart and separates the atria from the ventricles. It contains the coronary blood vessels and epicardial fat.

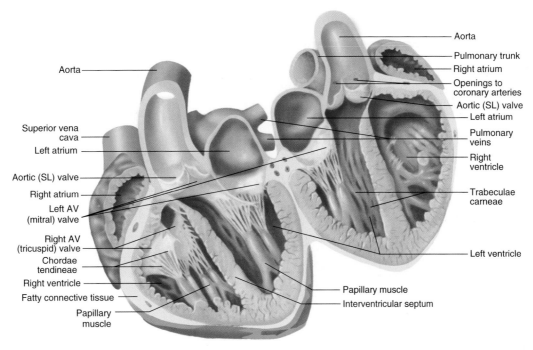

Fig. 1.10 Interior of the heart. This illustration shows the heart as it would appear if it were cut along a frontal plane and opened like a book. The front portion of the heart lies to the reader's right; the back portion of the heart lies to the reader's left. The four chambers of the heart—two atria and two ventricles—are easily seen. *AV,* Atrioventricular; *SL,* semilunar. (From Patton KT, Thibodeau GA: *Anatomy & physiology,* ed 9, St. Louis, 2016, Mosby.)

ATRIA

[Objective 5]

The two upper chambers of the heart are the right and left **atria** (singular, *atrium*) (Fig. 1.10). An earlike flap called an *auricle* (meaning "little ear") protrudes from each atrium.

The purpose of the atria is to *receive* blood. The right atrium receives blood low in oxygen from the superior vena cava (which carries blood from the head and upper extremities), the inferior vena cava (which carries blood from the lower body), and the coronary sinus (which is the largest vein that drains the heart). The left atrium receives freshly oxygenated blood from the lungs via the right and left pulmonary veins.

The four chambers of the heart vary in muscular wall thickness, reflecting the degree of pressure each chamber must generate to pump blood. For example, the atria encounter little resistance when pumping blood to the ventricles. As a result, the atria have a thin myocardial layer. The wall of the right atrium is about 2 mm thick, and the wall of the left atrium is about 3 mm thick. Blood is pumped from the atria through an **atrioventricular (AV)** valve and into the ventricles. The valves of the heart are discussed later in this chapter.

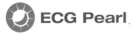 **ECG Pearl**

Think of the atria as holding tanks or reservoirs for blood.

VENTRICLES

[Objective 5]

The heart's two lower chambers are the right and left ventricles. Their purpose is to *pump* blood. The right ventricle pumps blood to the lungs. The left ventricle pumps blood out to the body. Because the ventricles must pump blood either to the lungs (the right ventricle) or to the rest of the body (the left ventricle), the ventricles have a much thicker myocardial layer than the atria. Because the right ventricle moves blood only through the blood vessels of the lungs and then into the left atrium, it has one sixth of the muscle mass and one third of the wall thickness of the left ventricle, which must propel blood to most vessels of the body (Hutchison & Rudakewich, 2009) (Fig. 1.11).

CLINICAL CORRELATIONS

When the left ventricle contracts, it normally produces an impulse that can be felt at the apex of the heart (*apical impulse*). This occurs because as the left ventricle contracts, it rotates forward. In a normal heart, this causes the apex of the left ventricle to hit the chest wall. You may be able to see the apical impulse in thin individuals. The apical impulse is also called the *point of maximal impulse* because it is the site where the left ventricular contraction is most strongly felt.

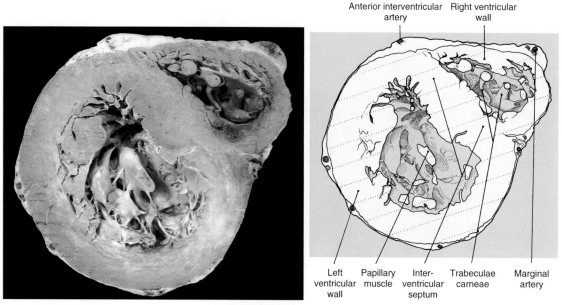

Fig. 1.11 Section through the heart showing the apical portions of the left and right ventricles. (From Gosling JA: *Human anatomy: color atlas and text,* ed 4, London, 2002, Mosby.)

Heart Valves

The heart has a skeleton, which is made up of four rings of thick connective tissue. This tissue surrounds the bases of the pulmonary trunk, the aorta, and the heart valves. The inside of the rings provides secure attachments for the heart valves. The outside of the rings provides for the attachment of the cardiac muscle of the myocardium (Fig. 1.12). The heart's skeleton also helps form the partitions (septa) that separate the atria from the ventricles.

There are four one-way valves in the heart: two sets of AV valves and two sets of **semilunar (SL)** valves. The valves open and close in a specific sequence and assist in producing the pressure gradient needed between the chambers to ensure a smooth flow of blood through the heart and prevent the backflow of blood.

ATRIOVENTRICULAR VALVES

[Objectives 6, 7]

Atrioventricular valves separate the atria from the ventricles. The two AV valves consist of tough, fibrous rings (annuli fibrosi); flaps (leaflets or cusps) of endocardium; chordae tendineae; and papillary muscles.

The tricuspid valve is the AV valve that lies between the right atrium and right ventricle. It consists of three separate cusps or flaps (Fig. 1.13). It is larger in diameter and thinner than the mitral valve. The mitral valve, which is also called the *bicuspid valve,* has only two cusps and lies between the

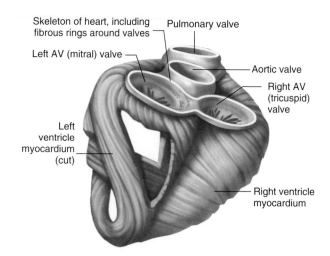

Fig. 1.12 Skeleton of the heart. This posterior view shows part of the ventricular myocardium with the heart valves still attached. The rim of each heart valve is supported by a fibrous structure, called the *skeleton of the heart,* which encircles all four valves. *AV,* Atrioventricular. (From Patton KT, Thibodeau GA: *Anatomy & physiology,* ed 9, St. Louis, 2016, Mosby.)

left atrium and left ventricle (Fig. 1.14). The mitral valve is so named because of its resemblance to a miter, which is a double-cusp bishop's hat, when open.

The AV valves open when a forward pressure gradient forces blood in a forward direction. They close when a backward pressure gradient pushes blood backward. The

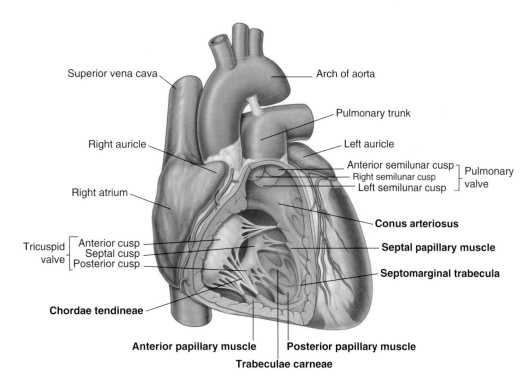

Fig. 1.13 Internal view of the right ventricle. (From Drake R, Vogl AW, Mitchell AWM: *Gray's anatomy for students,* ed 3, New York, 2015, Churchill Livingstone.)

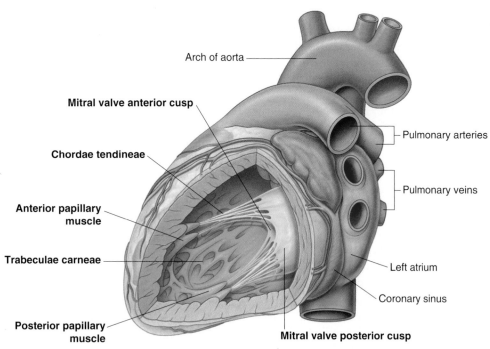

Fig. 1.14 Internal view of the left ventricle. (From Drake R, Vogl AW, Mitchell AWM: *Gray's anatomy for students,* ed 3, New York, 2015, Churchill Livingstone.)

AV valves require almost no backflow to cause closure (Hall, 2016).

The flow of blood from the superior and inferior venae cavae into the atria is normally continuous. About 70% of this blood flows directly through the atria and into the ventricles before the atria contract; this is called *passive filling*. As the atria fill with blood, the pressure within the atrial chamber rises. This pressure forces the tricuspid and mitral valves open, and the ventricles begin to fill, gradually increasing the pressure within the ventricles. When the atria contract, an additional 10% to 30% of the returning blood is added to filling of the ventricles. This additional contribution of blood resulting from atrial contraction is called **atrial kick**. On the right side of the heart, blood low in oxygen empties into the right ventricle. On the left side of the heart, freshly oxygenated blood empties into the left ventricle. When the ventricles then contract (i.e., systole), the pressure within the ventricles rises sharply. The tricuspid and mitral valves completely close when the pressure within the ventricles exceeds that of the atria.

Chordae tendineae (tendinous cords) are thin strands of connective tissue. On one end, they are attached to the underside of the AV valves. On the other end, they are attached to small mounds of myocardium called **papillary muscles**. Papillary muscles project inward from the lower portion of the ventricular walls. When the ventricles contract and relax, so do the papillary muscles. The papillary muscles adjust their tension on the chordae tendineae, preventing them from bulging too far into the atria. For example, when the right ventricle contracts, the papillary muscles of the right ventricle pull on the chordae tendineae. The chordae tendineae prevent the flaps of the tricuspid valve from bulging too far into the right atrium. Thus, the chordae tendineae and papillary muscles serve as anchors. Because the chordae tendineae are thin and string-like, they are sometimes called "heart strings."

SEMILUNAR VALVES

[Objective 6]

The pulmonic and aortic valves are SL valves. The SL valves prevent the backflow of blood from the aorta and pulmonary arteries into the ventricles. The SL valves have three cusps shaped like half-moons. The openings of the SL valves are smaller than the openings of the AV valves, and the flaps of the SL valves are smaller and thicker than the AV valves. Unlike the AV valves, the SL valves are not attached to chordae tendineae.

When the ventricles contract, the SL valves open, allowing blood to flow out of the ventricles. When the right ventricle contracts, blood low in oxygen flows through the pulmonic valve into the pulmonary trunk, which divides into the right and left pulmonary arteries. When the left ventricle contracts, freshly oxygenated blood flows through the aortic valve into the aorta and out to the body (Fig. 1.15). The SL valves close as ventricular contraction ends and the pressure in the pulmonary artery and aorta exceeds that of the ventricles.

CLINICAL CORRELATIONS

Improper valve function can hamper blood flow through the heart. *Valvular heart disease* is the term used to describe a malfunctioning heart valve. Types of valvular heart disease include the following:

- *Valvular prolapse.* If a valve flap inverts, it is said to have *prolapsed.* Prolapse can occur if one valve flap is larger than the other. It can also occur if the chordae tendineae stretch markedly or rupture.
- *Valvular regurgitation.* Blood can flow backward, or regurgitate, if one or more of the heart's valves does not close properly. Valvular regurgitation is also known as *valvular incompetence* or *valvular insufficiency.*
- *Valvular stenosis.* If a valve narrows, stiffens, or thickens, it is said to be *stenosed.* The heart must work harder to pump blood through a stenosed valve.

Papillary muscles receive their blood supply from the coronary arteries. If a papillary muscle ruptures because of an inadequate blood supply (as in myocardial infarction), the attached valve cusps will not completely close and may result in a *murmur.* If a papillary muscle in the left ventricle ruptures, the leaflets of the mitral valve may invert (i.e., prolapse). This may result in blood leaking from the left ventricle into the left atrium (e.g., regurgitation) during ventricular contraction. Blood flow to the body (i.e., cardiac output) could decrease as a result.

HEART SOUNDS

Heart sounds occur because of vibrations in the tissues of the heart caused by the closing of the heart's valves. Vibrations are created as blood flow is suddenly increased or slowed with the contraction and relaxation of the heart chambers and with the opening and closing of the valves.

Normal heart sounds are called *S1* and *S2*. The first heart sound ("lubb") occurs during ventricular contraction when the tricuspid and mitral (AV) valves are closing. The second heart sound ("dupp") occurs during ventricular relaxation as the pulmonic and aortic (SL) valves close. A third heart sound is produced by ventricular filling. In those younger than 40 years of age, the left ventricle normally permits rapid filling. The more rapid the ventricular filling, the greater the likelihood of hearing a third heart sound. A third heart sound (S3) heard in people older than 40 years of age is considered abnormal. An abnormal third heart sound is frequently associated with heart failure. An S1–S2–S3 sequence is called a *ventricular gallop* or gallop rhythm. It sounds like "Kentucky"—*Ken* (S1) *-tuck* (S2) *-y* (S3). The location of the

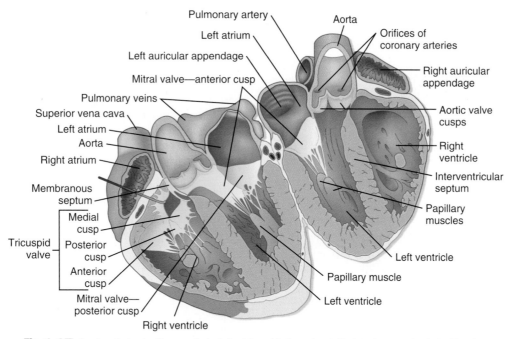

Fig. 1.15 Drawing of a heart split perpendicular to the interventricular septum to illustrate the anatomic relationships of the leaflets of the atrioventricular and aortic valves. (From Koeppen BM, Stanton BA: *Berne & Levy physiology,* ed 6, St. Louis, 2010, Mosby.)

heart's AV and SL valves for auscultation is shown in Fig. 1.16. A summary of the heart's valves and auscultation points for heart sounds appears in Table 1.2.

 CLINICAL CORRELATIONS

In people younger than 40 years of age, the left ventricle normally permits rapid filling. The more rapid the ventricular filling, the greater the likelihood of hearing a third heart sound. A third heart sound (S3) heard in those older than 40 years of age is considered abnormal. An abnormal third heart sound is frequently associated with heart failure. An S1–S2–S3 sequence is called a *ventricular gallop* or *gallop rhythm*. It sounds like *Ken* (S1) *-tuck* (S2) *-y* (S3).

Turbulent blood flow within the cardiac chambers and vessels can produce *heart murmurs*. An inflamed pericardium can produce a *pericardial friction rub*, which sounds like rough sandpaper.

The Heart's Blood Supply

The coronary circulation consists of coronary arteries and veins. The right and left coronary arteries encircle the myocardium like a crown, or corona.

CORONARY ARTERIES

[Objective 8]

The main coronary arteries lie on the outer (epicardial) surface of the heart. Coronary arteries that run on the surface of

the heart are called *epicardial coronary arteries*. They branch into progressively smaller vessels, eventually becoming arterioles, and then capillaries. Thus, the epicardium has a rich blood supply to draw from. Branches of the main coronary arteries penetrate into the heart's muscle mass and supply the subendocardium with blood. The diameter of these "feeder branches" (i.e., collateral circulation) is much narrower. The tissues supplied by these branches get enough blood and oxygen to survive, but they do not have much extra blood flow.

The work of the heart is important. To ensure that it has an adequate blood supply, the heart makes sure to provide itself with a fresh supply of oxygenated blood before supplying the rest of the body. This freshly oxygenated blood is supplied mainly by the branches of two vessels: the right and left coronary arteries.

The right and left coronary arteries are the very first branches off the base of the aorta. The openings to these vessels lie just beyond the cusps of the aortic SL valve. When the left ventricle contracts (systole), the force of the pressure within the left ventricle pushes blood into the arteries that branch from the aorta. This causes the arteries to fill. However, the heart's blood vessels (i.e., the coronary arteries) are compressed during ventricular contraction, reducing blood flow to the tissues of the heart. Thus, the coronary arteries fill when the aortic valve is closed and the left ventricle is relaxed (i.e., diastole).

The three major epicardial coronary arteries include the left anterior descending (LAD) artery, circumflex (Cx) artery, and right coronary artery (RCA). A person is said to have coronary

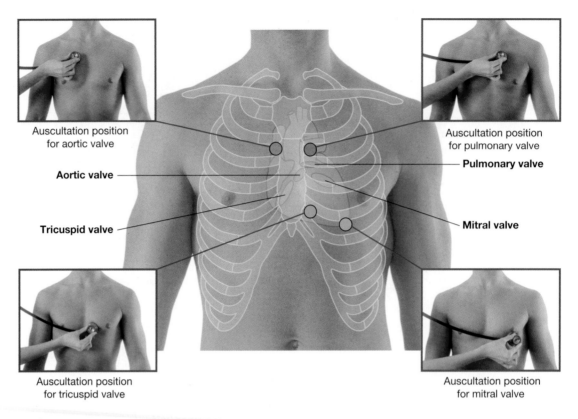

Auscultation position
for aortic valve

Aortic valve

Tricuspid valve

Auscultation position
for tricuspid valve

Auscultation position
for pulmonary valve

Pulmonary valve

Mitral valve

Auscultation position
for mitral valve

Fig. 1.16 Anterior view of the chest showing the heart, the location of the heart's valves, and where to listen to heart sounds. (From Drake R, Vogl AW, Mitchell AWM: *Gray's anatomy for students,* ed 3, New York, 2015, Churchill Livingstone.)

TABLE 1.2	Heart Valves and Auscultation Points		
Valve Name	**Valve Type**	**Location**	**Auscultation Point**
Tricuspid	Atrioventricular	Separates the right atrium and right ventricle	Just to the left of the lower part of the sternum near the fifth intercostal space
Mitral (bicuspid)	Atrioventricular	Separates the left atrium and left ventricle	Heart apex in the left fifth intercostal space at the midclavicular line
Pulmonic (pulmonary)	Semilunar	Between the right ventricle and pulmonary artery	Left second intercostal space close to the sternum
Aortic	Semilunar	Between the left ventricle and aorta	Right second intercostal space close to the sternum

artery disease (CAD) if there is more than 50% diameter narrowing (i.e., stenosis) in one or more of these vessels.

 CLINICAL CORRELATIONS

Because a heart attack, which is also called a *myocardial infarction*, is usually caused by a blocked coronary artery, it is worthwhile to become familiar with the arteries that supply the heart. When myocardial ischemia or infarction is suspected, an understanding of coronary artery anatomy and the areas of the heart that each vessel supplies helps you predict which coronary artery is blocked and anticipate problems associated with blockage of that vessel.

Right Coronary Artery

The RCA originates from the right side of the aorta (Fig. 1.17). It travels along the groove between the right atrium and right ventricle. A branch of the RCA supplies the following structures:

- Right atrium
- Right ventricle
- Inferior surface of the left ventricle in about 85% of individuals
- Posterior surface of the left ventricle in 85%
- Sinoatrial (SA) node in about 60%
- AV bundle in 85% to 90%

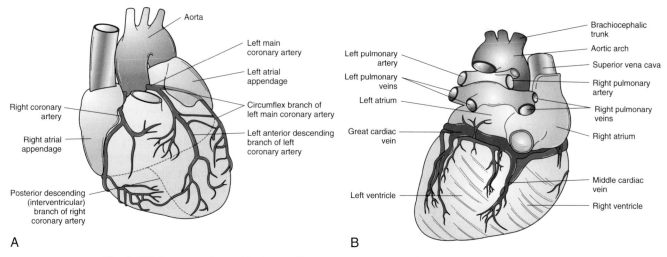

Fig. 1.17 Coronary arteries supplying the heart. The right coronary artery supplies the right atrium, ventricle, and posterior aspect of the left ventricle in most individuals. The left coronary artery divides into the left anterior descending and circumflex arteries, which perfuse the left ventricle. A, Anterior view. B, Posterior view. (From Copstead-Kirkhorn L, Banasik JL: *Pathophysiology,* ed 5, Philadelphia, 2013, Elsevier.)

Left Coronary Artery

The left coronary artery (LCA) originates from the left side of the aorta (see Fig. 1.17). The first segment of the LCA is called the *left main coronary artery*. It is about the diameter of a soda straw and less than 1 inch (2.5 cm) long. Blockage of the proximal LAD coronary artery has been referred to as the "widow maker" because of its association with sudden cardiac arrest when it is blocked.

The left main coronary artery supplies oxygenated blood to its two primary branches: the LAD, which is also called the *anterior interventricular artery*, and the Cx. These vessels are slightly smaller than the left main coronary artery.

The LAD is on the outer (i.e., epicardial) surface on the front of the heart. It travels along the groove that lies between the right and left ventricles (i.e., the anterior interventricular sulcus) toward the heart's apex. In most patients, the LAD travels around the apex of the left ventricle and ends along the left ventricle's inferior surface. In the remaining patients, the LAD does not reach the inferior surface. Instead, it stops at or before the heart's apex. The major branches of the LAD are the septal and diagonal arteries. The LAD supplies blood to the following:

- The anterior surface of the left ventricle
- Part of the lateral surface of the left ventricle
- The anterior two thirds of the interventricular septum

The Cx coronary artery circles around the left side of the heart in a groove on the back of the heart that separates the left atrium from the left ventricle called the *coronary sulcus* (see Fig. 1.17). The Cx supplies blood to the following:

- The left atrium
- Part of the lateral surface of the left ventricle
- The inferior surface of the left ventricle in about 15% of individuals
- The posterior surface of the left ventricle in 15%
- The SA node in about 40%
- The AV bundle in 10% to 15%

A summary of the areas of the heart supplied by the three major coronary arteries is shown in Table 1.3.

Coronary Artery Dominance

In about 85% of people the RCA forms the posterior descending artery, and in about 10% of people the circumflex artery forms the posterior descending artery (Lohr & Benjamin, 2016). The coronary artery that forms the posterior descending artery is considered the *dominant* coronary artery. If a branch of the RCA becomes the posterior descending artery, the coronary artery arrangement is described as a *right-dominant system*. If the Cx branches and ends at the posterior descending artery, the coronary artery arrangement is described as a *left-dominant system*. In some people, neither coronary artery is dominant. If damage to the posterior wall of the left ventricle is suspected, a cardiac catheterization usually is necessary to determine which coronary artery is involved.

ACUTE CORONARY SYNDROMES

[Objectives 9, 10]

Acute coronary syndrome (ACS) is a term that refers to distinct conditions caused by a similar sequence of pathologic events involving abruptly reduced coronary artery blood flow. This sequence of events results in conditions that range from myocardial ischemia or injury to death (i.e., necrosis) of the heart muscle. The usual cause of an ACS is the rupture of an atherosclerotic plaque. *Arteriosclerosis* is a chronic disease of the arterial system characterized by abnormal thickening and hardening of the vessel walls. *Atherosclerosis* is a form of arteriosclerosis in which the thickening and hardening of the vessel walls are caused by a buildup of fat-like deposits (e.g., plaque) in the inner lining of large and middle-sized muscular arteries. As the fatty deposits build up, the opening of the artery slowly narrows, and blood flow to the muscle decreases (Fig. 1.18).

The complete blockage of a coronary artery may cause a **myocardial infarction (MI)**. However, because a plaque usually increases in size over months and years, other vascular pathways may enlarge as portions of a coronary artery become blocked. These vascular pathways (i.e., collateral circulation) serve as an alternative route for blood flow around the blocked artery to the heart muscle; thus, the presence of collateral arteries may prevent infarction despite complete blockage of the primary artery.

 ### Did You Know? _____

Any artery in the body can develop atherosclerosis. If the coronary arteries are involved (i.e., coronary artery disease) and if blood flow to the heart is decreased, angina pectoris or more serious signs and symptoms may result. If the arteries in the leg are involved (i.e., peripheral vascular disease), leg pain (i.e., claudication) may result. If the arteries supplying the brain are involved (i.e., carotid artery disease), a stroke or transient ischemic attack may result.

Angina pectoris is chest discomfort or other related symptoms that occur suddenly when the increased oxygen demand of the heart temporarily exceeds the blood supply. Angina is a symptom of myocardial ischemia, and it most often occurs in patients with CAD that involves at least one coronary artery. However, it can be present in patients with normal coronary arteries. Angina also occurs in people with uncontrolled high blood pressure or valvular heart disease. Possible causes of myocardial ischemia are shown in Box 1.1.

The term *angina* refers to squeezing or tightening rather than pain. The discomfort that is associated with angina occurs because of the stimulation of nerve endings by lactic acid and carbon dioxide that builds up in ischemic tissue. Examples of common words and phrases used by patients experiencing angina to describe the sensation they are feeling include "heaviness," "squeezing," "a band across my chest," "a weight in the center of my chest," and "a vise tightening around my chest."

TABLE **1.3** Coronary Arteries		
Coronary Artery	**Portion of Myocardium Supplied**	**Portion of Conduction System Supplied**
Right	• Right atrium • Right ventricle • Inferior surface of left ventricle (about 85%)* • Posterior surface of left ventricle (85%)*	• Sinoatrial (SA) node (about 60%)* • Atrioventricular (AV) bundle (85% to 90%)*
Left anterior descending	• Anterior surface of left ventricle • Part of lateral surface of left ventricle • Anterior two thirds of interventricular septum	• Most of right bundle branch • Part of left bundle branch
Circumflex	• Left atrium • Part of lateral surface of left ventricle • Inferior surface of left ventricle (about 15%)* • Posterior surface of left ventricle (15%)*	• SA node (about 40%)* • AV bundle (10% to 15%)*

*Of population.

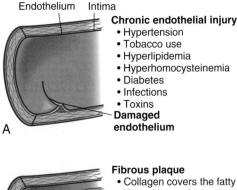
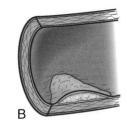
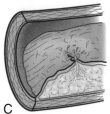
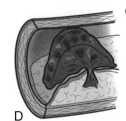

Fig. 1.18 Pathogenesis of atherosclerosis. A, Damaged endothelium. B, Fatty streak and lipid core formation. C, Fibrous plaque. Raised plaques are visible: some are yellow; others are white. D, Complicated lesion: thrombus is *red*; collagen is *blue*. Plaque is complicated by red thrombus deposition. (From Lewis, SL, Bucher L, Heitkemper MM, Harding MM: *Medical-surgical nursing: assessment and management of clinical problems,* ed 10, St. Louis, 2017, Elsevier.)

Chest discomfort associated with myocardial ischemia usually begins in the central or left chest and then radiates to the arm (especially the little finger [ulnar] side of the left arm), the wrist, the jaw, the epigastrium, the left shoulder, or between the shoulder blades. Ischemic chest discomfort is usually not sharp, is not worsened by deep inspiration, is not affected by moving muscles in the area where the discomfort is localized, and is not positional in nature. Other symptoms associated with ACSs include shortness of breath, sweating, nausea, vomiting, dizziness, and discomfort in other areas of the upper body (O'Connor, et al., 2010).

Not all patients experiencing an ACS present similarly. **Atypical presentation** refers to the uncharacteristic signs and symptoms that are experienced by some patients. Atypical chest discomfort is localized to the chest area but may have musculoskeletal, positional, or pleuritic features. Patients experiencing an ACS who are most likely to present atypically include older adults, individuals with diabetes, women, patients with prior cardiac surgery, and patients in the immediate postoperative period after noncardiac surgery (Karve, Bossone, & Mehta, 2007). Older adults may have atypical symptoms such as dyspnea, shoulder or back pain, weakness, fatigue, mental status changes, syncope, unexplained nausea, and abdominal or epigastric discomfort. They are also more likely than younger patients to present with more severe preexisting conditions, such as hypertension, heart failure, or a previous acute MI. Individuals with diabetes may present atypically because of autonomic dysfunction. Common signs and symptoms include generalized weakness, syncope, lightheadedness, or a change in mental status. Women who experience an ACS report acute symptoms including chest discomfort, unusual fatigue, sleep disturbances, dyspnea, nausea or vomiting, indigestion, dizziness or fainting, sweating, arm or shoulder pain, and weakness. The location of the discomfort is often in the back, arm, shoulder, or neck. Some women have vague chest discomfort that tends to come and go with no known aggravating factors.

 ECG Pearl

The extent of arterial narrowing and the amount of reduction in blood flow are critical determinants of coronary artery disease.

Ischemia can occur because of increased myocardial oxygen demand (demand ischemia), reduced myocardial oxygen supply (supply ischemia), or both. If the cause of the ischemia is not reversed and blood flow restored to the affected area of the heart muscle, ischemia may lead to cellular injury and, ultimately, infarction. Ischemia can quickly resolve by reducing the heart's oxygen demand, resting or slowing the heart rate (HR) with medications such as beta-blockers, or increasing blood flow by dilating the coronary arteries with drugs such as nitroglycerin (NTG).

Ischemia prolonged by more than just a few minutes causes myocardial *injury. Myocardial injury* refers to myocardial tissue that has been cut off from or experienced a severe reduction in its blood and oxygen supply. Injured myocardial cells are still alive but will die (i.e., *infarct*) if the ischemia is not quickly corrected. An MI occurs when blood flow to the heart muscle stops or is suddenly decreased long enough to cause cell death. The symptoms that accompany an MI are often more intense than those associated with angina and last more than 15 to 20 minutes.

If the blocked coronary vessel is quickly opened to restore blood flow and oxygen to the injured area, no tissue death occurs. Methods of restoring blood flow may include giving clot-busting drugs (i.e., fibrinolytics), performing coronary angioplasty, or performing a coronary artery bypass graft (CABG), among others.

| Box **1.1** | Possible Causes of Myocardial Ischemia |

Inadequate Oxygen Supply	**Increased Myocardial Oxygen Demand**
• Anemia	• Aortic stenosis
• Coronary artery narrowing caused by a clot, vessel spasm, or rapid progression of atherosclerosis	• Cocaine, amphetamines
	• Eating a heavy meal
	• Emotional stress
• Hypoxemia	• Exercise
	• Exposure to cold weather
	• Fever
	• Heart failure
	• Hypertension
	• Obstructive cardiomyopathy
	• Pheochromocytoma
	• Rapid heart rate
	• Smoking
	• Thyrotoxicosis

CLINICAL CORRELATIONS

When myocardial cells die, such as during a myocardial infarction, substances in intracardiac cells pass through broken cell membranes and leak into the bloodstream. These substances, which are called *inflammatory markers*, *cardiac biomarkers*, or *serum cardiac markers*, include creatine kinase myocardial band (CK-MB), myoglobin, troponin I, and troponin T. To verify that an infarction has occurred, blood tests can measure the levels of these substances in the blood. The diagnosis of an acute coronary syndrome is made on the basis of the patient's assessment findings and his or her symptoms and history, the presence of cardiovascular risk factors, serial electrocardiogram results, blood test results (i.e., cardiac biomarkers), and other diagnostic test results.

CORONARY VEINS

The coronary (cardiac) veins travel alongside the arteries. Blood that has passed through the myocardial capillaries is drained by branches of the cardiac veins that join the coronary sinus. The coronary sinus is the largest vein that drains the heart (see Fig. 1.17). It lies in the groove (sulcus) that separates the atria from the ventricles. The coronary sinus receives blood from the great, middle, and small cardiac veins; a vein of the left atrium; and the posterior vein of the left ventricle. The coronary sinus drains into the right atrium. The anterior cardiac veins do not join the coronary sinus but empty directly into the right atrium.

The Heart's Nerve Supply

[Objective 11]

The myocardium is able to produce its own electrical impulses without signals from an outside source, such as a nerve. Because there are times when the body needs to increase or decrease its HR and/or force of contraction, it is beneficial that both divisions of the autonomic nervous system send fibers to the heart (Fig. 1.19). The sympathetic division prepares the body to function under stress (i.e., the "fight-or-flight" response). The parasympathetic division conserves and restores body resources (i.e., the "rest and digest" response).

SYMPATHETIC STIMULATION

Sympathetic (accelerator) nerves innervate specific areas of the heart's electrical system, atrial muscle, and the ventricular myocardium. When sympathetic nerves are stimulated, the neurotransmitters norepinephrine and epinephrine are released. Remember: The job of the sympathetic division is to prepare the body for emergency or stressful situations. Therefore, the release of norepinephrine and epinephrine results in the following predictable actions:
- Dilation of pupils
- Dilation of smooth muscles of bronchi to improve oxygenation

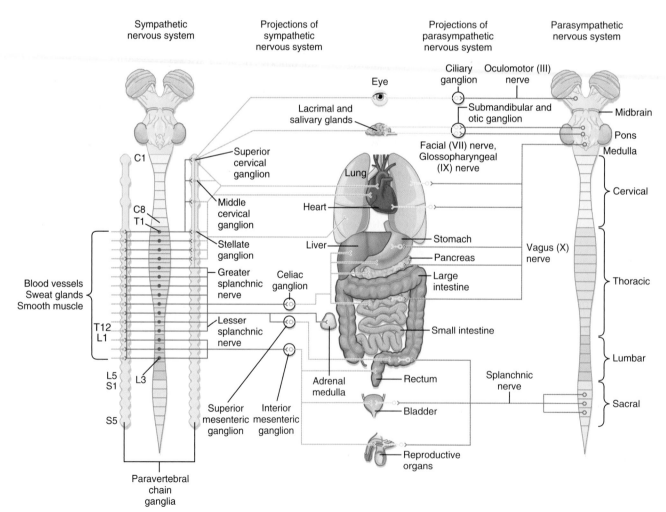

Fig. 1.19 Schematic showing the sympathetic and parasympathetic pathways. Sympathetic pathways are shown in *red* and parasympathetic pathways in *blue*. (From Koeppen BM, Stanton BA: *Berne & Levy physiology*, ed 6, St. Louis, 2010, Mosby.)

- Increased HR, force of contraction, conduction velocity, blood pressure, and cardiac output (CO)
- Increased sweating
- Mobilization of stored energy to ensure an adequate supply of glucose for the brain and fatty acids for muscle activity
- Shunting of blood from skin and blood vessels of internal organs to skeletal muscle

Sympathetic (adrenergic) receptors are located in different organs and have different physiologic actions when stimulated. There are five main types of sympathetic receptors: $alpha_1$, $alpha_2$, $beta_1$, $beta_2$, and $beta_3$.

- $Alpha_1$ receptors are found in the eyes, blood vessels, bladder, and male reproductive organs. Stimulation of $alpha_1$ receptor sites results in constriction.
- $Alpha_2$ receptor sites are found in parts of the digestive system and on presynaptic nerve terminals in the peripheral nervous system. Stimulation results in decreased secretions, peristalsis, and suppression of norepinephrine release.
- Beta receptor sites are divided into $beta_1$, $beta_2$, and $beta_3$. $Beta_1$ receptors are found in the heart and kidneys. Stimulation of $beta_1$ receptor sites in the heart results in increased HR, contractility, and, ultimately, irritability of cardiac cells (Fig. 1.20). Stimulation of $beta_1$ receptor sites in the kidneys results in the release of renin into the blood. Renin promotes the production of angiotensin, a powerful vasoconstrictor. $Beta_2$ receptor sites are found in the arterioles of the heart, lungs, and skeletal muscle. Stimulation results in dilation. $Beta_3$ receptor sites are found in fat cells. When

stimulated, they are thought to promote the breakdown of fats and other lipids.

 ECG Pearl

Remember: $Beta_1$ receptors affect the heart (you have one heart); $beta_2$ receptors affect the lungs (you have two lungs).

PARASYMPATHETIC STIMULATION

Parasympathetic (inhibitory) nerve fibers innervate the SA node, the atrial muscle, and the AV bundle of the heart by the vagus nerves. Acetylcholine (ACh) is a chemical messenger (neurotransmitter) released when parasympathetic nerves are stimulated. ACh binds to parasympathetic receptors. The two main types of cholinergic receptors are nicotinic and muscarinic receptors. Nicotinic receptors are located in skeletal muscle. Muscarinic receptors are located in smooth muscle. Parasympathetic stimulation has the following actions:

- Slows the rate of discharge of the SA node (Fig. 1.21)
- Slows conduction through the AV node
- Decreases the strength of atrial contraction
- Can cause a small decrease in the force of ventricular contraction

BARORECEPTORS AND CHEMORECEPTORS

Baroreceptors are specialized nerve tissue (sensors). They are found in the internal carotid arteries and the aortic arch. These sensory receptors detect changes in blood pressure. When they are stimulated, they cause a reflex

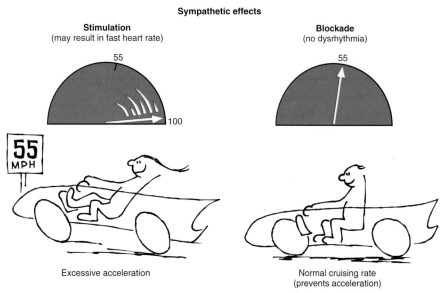

Fig. 1.20 Effects of sympathetic stimulation on the heart. (From Wiederhold R: *Electrocardiography: the monitoring and diagnostic leads,* ed 2, Philadelphia, 1999, Saunders.)

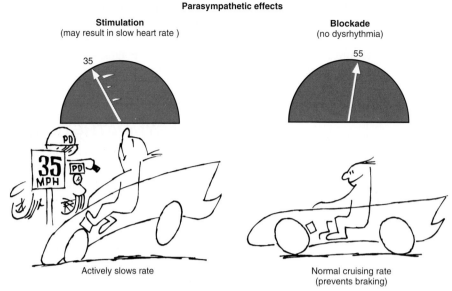

Parasympathetic effects

Stimulation
(may result in slow heart rate)

Blockade
(no dysrhythmia)

35

55

Actively slows rate

Normal cruising rate
(prevents braking)

Fig. 1.21 Effects of parasympathetic stimulation on the heart. (From Wiederhold R: *Electrocardiography: the monitoring and diagnostic leads,* ed 2, Philadelphia, 1999, Saunders.)

TABLE **1.4**	Review of the Autonomic Nervous System	
	Sympathetic Division	**Parasympathetic Division**
General effect	Fight or flight	Feed and breed; rest and digest
Primary neurotransmitter	Norepinephrine, epinephrine	Acetylcholine
Effects of Stimulation		
Abdominal blood vessels	Constriction (alpha receptors)	No effect
Adrenal medulla	Increased secretion of epinephrine	No effect
Bronchioles	Dilation (beta receptors)	Constriction
Blood vessels of skin	Constriction (alpha receptors)	No effect
Blood vessels of skeletal muscle	Dilation (beta receptors)	No effect
Cardiac muscle	Increased rate and strength of contraction (beta receptors)	Decreased rate; decreased strength of atrial contraction, little effect on strength of ventricular contraction
Coronary blood vessels	Constriction (alpha receptors) Dilation (beta receptors)	Dilation

response in either the sympathetic or the parasympathetic divisions of the autonomic nervous system. For example, if the blood pressure decreases, the body will attempt to compensate by:

• Constricting peripheral blood vessels
• Increasing the HR (chronotropy)
• Increasing the force of myocardial contraction (inotropy)

These compensatory responses occur because of a response by the sympathetic division. This is called a *sympathetic or adrenergic response*. If the blood pressure increases, the body will decrease sympathetic stimulation and increase the response by the parasympathetic division. This is called a *parasympathetic*

or cholinergic response. The baroreceptors will adjust to a new normal after a few days of exposure to a specific pressure.

Chemoreceptors in the internal carotid arteries and aortic arch detect changes in the concentration of hydrogen ions (pH), oxygen, and carbon dioxide in the blood. The response to these changes by the autonomic nervous system can be sympathetic or parasympathetic.

A review of the autonomic nervous system can be found in Table 1.4. **Chronotropy, inotropy,** and **dromotropy** are terms used to describe effects on HR, myocardial contractility, and speed of conduction through the AV node. These terms are explained in Box 1.2.

Terminology

Chronotropic Effect
- Refers to a change in heart rate.
- A positive chronotropic effect refers to an increase in heart rate.
- A negative chronotropic effect refers to a decrease in heart rate.

Inotropic Effect
- Refers to a change in myocardial contractility.
- A positive inotropic effect results in an increase in myocardial contractility.
- A negative inotropic effect results in a decrease in myocardial contractility.

Dromotropic Effect
- Refers to the speed of conduction through the atrioventricular (AV) junction.
- A positive dromotropic effect results in an increase in AV conduction velocity.
- A negative dromotropic effect results in a decrease in AV conduction velocity.

THE HEART AS A PUMP

The right and left sides of the heart are separated by an internal wall of connective tissue called a **septum**. The *interatrial septum* separates the right and left atria. The *interventricular septum* separates the right and left ventricles. The septa separate the heart into two functional pumps. The right atrium and right ventricle make up one pump. The left atrium and left ventricle make up the other (Fig. 1.22).

The right side of the heart is a low-pressure system whose job is to pump unoxygenated blood from the body to and through the lungs to the left side of the heart. This is called the *pulmonary circulation*. The pressure within the right atrium is normally between 2 and 6 mm Hg. The pressure within the right ventricle is normally between 0 and 8 mm Hg when the chamber is at rest (diastole) and between 15 and 25 mm Hg during contraction (systole).

The job of the left side of the heart is to receive oxygenated blood from the lungs and pump it out to the rest of the body. This is called the *systemic circulation*. The left side of the heart is a high-pressure pump. The pressure within the left atrium is normally between 8 and 12 mm Hg. Blood is carried from the heart to the organs of the body through arteries, arterioles, and capillaries. Blood is returned to the right side of the heart through venules and veins.

The left ventricle is a high-pressure chamber. Its wall is much thicker than the right ventricle (the right ventricle is about 3 to 5 mm thick; the left ventricle is about 13 to 15 mm). This is because the left ventricle must overcome a lot of pressure and resistance from the arteries and contract forcefully in order to pump blood out to the body. The pressure within the left ventricle is normally between 8 and 12 mm Hg when the chamber is at rest (diastole) and between 110 and 130 mm Hg during contraction (systole). Because the wall of the left ventricle is much thicker than the right, the interventricular septum normally bulges to the right.

Cardiac Cycle
[Objectives 12, 13]

The cardiac cycle refers to a repetitive pumping process that includes all of the events associated with blood flow through the heart. The cycle has two phases for each heart chamber: systole and diastole. **Systole** is the period during which the chamber contracts and blood is ejected. **Diastole** is the period of relaxation during which the chambers are allowed

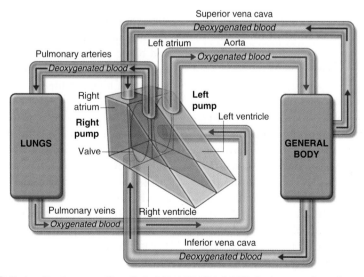

Fig. 1.22 The heart has two pumps. (From Drake R, Vogl AW, Mitchell AWM: *Gray's anatomy for students,* ed 3, New York, 2015, Churchill Livingstone.)

to fill. The myocardium receives its fresh supply of oxygenated blood from the coronary arteries during ventricular diastole.

The cardiac cycle depends on the ability of the cardiac muscle to contract and on the condition of the heart's conduction system. The efficiency of the heart as a pump may be affected by abnormalities of the cardiac muscle, the valves, or the conduction system.

During the cardiac cycle, the pressure within each chamber of the heart rises in systole and falls in diastole. The heart's valves ensure that blood flows in the proper direction. Blood flows from one heart chamber to another from higher to lower pressure. These pressure relationships depend on the careful timing of contractions. The heart's conduction system (discussed in Chapter 2) provides the necessary timing of events between atrial and ventricular systole.

ATRIAL SYSTOLE AND DIASTOLE

Blood from the tissues of the head, neck, and upper extremities is emptied into the superior vena cava. Blood from the lower body is returned to the inferior vena cava. During atrial diastole, blood from the superior and inferior venae cavae and the coronary sinus enters the right atrium. The amount of blood flowing into the right heart from the systemic circulation is called **venous return**. The right atrium fills and distends. This pushes the tricuspid valve open, and the right ventricle fills.

The left atrium receives oxygenated blood from the four pulmonary veins (two from the right lung and two from the left lung). The flaps of the mitral valve open as the left atrium fills. This allows blood to flow into the left ventricle.

The ventricles are 70% filled before the atria contract. Contraction of the atria forces additional blood (about 10% to 30% of the ventricular capacity) into the ventricles (the atrial kick). Thus the ventricles fill completely with blood during atrial systole. The atria then enter a period of atrial diastole, which continues until the start of the next cardiac cycle.

VENTRICULAR SYSTOLE AND DIASTOLE

Ventricular systole occurs as atrial diastole begins. As the ventricles contract, blood is propelled through the systemic and pulmonary circulation and toward the atria. The term *isovolumetric* (meaning "having the same volume") *contraction* describes the brief period between the start of ventricular systole and the opening of the SL valves. During this period, the ventricular volume remains constant as the pressure within the chamber rises sharply.

When the right ventricle contracts, the tricuspid valve closes. The right ventricle expels the blood through the pulmonic valve into the pulmonary trunk. The pulmonary trunk divides into a right and left pulmonary artery, each of which carries blood to one lung (i.e., the pulmonary circuit).

Blood flows through the pulmonary arteries to the lungs. Blood low in oxygen passes through the pulmonary capillaries. There it comes in direct contact with the alveolar-capillary membrane, where oxygen and carbon dioxide are exchanged. Blood then flows into the pulmonary veins and then to the left atrium.

When the left ventricle contracts, the mitral valve closes to prevent backflow of blood. Blood leaves the left ventricle through the aortic valve to the aorta, which is the main vessel of the systemic arterial circulation. Blood is distributed throughout the body (i.e., the systemic circuit) through the aorta and its branches. Blood continues to move in one direction because pressure pushes it from the high-pressure (i.e., arterial) side, and valves in the veins prevent backflow on the lower pressure (i.e., venous) side as blood returns to the heart.

 Did You Know? _____

The aorta is composed of four primary parts: the ascending aorta, the aortic arch, the thoracic portion of the descending aorta, and the abdominal portion of the descending aorta.

When the SL valves close, the heart begins a period of ventricular diastole. During ventricular diastole, the ventricles are relaxed and begin to fill passively with blood. The cardiac cycle begins again with atrial systole and the completion of ventricular filling. The cardiac cycle and blood flow through the heart are shown in Fig. 1.23.

 Did You Know? _____

Both the atria and ventricles have a systolic and diastolic phase. When the term *systole* or *diastole* is used but the area of the heart is not specified, however, you can assume that the term refers to *ventricular* systole or diastole.

Blood Pressure

[Objective 14]

The mechanical activity of the heart is reflected by the pulse and blood pressure. **Blood pressure** is the force exerted by the circulating blood volume on the walls of the arteries. The volume of blood in the arteries is directly related to arterial blood pressure.

Blood pressure is equal to CO × peripheral resistance. CO is discussed later. **Peripheral resistance** is the resistance to the flow of blood determined by blood vessel diameter and the tone of the vascular musculature. **Tone** is a term that may be used when referring to the normal state of balanced tension in body tissues.

Blood pressure is affected by conditions or medications that affect peripheral resistance or CO (Fig. 1.24). For example, an increase in either CO or peripheral resistance typically results in an increase in blood pressure. Conversely, a decrease in either will result in a decrease in blood pressure.

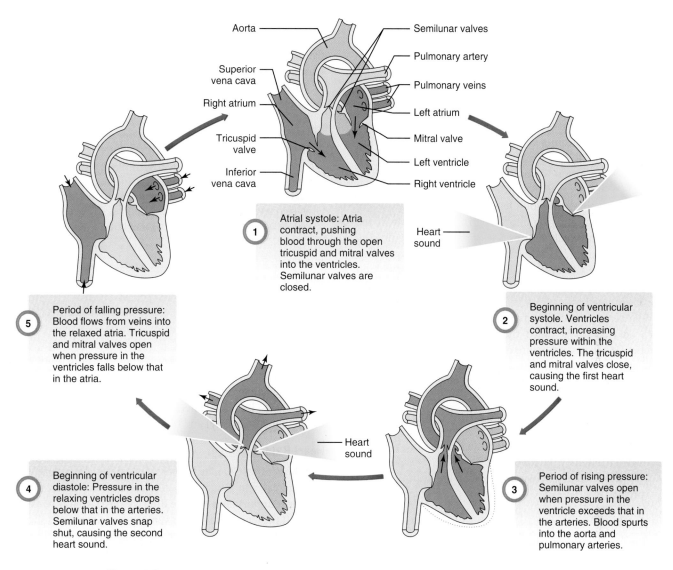

1 Atrial systole: Atria contract, pushing blood through the open tricuspid and mitral valves into the ventricles. Semilunar valves are closed.

Heart sound

5 Period of falling pressure: Blood flows from veins into the relaxed atria. Tricuspid and mitral valves open when pressure in the ventricles falls below that in the atria.

2 Beginning of ventricular systole. Ventricles contract, increasing pressure within the ventricles. The tricuspid and mitral valves close, causing the first heart sound.

Heart sound

4 Beginning of ventricular diastole: Pressure in the relaxing ventricles drops below that in the arteries. Semilunar valves snap shut, causing the second heart sound.

3 Period of rising pressure: Semilunar valves open when pressure in the ventricle exceeds that in the arteries. Blood spurts into the aorta and pulmonary arteries.

Aorta
Semilunar valves
Pulmonary artery
Superior vena cava
Pulmonary veins
Right atrium
Left atrium
Tricuspid valve
Mitral valve
Left ventricle
Inferior vena cava
Right ventricle

Fig. 1.23 Blood flow through the heart during the cardiac cycle. (From Solomon E: *Introduction to human anatomy and physiology,* ed 4, St. Louis, 2016, Saunders.)

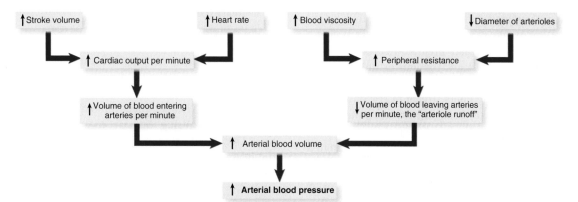

↑Stroke volume ↑Heart rate ↑Blood viscosity ↓Diameter of arterioles

↑ Cardiac output per minute ↑ Peripheral resistance

↑Volume of blood entering arteries per minute ↓Volume of blood leaving arteries per minute, the "arteriole runoff"

↑ Arterial blood volume

↑ **Arterial blood pressure**

Fig. 1.24 Relationship between arterial blood volume and blood pressure. Arterial blood pressure is directly proportional to arterial blood volume. Cardiac output (CO) and peripheral resistance (PR) are directly proportional to arterial blood volume but for opposite reasons: CO affects blood entering the arteries, and PR affects blood leaving the arteries. If cardiac output increases, the amount of blood entering the arteries increases and tends to increase the volume of blood in the arteries. If peripheral resistance increases, it decreases the amount of blood leaving the arteries, which tends to increase the amount of blood left in them. Thus, an increase in either CO or PR results in an increase in arterial blood volume, which increases arterial blood pressure. (From Patton KT, Thibodeau GA: *Anatomy & physiology,* ed 9, St. Louis, 2016, Mosby.)

CARDIAC OUTPUT

[Objective 14]

Each ventricle holds about 150 mL of blood when it is full. They normally eject about half this volume (70–80 mL) with each contraction. **Cardiac output (CO)** is the amount of blood pumped into the aorta each minute by the heart. It is defined as the **stroke volume (SV)**, which is the amount of blood ejected from a ventricle with each heartbeat, multiplied by the HR. In a healthy average adult, the CO at rest is about 5 L/min (an SV of 70 mL multiplied by an HR of 70 beats/min). Because the cardiovascular system is a closed system, the volume of blood leaving one part of the system must equal that entering another part. For example, if the left ventricle normally pumps 5 L/min, the volume flowing through the arteries, capillaries, and veins must equal 5 L/min. Thus, the CO of the right ventricle (pulmonary blood flow) is normally equal to that of the left ventricle on a minute-to-minute basis.

The *percentage* of blood pumped out of a ventricle with each contraction is called the **ejection fraction**. Ejection fraction is used as a measure of ventricular function. A normal ejection fraction is between 50% and 65%. A person is said to have impaired ventricular function when the ejection fraction is less than 40%.

Stroke Volume

Cardiac output may be increased by an increase in SV *or* HR. SV is determined by the following:

- The degree of ventricular filling when the heart is relaxed (preload)
- The pressure against which the ventricle must pump (afterload)
- The myocardium's contractile state (contracting or relaxing)

Preload, which is also called the *end-diastolic volume*, is the force exerted on the walls of the ventricles at the end of diastole. The volume of blood returning to the heart influences preload. More blood returning to the right atrium (e.g., increased venous return) increases preload. Less blood returning decreases preload. According to the Frank-Starling law of the heart, the greater the stretch of the cardiac muscle (within limits), the greater the resulting contraction. Heart muscle fibers stretch in response to the increased volume (preload) before contracting. Stretching of the muscle fibers allows the heart to eject the additional volume with increased force, thereby increasing SV. So in a normal heart, the greater the preload, the greater the force of ventricular contraction and the greater the SV, resulting in increased CO.

This ability to adjust is important so that the heart can alter its pumping capacity in response to changes in venous return. For example, during exercise, the heart muscle fibers stretch in response to increased volume (preload) before contracting. If, however, the ventricle is stretched beyond its physiologic limit, CO may fall because of volume overload and overstretching of the muscle fibers. **Heart failure**

is a condition in which the heart is unable to pump enough blood to meet the metabolic needs of the body. It may result from any condition that impairs preload, afterload, cardiac contractility, or HR.

Afterload is the pressure or resistance against which the ventricles must pump to eject blood. Afterload is influenced

CLINICAL CORRELATIONS

Abnormal heart rhythms (**dysrhythmias**), such as atrial flutter and atrial fibrillation (discussed in Chapter 4), impede normal atrial contraction. Ineffectual atrial contraction can result in a loss of atrial kick, decreased stroke volume, and a subsequent decrease in cardiac output.

by the following:

- Arterial blood pressure
- The ability of the arteries to become stretched (arterial distensibility)
- Arterial resistance

The lower the resistance (lower afterload), the more easily blood can be ejected. Increased afterload (increased resistance) increases the heart's workload. Conditions that contribute to increased afterload include increased thickness of the blood (viscosity) and high blood pressure.

Heart Rate

Remember that CO may be increased by an increase in SV *or* HR. Increases in HR shorten all phases of the cardiac cycle. The most important is that the time the heart spends relaxing is less. If the length of time for ventricular relaxation is shortened, there is less time for them to fill adequately with blood. If the ventricles do not have time to fill, the following occur:

- The amount of blood sent to the coronary arteries is reduced.
- The amount of blood pumped out of the ventricles will decrease (i.e., CO).
- Signs of myocardial ischemia may be seen.

The concentrations of extracellular ions also affect HR. Excess potassium (i.e., hyperkalemia) causes the heart to become dilated and flaccid (limp), slows the HR, and can dramatically alter conduction. An increase in calcium (i.e., hypercalcemia) has an effect almost exactly opposite that of potassium, causing the heart to go into spastic contraction. Decreased calcium levels (i.e., hypocalcemia) make the heart flaccid, similar to the effect of increased potassium levels.

Other factors that influence HR include hormone levels (e.g., epinephrine, norepinephrine), medications, stress, anxiety, fear, and body temperature. HR increases when body temperature increases and decreases when body temperature decreases.

An increase in the force of the heart's contractions (and, subsequently, SV) may occur because of many conditions, including norepinephrine and epinephrine release from

Box **1.3**	Signs and Symptoms of Decreased Cardiac Output

- Acute changes in blood pressure
- Acute changes in mental status
- Cold, clammy skin
- Color changes in the skin and mucous membranes
- Crackles (rales)
- Dyspnea
- Dysrhythmias
- Fatigue
- Orthopnea
- Restlessness

the adrenal medulla, insulin and glucagon release from the pancreas, and medications (e.g., calcium, digitalis, dopamine, dobutamine). A decrease in the force of contraction may result from many conditions, including severe hypoxia, decreased pH, elevated carbon dioxide levels (hypercapnia), and medications (e.g., calcium channel blockers, beta-blockers).

Cardiac output varies depending on hormone balance, an individual's activity level and body size, and the body's metabolic needs. Factors that increase CO include increased body metabolism, exercise, and the age and size of the body. Factors that may decrease CO include shock, hypovolemia, and heart failure. Signs and symptoms of decreased CO appear in Box 1.3. Heart failure may result from any condition that impairs preload, afterload, cardiac contractility, or HR. As the heart begins to fail, the body's compensatory mechanisms attempt to improve CO by manipulating one or more of these factors.

Now that we have discussed CO, SV, and HR, let us review an important point. Remember that CO may be increased by an increase in HR *or* SV. Consider the following examples:

1. A patient has an SV of 80 mL/beat. His HR is 70 beats/min. Is his CO normal, decreased, or increased? Substitute numbers into the formula you already learned: CO = SV × HR. 5600 mL/min = 80 mL/beat × 70 beats/min. CO is normally between 4 and 8 L/min. This patient's CO is within normal limits.

2. Now, let us see what an increase in HR will do. If the patient's HR increases to 180 beats/min and his SV remains at 80 mL/beat, what happens to his CO? Using our formula again (CO = SV × HR) and substituting numbers, we end up with 14,400 mL/min = 80 mL/beat × 180 beats/min. This patient's CO is increased.

3. What happens to CO if the patient's HR is 70 beats/min but his SV drops to 50 mL/beat? Using our formula one more time (CO = SV × HR) and substituting numbers, we end up with 3500 mL/min = 50 mL/beat × 70 beats/min. This patient's CO is decreased. If the patient's HR increased to 90 beats/min to try to compensate for his failing pump, what would happen to his CO? (4500 mL/min = 50 mL/beat × 90 beats/min). According to our example, the patient's CO would increase—at least temporarily.

STOP & REVIEW

Multiple Choice

Identify the choice that best completes the statement or answers the question.

_____ 1. The area in the middle of the thoracic cavity in which the heart lies is the
   a. mediastinum.
   b. pleural cavity.
   c. parietal cavity.
   d. visceral cavity.

_____ 2. The inferior surface of the heart is formed by the
   a. right and left atria.
   b. right and left ventricles.
   c. left atrium and left ventricle.
   d. right atrium and right ventricle.

_____ 3. Which of the following statements is correct?
   a. The circumflex artery is a branch of the right coronary artery.
   b. A branch of the right coronary artery supplies the right atrium and right ventricle.
   c. The major branches of the right coronary artery are the septal and diagonal arteries.
   d. The left main coronary artery is another name for the left anterior descending artery.

_____ 4. The right atrium
   a. pumps blood to the lungs.
   b. pumps blood to the systemic circulation.
   c. receives blood from the right and left pulmonary veins.
   d. receives blood from the superior and inferior vena cavae and the coronary sinus.

_____ 5. Although about 70% of ventricular filling occurs passively, __ contributes an additional 10% to 30% of blood flow to ventricular filling.
   a. atrial kick
   b. SV
   c. CO
   d. ventricular systole

_____ 6. Which of the following is the innermost layer of the heart that lines its inner chambers and valves and is continuous with the innermost layer of the arteries, veins, and capillaries of the body?
   a. Epicardium
   b. Myocardium
   c. Pericardium
   d. Endocardium

_____ 7. When a ventricle relaxes in the normal heart, blood is prevented from flowing back into it by
   a. the mitral valve.
   b. an SL valve.
   c. the tricuspid valve.
   d. an AV valve.

_____ 8. The right ventricle
   a. pumps oxygenated blood into the systemic circulation.
   b. pumps unoxygenated blood into the pulmonary circulation.
   c. receives unoxygenated blood from the systemic circulation.
   d. receives oxygenated blood from the pulmonary circulation.

_____ 9. The __ pericardium is the inner layer of the pericardium, which is also the outer layer of the heart wall called the __.
   a. parietal, myocardium
   b. visceral, epicardium
   c. parietal, endocardium
   d. visceral, endocardium

_____ 10. Which of the following conditions are potentially reversible?
   a. Myocardial ischemia and myocardial injury
   b. Myocardial injury and MI
   c. Myocardial ischemia and MI

_____ 11. Which of the following statements is true regarding CO?
   a. The higher the afterload, the more easily blood is ejected from a ventricle.
   b. SV is the percentage of blood pumped out of a ventricle with each contraction.
   c. An inverse relationship exists between venous return and preload; increased venous return decreases preload.
   d. Within limits, the more blood that is returned to the heart, the greater the volume of blood pumped during the next contraction.

Questions 12 through 14 pertain to the following scenario.
A 65-year-old man presents with a sudden onset of substernal chest pain that radiates to his left arm and jaw and nausea. He states that his symptoms began while at rest. The patient has a history of coronary artery disease and had a three-vessel coronary artery bypass graft last year. His medications include diltiazem (Cardizem) and nitroglycerin. He has no known allergies.

_____ 12. On the basis of the information presented, this patient is most likely experiencing a(n)
   a. stroke.
   b. cardiac arrest.
   c. valvular prolapse.
   d. ACS.

_____ **13.** Your assessment reveals that the patient is anxious, his skin is pale and sweaty, and his heart rate is faster than normal for his age. The patient's assessment findings are most likely
   a. the result of a blocked cerebral blood vessel.
   b. the result of the improper closure of one or more heart valves.
   c. caused by sympathetic stimulation and the release of norepinephrine.
   d. caused by parasympathetic stimulation and the release of acetylcholine.

_____ **14.** This patient's heart rate is faster than normal for his age. Why might this finding be a cause for concern?
   a. Rapid heart rates predispose the patient to valvular heart disease.
   b. Rapid heart rates shorten diastole and can result in decreased CO.
   c. Rapid heart rates lengthen systole but decrease myocardial contractility, which can lead to shock.
   d. Rapid heart rates are usually accompanied by pulmonary congestion, which leads to heart failure.

Matching

Match the terms below with their descriptions by placing the letter of each correct answer in the space provided.

a. Right coronary artery
b. Arteriosclerosis
c. Septum
d. Atria
e. Endocardium
f. Atrioventricular
g. Contracts
h. Half moon

i. SV
j. Aortic
k. Ventricles
l. Pericardium
m. Ischemia
n. Angina pectoris
o. Ejection fraction

_____ **15.** A double-walled sac that encloses the heart
_____ **16.** An SL valve is shaped like a __.
_____ **17.** Decreased supply of oxygenated blood to a body part or organ
_____ **18.** Innermost layer of the heart
_____ **19.** Lower heart chambers
_____ **20.** This type of heart valve separates an atrium and ventricle.
_____ **21.** Chest discomfort or other related symptoms of sudden onset that may occur because the increased oxygen demand of the heart temporarily exceeds the blood supply
_____ **22.** Coronary artery that supplies the SA node and AV node in most of the population
_____ **23.** The amount of blood ejected from a ventricle with each heartbeat
_____ **24.** Upper chambers of the heart
_____ **25.** One of the SL valves
_____ **26.** The percentage of blood pumped out of a heart chamber with each contraction
_____ **27.** An internal wall of connective tissue
_____ **28.** When actin and myosin filaments slide together, the cardiac muscle cell __.
_____ **29.** A chronic disease of the arterial system characterized by abnormal thickening and hardening of the vessel walls

STOP & REVIEW / ANSWERS

1. A. The heart lies in the space between the lungs (i.e., the mediastinum) in the middle of the chest. The mediastinum contains the heart, great vessels, trachea, and esophagus, among other structures; it extends from the sternum to the vertebral column.
OBJ: Describe the location of the heart.

2. B. The heart's bottom (inferior) surface is formed by both the right and left ventricles, but mostly the left. The inferior surface of the heart is also called the *diaphragmatic surface*.
OBJ: Identify the surfaces of the heart.

3. B. A branch of the right coronary artery supplies the right atrium and right ventricle. The left main coronary artery supplies oxygenated blood to its two primary branches: the left anterior descending (LAD) artery and the circumflex artery. The major branches of the LAD are the septal and diagonal arteries.
OBJ: Name the primary branches and areas of the heart supplied by the right and left coronary arteries.

4. D. The right atrium receives blood low in oxygen from the superior vena cava (which carries blood from the head and upper extremities), the inferior vena cava (which carries blood from the lower body), and the coronary sinus (which is the largest vein that drains the heart). The left atrium receives freshly oxygenated blood from the lungs via the right and left pulmonary veins. The right ventricle pumps blood to the lungs. The left ventricle pumps blood to the systemic circulation.
OBJ: Identify and describe the chambers of the heart and the vessels that enter or leave each.

5. A. Although about 70% of ventricular filling occurs passively, atrial contraction (also known as the *atrial kick*) contributes an additional 10% to 30% of blood flow to ventricular filling.
OBJ: Explain atrial kick.

6. D. The endocardium is the heart's innermost layer. It lines the heart's inner chambers, valves, chordae tendineae (tendinous cords), and papillary muscles and is continuous with the innermost layer of the arteries, veins, and capillaries of the body, thereby creating a continuous, closed circulatory system.
OBJ: Identify the three cardiac muscle layers.

7. B. The SL valves prevent backflow of blood from the aorta and pulmonary arteries into the ventricles. When the right ventricle relaxes, blood is prevented from flowing back into it by the pulmonic valve. When the left ventricle relaxes, blood is prevented from flowing back into it by the aortic valve.
OBJ: Identify and describe the location of the atrioventricular and semilunar valves.

8. B. The right side of the heart is a low-pressure system whose job is to pump unoxygenated blood from the body to and through the lungs to the left side of the heart. The right ventricle receives blood low in oxygen from the right atrium and pumps the blood through the pulmonic valve into the pulmonary trunk, which divides into the right and left pulmonary arteries.
OBJ: Beginning with the right atrium, describe blood flow through the normal heart and lungs to the systemic circulation.

9. B. The visceral pericardium is the inner layer of the pericardium, which also attaches to the large vessels that enter and exit the heart and covers the outer surface of the heart muscle (i.e., the epicardium).
OBJ: Describe the structure and function of the coverings of the heart.

10. A. The sequence of events that occurs during an ACS results in conditions that range from myocardial ischemia or injury to death (i.e., necrosis) of heart muscle. Ischemia prolonged more than just a few minutes results in myocardial injury. *Myocardial injury* refers to myocardial tissue that has been cut off from or experienced a severe reduction in its blood and oxygen supply. Injured myocardial cells are still alive but will die (i.e., *infarct*) if the ischemia is not quickly corrected. An MI occurs when blood flow to the heart muscle stops or is suddenly decreased long enough to cause cell death.
OBJ: Discuss myocardial ischemia, injury, and infarction, indicating which conditions are reversible and which are not.

11. D. According to the Frank-Starling law of the heart, the greater the stretch of the cardiac muscle (within limits), the greater the resulting contraction. Preload (end-diastolic volume) is the force exerted on the walls of the ventricles at the end of diastole. In a normal heart, the greater the preload, the greater the force of ventricular contraction and the greater the SV, resulting in increased CO. Afterload is the pressure or resistance against which the ventricles must pump to eject blood. The lower the resistance (lower afterload), the more easily blood is ejected. The percentage of blood pumped out of a ventricle with each contraction is called the *ejection fraction*.
OBJ: Identify and explain the components of blood pressure and cardiac output.

12. D. On the basis of the information presented, this patient is most likely experiencing an ACS. ACS refers to distinct conditions caused by a similar sequence of pathologic events—a temporary or permanent blockage of a coronary artery. These conditions are characterized by an excessive demand or inadequate supply of oxygen and nutrients to the heart muscle associated with plaque disruption, thrombus formation, and vasoconstriction.
OBJ: Define and explain acute coronary syndromes.

13. C. This patient's assessment findings are typical of those experiencing an ACS and are most likely caused by sympathetic stimulation and the release of norepinephrine and epinephrine. The sympathetic division of the autonomic nervous system prepares the body to function under stress ("fight-or-flight" response). The effects of norepinephrine and epinephrine include an increased heart rate, force of contraction, blood pressure, and CO; increased sweating; and shunting of blood from the skin and blood vessels of internal organs to skeletal muscle.
OBJ: Compare and contrast the effects of sympathetic and parasympathetic stimulation of the heart.

14. B. The coronary arteries fill when the aortic valve is closed and the left ventricle is relaxed (i.e., diastole). If the length of time for ventricular relaxation is shortened (as with rapid heart rates), there is less time for them to fill adequately with blood. If the ventricles do not have time to fill, the amount of blood sent to the coronary arteries is reduced, the amount of blood pumped out of the ventricles will decrease (i.e., CO), and signs of myocardial ischemia may be seen.
OBJ: Identify and discuss each phase of the cardiac cycle.

15. L
16. H
17. M
18. E
19. K
20. F
21. N
22. A
23. I
24. D
25. J
26. O
27. C
28. G
29. B

REFERENCES

Anderson, M. E., & Roden, D. M. (2010). Basic cardiac electrophysiology and anatomy. In M. H. Crawford, J. P. DiMarco, & W. J. Paulus (Eds.), *Cardiology* (3rd ed.) (pp. 653–665). Philadelphia: Elsevier.

Hall, J. E. (2016). The heart. In *Guyton and Hall textbook of medical physiology* (13th ed.) (pp. 107–166). Philadelphia: Saunders.

Hutchison, S. J., & Rudakewich, G. (2009). Right ventricular infarction. In *Complications of myocardial infarction: Clinical diagnostic imaging atlas* (pp. 91–110). Philadelphia: Saunders.

Karve, A. M., Bossone, E., & Mehta, R. H. (2007). Acute ST-segment elevation myocardial infarction: critical care perspective. *Crit Care Clin, 23*(4), 685–707.

Lohr, N. L., & Benjamin, I. J. (2016). Structure and function of the normal heart and blood vessels. In I. J. Benjamin, R. C. Griggs, E. J. Wing, & J. G. Fitz (Eds.), *Andreoli and Carpenter's Cecil essentials of medicine* (9th ed.) (pp. 16–21). Philadelphia: Saunders.

O'Connor, R. E., Brady, W., Brooks, S. C., Diercks, D., Egan, J., Ghaemmaghami, C., & Yannopoulos, D. (2010). Part 10: Acute coronary syndromes: 2010 American Heart Association guidelines for cardiopulmonary resuscitation and emergency cardiovascular care. *Circulation, 122*(Suppl 3), S787–S817.

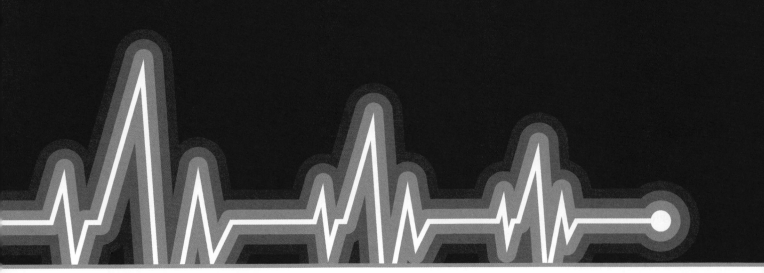

Basic Electrophysiology

2

LEARNING OBJECTIVES

After reading this chapter, you should be able to:
1. Describe the two basic types of cardiac cells in the heart, where they are found, and their function.
2. Describe the primary characteristics of cardiac cells.
3. Define the events comprising the cardiac action potential and correlate them with the waveforms produced on the electrocardiogram (ECG).
4. Define the terms *membrane potential, threshold potential, action potential, polarization, depolarization*, and *repolarization*.
5. List the most important ions involved in the cardiac action potential and their primary function in this process.
6. Define the absolute, effective, relative refractory, and supernormal periods and their locations in the cardiac cycle.
7. Describe the normal sequence of electrical conduction through the heart.
8. Describe the location, function, and, when appropriate, the intrinsic rate of the following structures: the sinoatrial node, the atrioventricular bundle, and the Purkinje fibers.
9. Differentiate the primary mechanisms responsible for producing cardiac dysrhythmias.
10. Describe reentry.
11. Explain the purpose of ECG monitoring.
12. Identify the limitations of the ECG.
13. Differentiate between the frontal plane and the horizontal plane leads.
14. Describe correct anatomic placement of the standard limb leads, the augmented leads, and the chest leads.
15. Relate the cardiac surfaces or areas represented by the ECG leads.
16. Identify the numeric values assigned to the small and to the large boxes on ECG paper.
17. Identify how heart rates, durations, and amplitudes can be determined from ECG recordings.
18. Define and describe the significance of each of the following as they relate to cardiac electrical activity: P wave, QRS complex, T wave, U wave, PR segment, TP segment, ST segment, PR interval, QRS duration, and QT interval.
19. Recognize the changes on the ECG that may reflect evidence of myocardial ischemia, injury, and infarction.
20. Define the term *artifact*, and explain methods used to minimize its occurrence.
21. Describe a systematic approach to the analysis and interpretation of cardiac dysrhythmias.

KEY TERMS

abnormal automaticity: A condition in which cardiac cells not normally associated with the property of automaticity begin to depolarize spontaneously or when escape pacemaker sites increase their firing rate beyond that considered normal

absolute refractory period (ARP): Corresponds with the onset of the QRS complex to approximately the peak of the T wave; during this period, cardiac cells cannot be stimulated to conduct an electrical impulse, no matter how strong the stimulus

accessory pathway: An extra bundle of working myocardial tissue that forms a connection between the atria and ventricles outside the normal conduction system

action potential: A five-phase cycle that reflects the difference in the concentration of charged particles across the cell membrane at any given time

amplitude: Height (voltage) of a waveform on the electrocardiogram

artifact: Distortion of an electrocardiographic tracing by electrical activity that is noncardiac in origin (e.g., electrical interference, poor electrical conduction, patient movement)

atrioventricular (AV) bundle: The bundle of His

atrioventricular (AV) node: A group of cells that conduct an electrical impulse through the heart; located in the floor of the right atrium immediately behind the tricuspid valve and near the opening of the coronary sinus; delays the electrical impulse in order to allow the atria to contract and complete filling of the ventricles

augmented limb lead: Leads aVR, aVL, and aVF; these leads record the difference in electrical potential at one location relative to zero potential rather than relative to the electrical potential of another extremity

automaticity: Ability of cardiac pacemaker cells to spontaneously initiate an electrical impulse without being stimulated from another source (such as a nerve)

axis: Imaginary line joining the positive and negative electrodes of a lead

baseline: Straight line recorded on electrocardiographic graph paper when no electrical activity is detected

biphasic: Waveform that is partly positive and partly negative

bipolar limb lead: Electrocardiographic lead consisting of a positive and negative electrode

bradycardia: Heart rate slower than 60 beats/min (from *brady*, meaning "slow")

bundle of His: Fibers located in the upper portion of the interventricular septum that receive an electrical impulse from the AV node and conduct the impulse to the right and left bundle branches

complex: Several waveforms

conduction system: A system of pathways in the heart composed of specialized electrical (pacemaker) cells

conductivity: Ability of a cardiac cell to receive an electrical stimulus and conduct that impulse to an adjacent cardiac cell

contractility: Ability of cardiac cells to shorten, causing cardiac muscle contraction in response to an electrical stimulus

current: The flow of electrical charge from one point to another

depolarization: Movement of ions across a cell membrane, causing the inside of the cell to become more positive; an electrical event expected to result in contraction

ectopic: Impulse(s) originating from a source other than the sinoatrial node

effective refractory period (ERP): Period of the cardiac action potential that includes the ARP and the first half of the relative refractory period

electrocardiogram (ECG): A graphic display of the heart's electrical activity

electrode: An adhesive pad that contains a conductive gel and is applied at specific locations on the patient's chest wall and extremities and connected by cables to an electrocardiogram machine

electrolytes: Elements or compounds that break into charged particles (ions) when melted or dissolved in water or another solvent

excitability: The ability of cardiac muscle cells to respond to an outside stimulus

ground electrode: Third ECG electrode (the first and second are the positive and negative electrodes), which minimizes electrical activity from other sources

His-Purkinje system: Portion of the conduction system consisting of the bundle of His, bundle branches, and Purkinje fibers

indicative changes: Electrocardiographic changes observed in leads that look directly at the affected area of the heart; indicative changes are significant when they are seen in two anatomically contiguous leads.

inherent: Natural, intrinsic

interval: Waveform and a segment; in pacing, the period, measured in milliseconds, between any two designated cardiac events

intrinsic rate: Rate at which a pacemaker of the heart normally generates impulses

ions: Electrically charged particles

isoelectric line: Absence of electrical activity; observed on the ECG as a straight line

J point: Point where the QRS complex and ST segment meet

lead: Electrical connection attached to the body to record electrical activity

membrane potential: Difference in electrical charge across the cell membrane

millivolt (mV): Difference in electrical charge between two points in a circuit

myocardial cells: Working cells of the myocardium that contain contractile filaments and form the muscular layer of the atrial walls and the thicker muscular layer of the ventricular walls

pacemaker cells: Specialized cells of the heart's electrical conduction system, capable of spontaneously generating and conducting electrical impulses

permeable: Ability of a membrane channel to allow passage of electrolytes when it is open

polarized state: Period after repolarization of a myocardial cell (also called the *resting state*) when the outside of the cell is positive and the interior of the cell is negative

PR interval: P wave plus the PR segment; reflects depolarization of the right and left atria (P wave) and the spread of the impulse through the AV node, AV bundle, right and left bundle branches, and the Purkinje fibers (PR segment)

Purkinje fibers: Fibers found in both ventricles that conduct an electrical impulse through the heart

P wave: First wave in the cardiac cycle; represents atrial depolarization and the spread of the electrical impulse throughout the right and left atria

QRS complex: Several waveforms (i.e., the Q wave, the R wave, and the S wave) that represent the spread of an electrical impulse through the ventricles (i.e., ventricular depolarization)

QT interval: The period from the beginning of the QRS complex to the end of the T wave

R wave: On an ECG, the first positive deflection in the QRS complex, representing ventricular depolarization; in pacing, R wave refers to the entire QRS complex, denoting an intrinsic ventricular event

reciprocal changes: Electrocardiographic changes observed in leads opposite the affected area of the heart; also called *mirror image changes*

reentry: Spread of an impulse through tissue already stimulated by that same impulse.

refractoriness: Period of recovery that cells need after being discharged before they are able to respond to a stimulus

relative refractory period (RRP): Corresponds with the downslope of the T wave; during this period, cardiac cells can be stimulated to depolarize if the stimulus is strong enough.

repolarization: Movement of ions across a cell membrane in which the inside of the cell is restored to its negative charge

segment: Line between waveforms; named by the waveform that precedes and follows it

sinoatrial (SA) node: Normal pacemaker of the heart that normally discharges at a rhythmic rate of 60 to 100 beats/min

ST segment: Portion of the ECG representing the end of ventricular depolarization (end of the R wave) and the beginning of ventricular repolarization (T wave)

supernormal period (SNP): Period during the cardiac cycle when a weaker than normal stimulus can cause cardiac cells to depolarize; extends from the end of phase 3 to the beginning of phase 4 of the cardiac action potential

T wave: Waveform that follows the QRS complex and represents ventricular repolarization

tachycardia: Heart rate greater than 100 beats/min (tachy, fast)

TP segment: Interval between two successive PQRST complexes during which electrical activity of the heart is absent; begins with the end of the T wave through the onset of the following P wave and represents the period from the end of ventricular repolarization to the onset of atrial depolarization

triggered activity: A disorder of impulse formation that occurs when escape pacemaker and myocardial working cells fire more than once after stimulation by a single impulse resulting in atrial or ventricular beats that occur alone, in pairs, in runs, or as a sustained ectopic rhythm.

unipolar lead: Lead that consists of a single positive electrode and a reference point

voltage: Difference in electrical charge between two points

waveform: Movement away from the baseline in either a positive or negative direction

CARDIAC CELLS

Types of Cardiac Cells

[Objective 1]

In general, cardiac cells have either a mechanical (i.e., contractile) or an electrical (i.e., pacemaker) function. **Myocardial cells** are also called *working cells* or *mechanical cells*, and they contain contractile filaments. When these cells are electrically stimulated, these filaments slide together and cause the myocardial cell to contract. These myocardial cells form the thin muscular layer of the atrial walls and the thicker muscular layer of the ventricular walls (i.e., the myocardium). These cells do not normally generate electrical impulses, and they rely on pacemaker cells for this function.

Pacemaker cells are also referred to as *conducting cells* or *automatic cells*. They are specialized cells of the electrical conduction system that are able to form electrical impulses spontaneously and to alter the speed of electrical conduction (Wagner, 2012).

Properties of Cardiac Cells

[Objective 2]

When a nerve is stimulated, a chemical (i.e., a neurotransmitter) is released. The chemical crosses the space between the end of the nerve and the muscle membrane (i.e., the neuromuscular junction). The chemical binds to receptor sites on the muscle membrane and stimulates the receptors. An electrical impulse develops and travels along the muscle membrane, resulting in contraction; thus, a skeletal muscle normally contracts only after it is stimulated by a nerve.

The heart is unique because it has pacemaker cells that can generate an electrical impulse without being stimulated by a nerve. The ability of cardiac pacemaker cells to create an electrical impulse without being stimulated from another source is called **automaticity**. Increased blood concentrations of calcium (Ca++) increase automaticity. Decreased concentrations of potassium (K+) in the blood decrease automaticity. The heart's normal pacemaker is the **sinoatrial (SA)** node because it is capable of self-excitation at a rate quicker than that of other pacemaker sites in the heart.

Cardiac muscle is electrically irritable because of an ionic imbalance across the membranes of cells. **Excitability** (i.e., irritability) is the ability of cardiac muscle cells to respond to an external stimulus, such as that from a chemical, mechanical, or electrical source. **Conductivity** is the ability of a cardiac cell to receive an electrical impulse and conduct it to an adjoining cardiac cell. All cardiac cells possess this characteristic. The intercalated disks present in the membranes of cardiac cells are responsible for the property of conductivity. They allow an impulse in any part of the myocardium to spread throughout the heart. The speed with which the impulse is conducted can be altered by factors such as sympathetic and parasympathetic stimulation and medications. **Contractility** (i.e., inotropy) is the ability of myocardial cells to shorten, thereby causing cardiac muscle contraction in response to an electrical stimulus.

The heart normally contracts in response to an impulse that begins in the SA node. The strength of the heart's contraction can be improved with certain medications, such as digitalis, dopamine, and epinephrine.

CARDIAC ACTION POTENTIAL

[Objectives 3, 4, 5]

Before the following discussion of the cardiac action potential, think about how a battery releases energy. A battery has two terminals; one terminal is positive, and the other is negative. Charged particles exert forces on each other, and opposite charges attract. Electrons, which are negatively charged particles, are produced by a chemical reaction inside the battery. If a wire is connected between the two terminals, the circuit is completed, and the stored energy is released, allowing electrons to flow quickly from the negative terminal along the wire to the positive terminal. If no wire is connected between the terminals, the chemical reaction does not take place, and no current flow occurs. **Current** is the flow of electrical charge from one point to another.

Separated electrical charges of opposite polarity (i.e., positive vs negative) have potential energy. The measurement of this potential energy is called **voltage**. Voltage is measured between two points. In the battery example, the current flow is caused by the voltage, or potential difference, between the two terminals. Voltage is measured in units of volts or millivolts.

Human body fluids contain **electrolytes**, which are elements or compounds that break into charged particles (i.e., **ions**) when melted or dissolved in water or another solvent. Differences in the composition of ions between the intracellular and extracellular fluid compartments are important for normal body function, including the activity of the heart. Body fluids that contain electrolytes conduct an electric current in much the same way as the wire in the battery example. Electrolytes move about in body fluids and carry a charge, just as electrons moving along a wire conduct a current.

 Did You Know?

The main electrolytes that affect the function of the heart are Na+, K+, Ca++, and chloride (Cl−). Disorders that affect the concentration of these important electrolytes can have serious consequences. For example, an imbalance of K+ can cause life-threatening disturbances in the heart's rhythm.

In the body, ions spend a lot of time moving back and forth across cell membranes (Fig. 2.1). When a pathway exists for transfer of a substance across a membrane, the membrane is said to be **permeable** to that substance (Aronson et al, 2012). As a result, a slight difference in the concentrations of charged particles across the membranes of cells is normal; thus, potential energy (i.e., voltage) exists because of the imbalance of charged particles, and this imbalance makes the cells excitable. The voltage (i.e., the difference in electrical charges) across the cell membrane is the **membrane potential**.

Electrolytes are quickly moved from one side of the cell membrane to the other by means of pumps (Fig. 2.2). These pumps require energy in the form of adenosine triphosphate (ATP) when movement occurs against a concentration gradient. The energy expended by the cells to move electrolytes across the cell membrane creates a flow of current. This flow of current is expressed in volts or **millivolts (mV)**. Voltage appears on an **electrocardiogram (ECG)** as spikes or waveforms; thus, an ECG is actually a sophisticated voltmeter.

Polarization

When a cell is at rest, K^+ leaks out of it. Large molecules such as proteins and phosphates remain inside the cell because they are too big to pass easily through the cell membrane. These large molecules carry a negative charge. This results in more negatively charged ions on the inside of the cell. When the inside of a cell is more negative than the outside, the cell is said to be in a *polarized state* (Fig. 2.3).

Depolarization

For a pacemaker cell to fire (i.e., produce an impulse), a flow of electrolytes across the cell membrane must exist. When a cell is stimulated, the cell membrane changes and becomes permeable to Na^+ and K^+, allowing the passage of electrolytes after it is open. Na^+ rushes into the cell through Na^+ channels. This causes the inside of the cell to become more positive relative

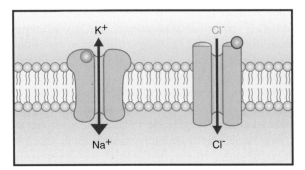

Fig. 2.1 Cell membranes contain pathways through which specific ions or other small, water-soluble molecules can cross. (From Urden LD, Stacy KM, Lough ME: *Critical care nursing,* ed 8, St. Louis, 2018, Mosby.)

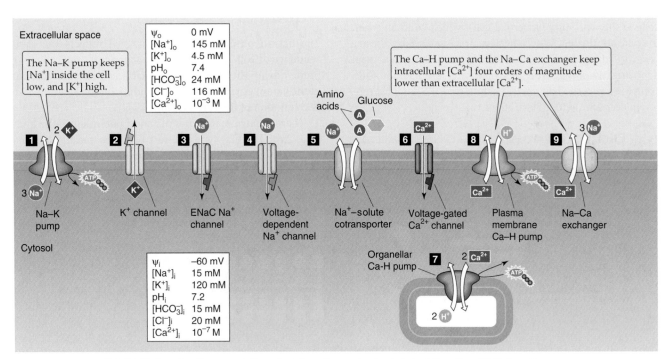

Fig. 2.2 Examples of ion concentrations, channels, and transporters in a typical cell. (From Boron WF, Boulpaep EL: *Medical physiology,* ed 3, Philadelphia, 2017, Saunders.)

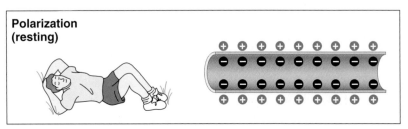

Fig. 2.3 Polarization. When the inside of a cell is more negative than the outside, the cell is said to be polarized. (From Herlihy B: The *human body in health and illness,* ed 5, St. Louis, 2014, Mosby.)

to the outside. A spike (i.e., a waveform) is then recorded on the ECG. The stimulus that alters the electrical charges across the cell membrane may be electrical, mechanical, or chemical.

As described in the battery example, when opposite charges come together, energy is released. When the movement of electrolytes changes the electrical charge of the inside of the cell from negative to positive, an impulse is generated. The impulse causes channels to open in the next cell membrane and then the next. The movement of charged particles across a cell membrane that causes the inside of the cell to become positive is called **depolarization** (Fig. 2.4). Depolarization occurs because of the movement of Na^+ into the cell and proceeds from the innermost layer of the heart (i.e., the endocardium) to the outermost layer (i.e., the epicardium). Depolarization, which is an electrical event, must take place before the heart can contract and pump blood, which is a mechanical event.

An impulse normally begins in the pacemaker cells found in the SA node of the heart. A chain reaction occurs from cell to cell in the heart's electrical conduction system until all the cells have been stimulated and depolarized. This chain reaction is a *wave of depolarization*. The chain reaction is made possible because of gap junctions that exist between the cells. Eventually, the impulse is spread from the pacemaker cells to the working myocardial cells, which contract when they are stimulated. When the atria are stimulated, a P wave is recorded on the ECG; thus, the P wave represents atrial depolarization. When the ventricles are stimulated, a QRS complex is recorded on the ECG; thus, the QRS complex represents ventricular depolarization.

? Did You Know?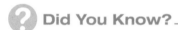

Depolarization is not the same as contraction. Depolarization is an electrical event that is expected to result in contraction, which is a mechanical event. It's possible to see organized electrical activity on the cardiac monitor even when the assessment of the patient reveals no palpable pulse. This clinical situation is called *pulseless electrical activity*.

Repolarization

After the cell depolarizes, it quickly begins to recover and restore its electrical charges to normal. The movement of charged particles across a cell membrane in which the inside of the cell is restored to its negative charge is called **repolarization**. The cell membrane stops the flow of Na^+ into the cell and allows K^+ to leave it. Negatively charged particles are left inside the cell; thus, the cell is returned to its resting state (Fig. 2.5). This causes contractile proteins in the working myocardial cells to separate (i.e., relax). The cell can be stimulated again if another electrical impulse arrives at the cell membrane. Repolarization proceeds from the epicardium to the endocardium. On the ECG, the ST segment and T wave represent ventricular repolarization.

Phases of the Cardiac Action Potential

The **action potential** of a cardiac cell reflects the rapid sequence of voltage changes that occur across the cell membrane during the electrical cardiac cycle. The configuration of the action potential varies depending on the location, size, and function of the cardiac cell.

There are two main types of action potentials in the heart (Fig. 2.6). The first type, the fast response action potential, occurs in normal atrial and ventricular myocardial cells and in the **Purkinje fibers**, which are specialized conducting fibers found in both ventricles that conduct an electrical impulse through the heart.

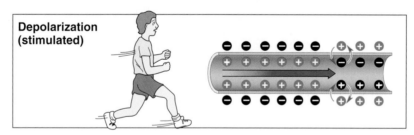

Fig. 2.4 Depolarization is the movement of ions across a cell membrane causing the inside of the cell to become more positive. (From Herlihy B: The *human body in health and illness*, ed 5, St. Louis, 2014, Mosby.)

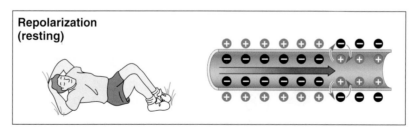

Fig. 2.5 Repolarization is the movement of charged particles across a cell membrane in which the inside of the cell is restored to its negative charge. (From Herlihy B: *The human body in health and illness*, ed 5, St. Louis, 2014, Mosby.)

The fast response action potential is divided into five phases. Phase 0, called the *upstroke*, *spike*, or *overshoot*, begins when the cell receives an impulse. Na⁺ moves rapidly into the cell through the Na⁺ channels, K⁺ leaves the cell, and Ca⁺⁺ moves slowly into the cell through Ca⁺⁺ channels (Fig. 2.7). The cell depolarizes and cardiac contraction begins. The upstroke is followed by a period of repolarization, which is divided into three phases. Phases 1, 2, and 3 have been referred to as *electrical systole*. During phase 1 (i.e., initial repolarization), the Na⁺

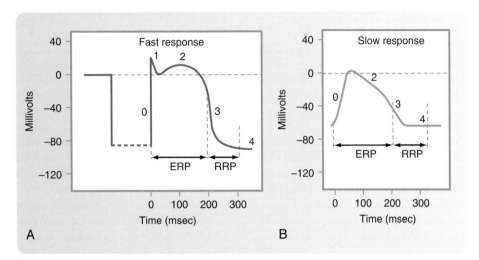

Fig. 2.6 Action potentials of fast-response A, and slow-response B, cardiac fibers. The phases of the action potentials are labeled. The effective refractory period (ERP) and the relative refractory period (RRP) are labeled. Note that when compared with fast-response fibers, the resting potential of slow fibers is less negative, the upstroke (phase 0) of the action potential is less steep, the amplitude of the action potential is smaller, phase 1 is absent, and the RRP extends well into phase 4 after the fibers have fully repolarized. (From Koeppen BM, Stanton BA: *Berne & Levy physiology,* ed 6, St. Louis, 2010, Mosby.)

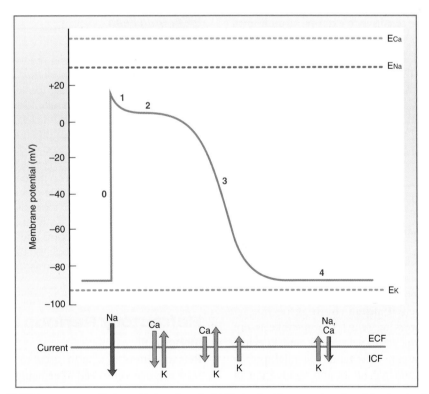

Fig. 2.7 Currents responsible for ventricular action potential. The length of the arrows shows the relative size of each ionic current. *E,* Equilibrium potential; *ECF,* extracellular fluid; *ICF,* intracellular fluid. (From Costanzo LS: *Physiology,* ed 5, Philadelphia, 2014, Saunders.)

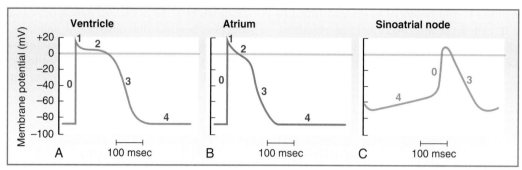

Fig. 2.8 A–C, Cardiac action potentials in the ventricle, atrium, and sinoatrial node. The numbers correspond to the phases of the action potentials. (From Costanzo LS: *Physiology,* ed 5, Philadelphia, 2014, Saunders.)

channels partially close, slowing the flow of Na$^+$ into the cell. At the same time, Cl$^-$ enters the cell, and K$^+$ leaves it through K$^+$ channels. The result is a decrease in the number of positive electrical charges within the cell. This produces a small negative deflection in the action potential. The cells of the atria, ventricles, and Purkinje fibers have many calcium channels. During phase 2 (i.e., the plateau phase), Ca^{++} slowly enters the cell through Ca^{++} channels. K$^+$ continues to leave the cell slowly through K$^+$ channels. Phase 3 (i.e., repolarization) begins with the downslope of the action potential. The cell rapidly completes repolarization as K$^+$ quickly flows out of the cell. Na$^+$ and Ca^{++} channels close, stopping the entry of Na$^+$ and Ca^{++}. The rapid movement of K$^+$ out of the cell causes the inside to become progressively more electrically negative. The cell gradually becomes more sensitive to external stimuli until its original sensitivity is restored. Repolarization is complete by the end of phase 3. Phase 4 is the resting membrane potential (i.e., return to resting state); this period is called *electrical diastole*. During phase 4, the Na$^+$/K$^+$ pump is activated to move Na$^+$ out of the cell and K$^+$ back into the cell. Relaxation of the cardiac muscle occurs mainly during phase 4. The cell will remain polarized (i.e., ready for discharge) until the cell membrane is reactivated by another stimulus.

The second type of cardiac action potential, the slow response action potential, occurs in the heart's normal pacemaker (i.e., the SA node) and in the **atrioventricular (AV) node**, which is the specialized conducting tissue that carries an electrical impulse from the atria to the ventricles (Fig. 2.8). The SA and AV nodes of the heart have relatively few sodium channels. Therefore, phase 0, the upstroke, of the slow response action potential is largely the result of the entry of Ca^{++} into the cell. (Calcium also triggers contraction in all myocardial working cells.) The upstroke is not as rapid or steep as in the atrial, ventricular, and Purkinje fibers. This finding indicates that the action potential spreads more slowly in the SA and AV nodes and conduction of the impulse is more likely to be blocked there than in fast-response cardiac tissue (Pappano, 2010). Phase 1 is absent in the slow-response action potential, and the transition

from the plateau phase to repolarization (i.e., phase 3) is less distinct. As in the other cardiac tissues, repolarization is dependent on K$^+$. Changes in the movement of K$^+$ and Ca^{++} produce activity in pacemaker cells during phase 4. For example, phase 4 is the longest portion of the SA node action potential and accounts for the ability of the cells in the SA node to spontaneously generate an action potential without requiring stimulation by a nerve (automaticity). The rate of phase 4 depolarization affects heart rate (Costanzo, 2014). For example, an increase in the rate of phase 4 depolarization results in the SA node firing more action potentials per time, increasing the heart rate. In contrast, a decrease in the rate of phase 4 depolarization results in the SA node firing fewer action potentials per time, decreasing the heart rate.

 Drug Pearl _____

Antiarrhythmic Agents

The heart typically beats at a regular rate and rhythm. If this pattern is interrupted, an abnormal heart rhythm can result. Health care professionals use the terms *arrhythmia* and *dysrhythmia* interchangeably to refer to an abnormal heart rhythm. Medications used to correct irregular heartbeats and slow down hearts that beat too fast are called *antiarrhythmics*. Although there is no universally accepted classification scheme for antiarrhythmic agents, a commonly used system is to classify the medications by their effects on the cardiac action potential. For example, class I antiarrhythmic medications such as procainamide and lidocaine block sodium channels, interfering with phase 0 depolarization. Class IV antiarrhythmics (Ca^{++} channel blockers) such as verapamil and diltiazem slow the rate at which calcium passes through the cells, interfering with phase 2 in the cells of the atria, ventricles, and Purkinje fibers.

Refractory Periods

[Objective 6]

Refractoriness is a term used to describe the period of recovery that cells need after being discharged before they are once again able to respond to a stimulus. During **absolute refractory period (ARP)**, the cell will not respond to further stimulation within itself (Fig. 2.9). This means that

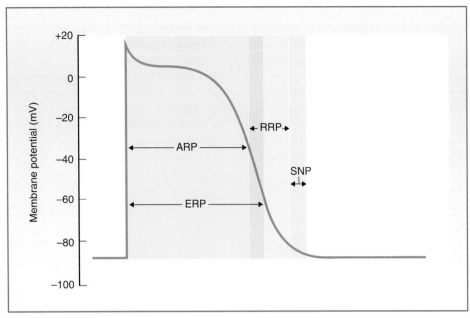

Fig. 2.9 Refractory periods of the ventricular action potential. Refractory periods of the ventricular action potential. The effective refractory period (ERP) includes the absolute refractory period (ARP) and the first half of the relative refractory period (RRP). The RRP begins when the absolute refractory period ends and includes the last portion of the ERP. The supernormal period (SNP) begins when the RRP ends. (From Costanzo LS: *Physiology*, ed 5, Philadelphia, 2014, Saunders.)

the myocardial working cells cannot contract and that the cells of the electrical conduction system cannot conduct an electrical impulse, no matter how strong the internal electrical stimulus. As a result, tetanic (i.e., sustained) contractions cannot be provoked in the cardiac muscle. The ARP corresponds to the time needed for the reopening of channels that allow the entry of sodium and calcium into the cell (Brashers & McCance, 2012). In a fast-response myocardial fiber, the ARP includes phases 0, 1, 2, and part of phase 3 of the cardiac action potential. Slow-response fibers become absolutely refractory at the beginning of the upstroke (Pappano, 2010). The **relative refractory period (RRP)** begins at the end of the ARP and ends when the cell membrane is almost fully repolarized. During the RRP, some cardiac cells have repolarized to their threshold potential and thus can be stimulated to respond (i.e., depolarize) to a stronger-than-normal stimulus.

The **effective refractory period (ERP)** includes the ARP and the first half of the RRP. "The distinction between the ARP and ERP is that *absolute* means *absolutely* no stimulus is large enough to generate another action potential; *effective* means that a *conducted* action potential cannot be generated (i.e., there is not enough inward current to conduct to the next site)" (Costanzo, 2014, p. 135).

A **supernormal period (SNP)** follows the RRP. A weaker-than-normal stimulus can cause cardiac cells to depolarize during this period. The SNP extends from the end of phase 3 to the beginning of phase 4 of the cardiac action potential. Because the cell is more excitable than normal, dysrhythmias can develop during this period (see Fig. 2.9).

 CLINICAL CORRELATIONS

The duration of the action potential determines the length of the refractory period. The longer the action potential, the longer the cell is refractory to firing another action potential (Costanzo, 2014). The action potential, and, consequently, the refractory period, in cells of the atria (i.e., 150 msec), ventricles (i.e., 250 msec), and Purkinje system (i.e., 300 msec) is long compared with other excitable tissues in the heart because of a sustained period of depolarization (i.e., plateau).

CONDUCTION SYSTEM

[Objectives 7, 8]

The specialized electrical (i.e., pacemaker) cells in the heart are arranged in a system of pathways called the **conduction system**. In the normal heart, the cells of the conduction system are interconnected. The conduction system makes sure that the chambers of the heart contract in a coordinated fashion.

Sinoatrial Node

The SA node is specialized conducting tissue located in the upper posterior part of the right atrium where the superior vena cava and the right atrium meet. Because the SA node is located in the right atrium, right atrial contraction begins and ends earlier than in the left atrium (Boulpaep, 2017). In an adult, the SA node is about 10 to 20 mm long and 2 to 3 mm thick (Rubart & Zipes, 2015). The SA node receives its blood supply from the

SA node artery that runs lengthwise through the center of the node. The SA node artery originates from the right coronary artery (RCA) in about 55% to 60% of people and from the circumflex (Cx) artery in the remaining 40% to 45% (Rubart & Zipes, 2015).

Two main types of cells exist within the SA node: (1) small, round cells that have few myofibrils and (2) slender, elongated cells that differ from the round cells and typical atrial myocardial cells. The round cells are thought to be pacemaker cells, and the others are thought to be responsible for conducting the electrical impulse within the SA node and to its borders. The SA node is richly supplied by sympathetic and parasympathetic nerve fibers.

The normal heartbeat is the result of an electrical impulse (i.e., an action potential) that begins in the SA node. Although the SA node is the smallest electrical region of the heart (Lederer, 2012), it is normally the primary pacemaker because it has the fastest firing rate (specifically, the fastest rate of phase 4 depolarization) of all of the heart's normal pacemaker sites (Fig. 2.10). The

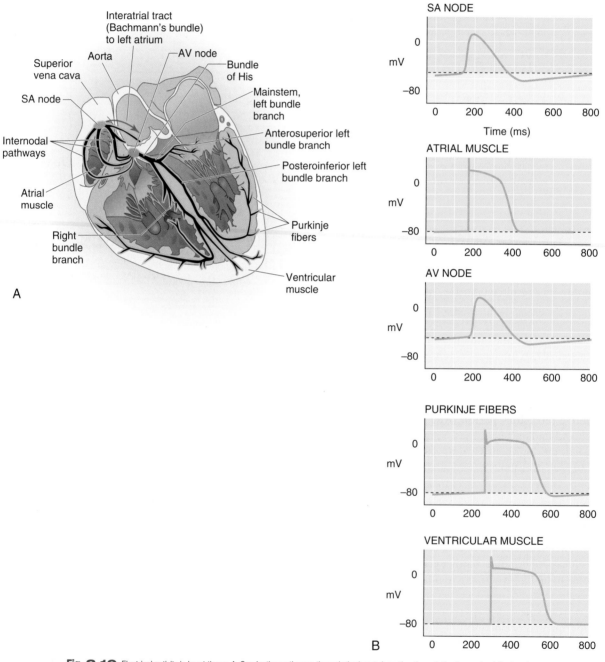

Fig. 2.10 Electrical activity in heart tissue. A, Conduction pathways through the heart. A section through the long axis of the heart is shown. B, Cardiac action potentials. The distinctive shapes of action potentials at five sites along the spread of excitation are shown. *AV,* Atrioventricular; *SA,* sinoatrial. (From Boron WF, Boulpaep EL: *Medical physiology,* ed 3, Philadelphia, 2017, Saunders.)

built-in (i.e., intrinsic) rate of the SA node is 60 to 100 beats/min. Although the SA node normally fires at a rate of 60 to 100 beats/min, this rate can increase to about 180 beats/min, primarily through sympathetic stimulation. Heart rates faster than 150 beats/min can be problematic because: (1) the duration of diastole shortens as heart rate increases, reducing ventricular filling time and, potentially, stroke volume, and (2) the heart's workload and oxygen requirements are increased, but the time for coronary artery filling, which occurs during diastole, is decreased (DeBeasi, 2003a).

As the impulse leaves the SA node, it spreads from cell to cell in wavelike form across the atrial muscle. As the impulse spreads, it stimulates the right atrium and the interatrial septum, and it travels along a special pathway called *Bachmann's bundle* to stimulate the left atrium. This results in contraction of the right and left atria at almost the same time. Because a fibrous skeleton separates the atrial myocardium from the ventricular myocardium, the electrical stimulus affects only the atria.

Areas of the heart other than the SA node can initiate beats (i.e., intrinsic automaticity) and assume pacemaker responsibility under special circumstances. The terms **ectopic**, which means "out of place," and *latent* are used to describe an impulse that originates from a source other than the SA node. Ectopic pacemaker sites include the cells of the AV junction and Purkinje fibers, although their intrinsic rates are slower than that of the SA node. Although an ectopic pacemaker normally is prevented from discharging because of the dominance of the SA node's rapidly firing pacemaker cells, an ectopic site may assume pacemaker responsibility in the following circumstances:

- The SA node fires too slowly because of vagal stimulation or suppression by medications.
- The SA node fails to generate an impulse because of disease or suppression by medications.
- The SA node action potential is blocked because of disease in conducting pathways, failing to activate the surrounding atrial myocardium.
- The firing rate of the ectopic site becomes faster than that of the SA node.

Although ectopic pacemakers supply a backup or safety mechanism in the event of SA node failure, such sites can be problematic if they fire while the SA node is still functioning. For example, ectopic sites may cause early (i.e., premature) beats or sustained rhythm disturbances.

Atrioventricular Node and Bundle

The AV node is a group of specialized conducting cells that is usually located in the floor of the right atrium immediately behind the tricuspid valve. In adults, the AV node typically measures about 5 to 7 mm in length and 2 to 5 mm in width; however, its size and shape are not uniform and vary greatly among individuals (Saksena et al, 2012). The AV node is supplied by a branch of the RCA in 85% to 90% of the population (Rubart & Zipes, 2015). In the remainder, a branch of the Cx artery provides the blood supply. The AV node is supplied by both sympathetic and parasympathetic nerve fibers.

Conduction through the AV node begins before atrial depolarization is completed. The AV node has been divided into three functional regions according to their action potentials and responses to electrical and chemical stimulation (Hwang et al, 2014) (Fig. 2.11):

- The atrionodal (AN) region (also called the *transitional zone*) located between the atrium and the rest of the node
- The nodal (N) region, the compact AV node where transitional cells merge with midnodal cells
- The nodal-His (NH) or lower region where the fibers of the AV node gradually merge with the bundle of His

As the impulse enters the AV node through the internodal pathways, conduction is markedly slowed in the N area of the AV node before the impulse reaches the ventricles (Issa et al, 2012) (Fig. 2.12). If this delay did not occur, the atria and the ventricles would contract at about the same time. The delay in conduction allows both atrial chambers to contract and empty blood into the ventricles before the next ventricular contraction begins. This

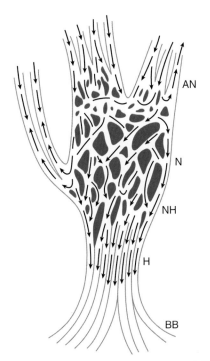

Fig. 2.11 The atrioventricular node and bundle. *AN,* Atrionodal; *BB,* bundle branches; *H,* bundle of His; *N,* nodal; *NH,* nodal-His. (From Clochesy J: *Critical care nursing,* ed 2, Philadelphia, 1996, Saunders.)

increases the amount of blood in the ventricles, increasing stroke volume.

Some people have two or more conduction pathways in the area of the AV node that conduct impulses at different speeds and recover at different rates (Zimetbaum, 2016). The pathways join into a final common pathway before impulses exiting the AV node continue to the bundle of His. The fast pathway (i.e., the beta pathway) conducts impulses rapidly but has a long refractory period (i.e., slow recovery time). The slow pathway (i.e., the alpha pathway) conducts impulses slowly but has a short refractory period (i.e., fast recovery time).

The **bundle of His**, also called the *common bundle* or the **AV bundle**, is a continuation of the AV node and connects the AV node with the bundle branches. The AV node and the bundle of His are called the *AV junction*. The lower portion of the NH area of the AV node is believed to possess pacemaker cells that have an intrinsic rate of 40 to 60 beats/min (see Fig. 2.11). Because this pacemaker rate is slower than that of the SA node, the AV junction is considered a secondary pacemaker (Lederer, 2012).

The term **His-Purkinje system**, or *His-Purkinje network*, refers to the bundle of His, bundle branches, and Purkinje fibers. In the heart's conduction system, the speed of impulse conduction is fastest in the His-Purkinje system and slowest in the SA and AV nodes.

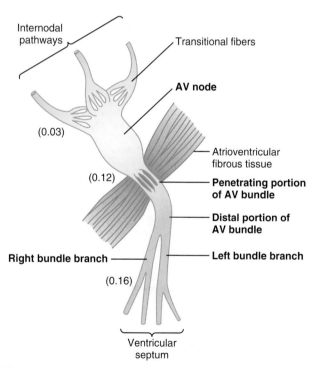

Fig. 2.12 *Organization of the atrioventricular (AV) node and AV bundle. The numbers represent the interval of time in fractions of a second from the origin of the impulse in the sinoatrial node. (From Hall JE:* Guyton and Hall textbook of medical physiology, *ed 13, Philadelphia, 2016, Saunders.)*

Normally, the atria and ventricles are separated by a continuous barrier of fibrous tissue, which acts as an insulator to prevent passage of an electrical impulse through any route other than the AV node and bundle. When the AV node and bundle are bypassed by an abnormal pathway, the abnormal route is called an **accessory pathway**.

 ECG Pearl _____

Abnormal cardiac rhythms that develop near or within the AV node are called *junctional dysrhythmias*. Those that develop above the bundle of His or activate the ventricles through an accessory pathway are called *supraventricular dysrhythmias*. Dysrhythmias that develop below the bundle of His are called *ventricular dysrhythmias*.

Right and Left Bundle Branches

The bundle of His passes down the right side of the interventricular septum for about 1 cm before dividing into the right and left bundle branches (Pappano, 2010). The upper portion of the interventricular septum is supplied with blood by branches of the anterior and posterior descending coronary arteries (Rubart & Zipes, 2015).

The right bundle branch is thin and travels to the apex of the right ventricle. The left bundle branch spreads the electrical impulse to the interventricular septum and left ventricle. The left bundle branch is thicker than the right and splits into divisions called *fascicles* on the subendocardial surface of the left side of the interventricular septum (Pappano, 2010).

Purkinje Fibers

The right and left bundle branches divide into smaller and smaller branches and then into a fibrous network called the *Purkinje fibers*, which spread out over the subendocardial surfaces of both ventricles. These fibers have pacemaker cells that have an intrinsic rate of 20 to 40 beats/min. Because this pacemaker rate is slower than that of the SA node and the AV junction, it is considered a tertiary pacemaker.

Purkinje fibers have a large diameter and an abundant concentration of gap junctions, enabling the rapid propagation of electrical impulses. It has been estimated that conduction time through the Purkinje system is about 150 times faster than conduction through the AV node (DeBeasi, 2003b). The spread of an electrical impulse through the Purkinje fibers proceeds from the endocardium, where the endocardial surfaces of both ventricles are rapidly activated, to the myocardium and ventricular muscle fibers, and then finally to the epicardial surface. A summary of the conduction system is shown in Table 2.1.

TABLE **2.1**	Summary of the Conduction System			
Structure	Location	Function	Intrinsic Pacemaker (beats/min)	Time Lapse from SA Node (sec)
Sinoatrial (SA) node	Right atrial wall just inferior to opening of superior vena cava	Primary pacemaker; initiates impulse that is normally conducted throughout the left and right atria	60 to 100	0
Atrioventricular (AV) node	Floor of the right atrium immediately behind the tricuspid valve and near the opening of the coronary sinus	Receives impulse from SA node and delays relay of the impulse to the bundle of His, allowing time for the atria to empty their contents into the ventricles before the onset of ventricular contraction		0.03
Bundle of His (AV bundle)	Superior portion of interventricular septum	Receives impulse from AV node and relays it to right and left bundle branches	40 to 60	0.04
Right and left bundle branches	Interventricular septum	Receives impulse from bundle of His and relays it to Purkinje fibers		0.17
Purkinje fibers	Ventricular myocardium	Receives impulse from bundle branches and relays it to ventricular myocardium	20 to 40	0.20 to 0.22

CAUSES OF DYSRHYTHMIAS

[Objective 9]

Dysrhythmias result from disorders of impulse formation, disorders of impulse conduction, or both.

Disorders of Impulse Formation
ABNORMAL AUTOMATICITY

Abnormal automaticity is a condition in which one of the following occurs: (1) Cardiac cells that are not normally associated with a pacemaker function begin to depolarize spontaneously *or* (2) a pacemaker site other than the SA node increases its firing rate beyond that which is considered normal.

Possible causes for abnormal automaticity include ischemia, hypoxia, electrolyte disorders, and exposure to chemicals or toxic substances, among others. Examples of rhythms associated with abnormal automaticity include premature beats, accelerated idioventricular rhythm, accelerated junctional rhythm, and some forms of ventricular tachycardia.

TRIGGERED ACTIVITY

Triggered activity results from abnormal electrical impulses that sometimes occur during repolarization, when cells are normally quiet. These abnormal electrical impulses are called *afterdepolarizations*. Triggered activity requires a stimulus to begin depolarization. It occurs when pacemaker cells from a site other than the SA node and myocardial working cells depolarize more than once after being stimulated by a single impulse.

Causes of triggered activity include hypoxia, excessive catecholamines, myocardial ischemia or injury, digitalis toxicity, and medications that prolong repolarization. Triggered activity can result in atrial or ventricular beats that occur alone, in pairs, in runs of three or more beats, or as a sustained ectopic rhythm.

Disorders of Impulse Conduction
CONDUCTION BLOCKS

Blockage of impulse conduction may be partial or complete. A block may occur because of trauma, drug toxicity, electrolyte disturbances, myocardial ischemia, or infarction. A partial conduction block may cause the impulse to become slowed or intermittent. In slowed conduction, all impulses are conducted, but it takes longer than normal to do so. When an intermittent block occurs, some (but not all) impulses are conducted. When a complete block exists, no impulses are conducted through the affected area. Examples of rhythms associated with disturbances in conduction include AV blocks.

REENTRY
[Objective 10]

An impulse normally spreads through the heart only once after it is initiated by pacemaker cells. **Reentry** is the spread of an impulse through tissue already stimulated by that same impulse. Reentry requires the following three conditions:

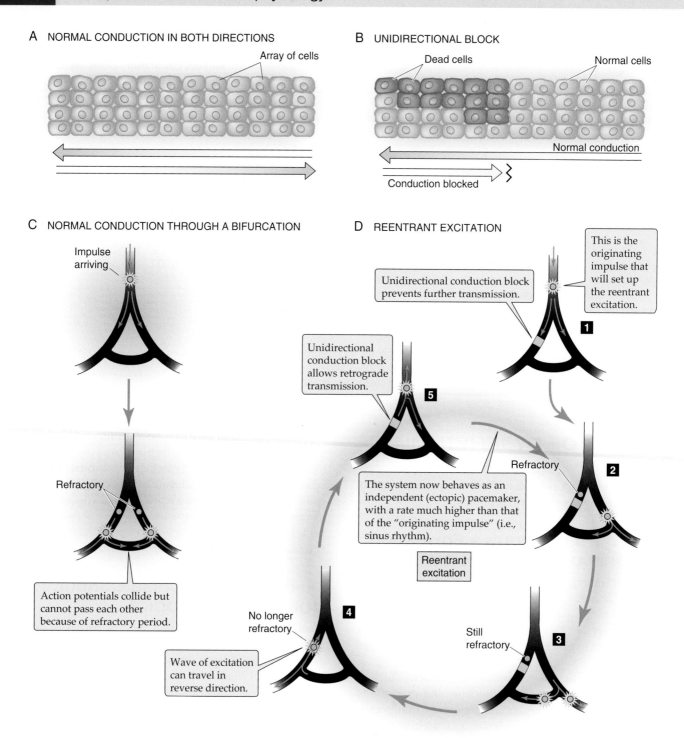

A NORMAL CONDUCTION IN BOTH DIRECTIONS

Array of cells

B UNIDIRECTIONAL BLOCK

Dead cells

Normal cells

Normal conduction

Conduction blocked

C NORMAL CONDUCTION THROUGH A BIFURCATION

Impulse arriving

Refractory

Action potentials collide but cannot pass each other because of refractory period.

No longer refractory

Wave of excitation can travel in reverse direction.

D REENTRANT EXCITATION

This is the originating impulse that will set up the reentrant excitation.

Unidirectional conduction block prevents further transmission.

1

Unidirectional conduction block allows retrograde transmission.

5

Refractory

2

The system now behaves as an independent (ectopic) pacemaker, with a rate much higher than that of the "originating impulse" (i.e., sinus rhythm).

Reentrant excitation

4

Still refractory

3

Fig. 2.13 Conduction. A, Normal conduction in both directions. B, Unidirectional block. C, Normal conduction through a bifurcation. D, Reentrant excitation. (From Boron WF, Boulpaep EL: *Medical physiology,* ed 3, Philadelphia, 2017, Saunders.)

(1) an area of unidirectional conduction block, (2) an area of delayed conduction, and (3) an area of unexcitable tissue (Peterson, 2009). When reentry occurs, an electrical impulse is delayed, blocked, or both, in one or more areas of the conduction system while the impulse is conducted normally through the rest of the conduction system (Fig. 2.13). This results in the delayed electrical impulse entering cardiac cells that have just been depolarized by the normally conducted impulse.

Macroreentry circuits and microreentry circuits are two main types of reentry circuits. If the reentry circuit involves conduction through a large area of the heart, such as the entire right or left atrium, it is called a *macroreentry circuit*. A reentry circuit involving conduction within a small area is called a *microreentry circuit*.

Possible causes of reentry include hyperkalemia, myocardial ischemia, some antiarrhythmic medications, and the presence of an accessory pathway. Examples of rhythms associated with reentry include AV nodal reentrant tachycardia, AV reentrant tachycardia, and atrial flutter.

THE ELECTROCARDIOGRAM

[Objectives 11, 12]

The ECG is a graphic display of the heart's electrical activity. The first ECG was introduced by Willem Einthoven, a Dutch physiologist, in the early 1900s. When electrodes are attached to the patient's limbs or chest and connected by cables to an ECG machine, the ECG machine functions as a voltmeter, detecting and recording the changes in voltage (i.e., action potentials) generated by depolarization and repolarization of the heart's cells. The voltage changes are displayed as specific waveforms and complexes (Fig. 2.14).

Electrocardiographic monitoring may be used for the following purposes:
- To monitor a patient's heart rate
- To evaluate the effects of disease or injury on heart function
- To evaluate pacemaker function
- To evaluate the response to medications (e.g., antiarrhythmics)

- To obtain a baseline recording before, during, and after a medical procedure
- To evaluate for signs of myocardial ischemia, injury, and infarction

The ECG *can* provide information about the following:
- The orientation of the heart in the chest
- Conduction disturbances
- Electrical effects of medications and electrolytes
- The mass of cardiac muscle
- The presence of ischemic damage

The ECG does *not* provide information about the mechanical (contractile) condition of the myocardium. To evaluate the effectiveness of the heart's mechanical activity, the patient's pulse and blood pressure are assessed.

Electrodes

Electrode refers to an adhesive pad containing a conductive substance in the center that is applied to the patient's skin (Fig. 2.15). The conductive media of the electrode conducts skin surface voltage changes through wires to a cardiac monitor (i.e., electrocardiograph). Electrodes are applied at specific locations on the patient's chest wall and extremities to view the heart's electrical activity from different angles and planes.

Remove oil and dead cells from the patient's skin before applying electrodes. There are a variety of techniques for doing so, such as a brisk dry rub of the skin. Many electrode manufacturers include an abrasive area on the disposable backing of the electrode for this purpose, but a gauze pad or terrycloth

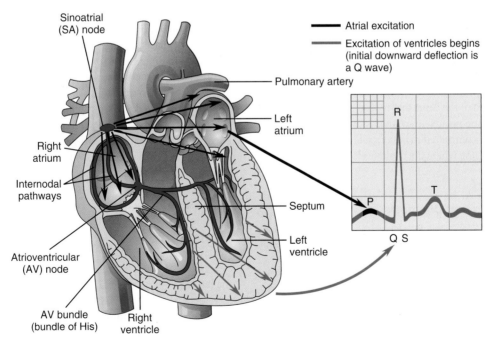

Fig. 2.14 Schematic drawing of the conducting system of the heart. An impulse normally is generated in the sinoatrial node and travels through the atria to the atrioventricular node, down the bundle of His and Purkinje fibers, and to the ventricular myocardium. Recording of the depolarizing and repolarizing currents in the heart with electrodes on the surface of the body produces characteristic waveforms. (From Copstead-Kirkhorn LE, Banasik JL: *Pathophysiology,* ed 5, St. Louis, 2013, Saunders.)

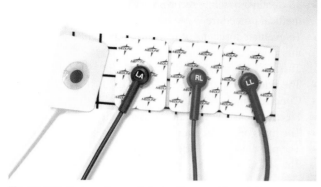

Fig. 2.15 Electrocardiogram electrodes. (Courtesy of Bruce R. Shade, EMT-P, EMS-I, AAS.)

washcloth works well too. In some circumstances, small areas may need to be shaved or chest hair cut if the electrode(s) will not stick. To minimize distortion (artifact), be sure the conductive jelly in the center of the electrode is not dry, and avoid placing the electrodes directly over bony areas.

One end of a monitoring cable, also called a *lead wire*, is attached to the electrode and the other to an ECG machine. The cable conducts current back to the cardiac monitor. ECG cables may be coded by color, symbol, or letter. However, colors are not standard and often vary.

Leads

[Objectives 13, 14, 15]

A **lead** is a record (i.e., tracing) of electrical activity, specifically the fluctuation in voltage differences, between positive and negative electrodes (Lederer, 2012). Each lead records the *average* current flow at a specific time in a portion of the heart. Leads allow for the viewing of the heart's electrical activity in the frontal and horizontal (transverse) planes.

Think of each positive electrode as an eye looking in at the heart. Because the position of the positive electrode on the body determines the area of the heart that is seen by each lead, accurate placement of the positive electrode is important. The view of each lead can be committed to memory, or it can be reasoned easily by remembering where the positive electrode is located.

 Lead In _____

ECG Monitoring and Diagnosis

Continuous patient monitoring is usually performed by means of bedside monitoring or telemetry, which is the electronic transmission of data to a distant location, such as a nurses' station. Continuous ECG monitoring may be performed using a single lead or, depending on equipment capability, three or even five leads may be used.

A 12-lead ECG provides views of the heart in both the frontal and horizontal planes and views the surfaces of the left ventricle from multiple angles. The 12-lead ECG is a useful diagnostic study you can obtain when there are changes in a patient's cardiac rhythm or condition. Indications for obtaining a 12-lead ECG are discussed in more detail in Chapter 9.

FRONTAL PLANE LEADS

Six leads view the heart in the frontal plane. Leads I, II, and III are called *standard limb leads*. Leads aVR, aVL, and aVF are called *augmented limb leads*.

A **bipolar lead** is an ECG lead that has a positive and negative electrode. Each lead records the difference in electrical potential (i.e., voltage) between two selected electrodes. Although all ECG leads are technically bipolar, leads I, II, and III use two distinct electrodes, one of which is connected to the positive input of the ECG machine and the other to the negative input (Wagner et al, 2009).

Standard Limb Leads

Leads I, II, and III make up the standard limb leads (Fig. 2.16). If an electrode is placed on the right arm, left arm, and left leg, three leads are formed. The positive electrode is located at the left wrist in lead I, and leads II and III both have their positive electrode located at the left foot. The difference in electrical potential between the positive pole and its corresponding negative pole is measured by each lead.

An imaginary line that joins the positive and negative electrodes of a lead is called the **axis** of the lead. The axes of these three limb leads form an equilateral triangle with the heart at the center, which is called *Einthoven's triangle*. Einthoven's triangle is a way of showing that the two arms and the left leg form apices of a triangle surrounding the heart (see Fig. 2.16). The two apices at the upper part of the triangle represent the points at which the two arms connect electrically with the fluids around the heart. The lower apex is the point at which the left leg connects with the fluids (Hall, 2016). Over the years, electrode placement for leads I, II, and III has been altered and moved to the patient's chest to allow for patient movement and to minimize distortion on the ECG tracing. However, proper electrode positioning for the limb leads includes placement near the patient's wrists and ankles or, at a minimum, distal to the patient's shoulders and hips (Mirvis & Goldberger, 2015).

Lead I records the difference in electrical potential between the left arm (+) and right arm (−) electrodes. Lead I views the lateral surface of the left ventricle. With normal depolarization, waveforms observed in this lead are usually positive. If negative P waves and primarily negative QRS complexes and T waves are observed in lead I, take a moment to recheck the lead wires connected to the right and left arm electrodes; it is likely that the lead wires have been reversed (Harrigan et al, 2014).

Lead II records the difference in electrical potential between the left leg (+) and right arm (−) electrodes. Lead II views the inferior surface of the left ventricle. This lead is commonly used for cardiac monitoring because positioning of the positive and negative electrodes in this lead most closely resembles the normal pathway of current flow in the heart.

Lead III records the difference in electrical potential between the left leg (+) and left arm (−) electrodes. Waveforms observed in this lead are usually positive. Lead

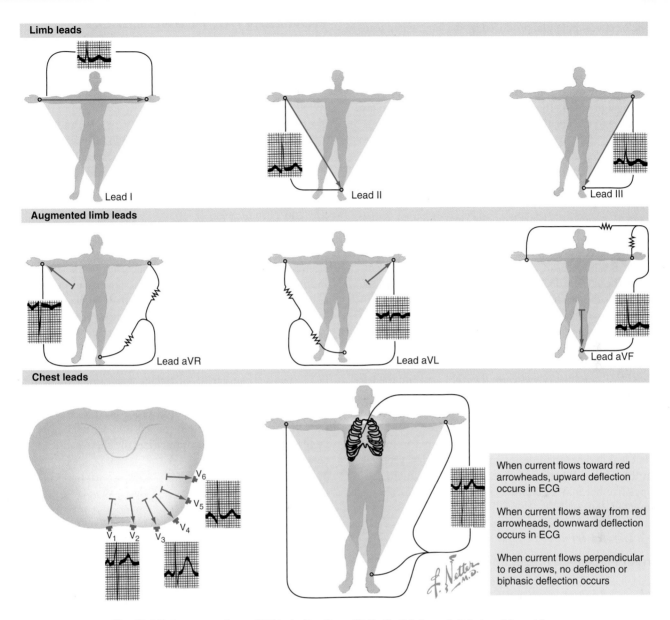

Fig. 2.16 The electrocardiogram (ECG) leads. (From Runge MS, Stouffer G, Patterson C: *Netter's cardiology,* ed 2, Philadelphia, 2010, Saunders.)

III views the inferior surface of the left ventricle. A summary of the standard limb leads appears in Table 2.2.

Augmented Limb Leads

Leads aVR, aVL, and aVF are limb leads that record measurements at a specific electrode with respect to a reference electrode. Frank Norman Wilson and colleagues used the term *central terminal* to describe a reference point that is the average of the limb lead electrical potentials. In the augmented leads, the Wilson central terminal (WCT) is calculated by the ECG machine's computer as an average potential of the electrical currents from the two electrodes other than the one being used as the positive electrode. For example, in lead aVL, the positive electrode is located on the patient's left arm. The ECG machine's computer calculates the central terminal by joining the electrical currents obtained from the electrodes on the patient's right arm and left leg. Lead aVL therefore represents the difference in electrical potential between the left arm and the central terminal. The electrical potential of the central terminal is essentially zero.

TABLE 2.2	Standard Limb Leads		
Lead	Positive Electrode	Negative Electrode	Heart Surface Viewed
I	Left arm	Right arm	Lateral
II	Left leg	Right arm	Inferior
III	Left leg	Left arm	Inferior

The electrical potential produced by the augmented leads is normally relatively small. The ECG machine augments (i.e., magnifies) the amplitude of the electrical potentials detected at each extremity by about 50% over those recorded at the standard limb leads. The "a" in aVR, aVL, and aVF refers to augmented. The "V" refers to voltage, and the last letter refers to the position of the positive electrode. The "R" refers to the right arm, the "L" to left arm, and the "F" to left foot (i.e., leg). Therefore, the positive electrode in aVR is located on the right arm, aVL has a positive electrode at the left arm, and aVF has a positive electrode positioned on the left leg (see Fig. 2.16).

Lead aVR views the heart from the right shoulder, which is the positive electrode. Because the wave of depolarization is moving away from lead aVR, waveforms in this lead are typically negative. Lead aVR has been called "the forgotten lead" because it does not view any single surface of the heart. Many clinicians believe that lead aVR reflects reciprocal (i.e., mirror image) changes from leads aVL, II, V_5, and V_6 (Gorgels et al, 2001). Research has shown value in the use of lead aVR in differentiating atrial tachydysrhythmias (Vorobiof & Ellestad, 2011).

Lead aVL combines views from the right arm and the left leg, with the view being from the left arm and oriented to the lateral wall of the left ventricle. Waveforms observed in this lead are usually positive but may be biphasic. Lead aVF combines views from the right arm and the left arm toward the left leg; it views the inferior surface of the left ventricle from the left leg. Waveforms observed in this lead are usually positive but may be biphasic. Table 2.3 summarizes the augmented limb leads.

 Lead In _____

Correct Placement of Electrodes

Leads I, II, III, aVR, aVL, and aVF are obtained from electrodes placed on the patient's arms and legs. The deltoid area is suitable for electrodes attached to the arms and is easily accessible. Either the thigh or lower leg is suitable for the leg electrodes. Use the more convenient site but keep the electrodes in a similar position. For example, keep the upper extremity electrodes on the deltoids rather than placing one on the upper arm and one on the inner arm. Be sure that the patient's limbs are resting on a supportive surface. This decreases muscle tension in the patient's arms and legs and helps minimize distortion of the electrocardiogram tracing (i.e., artifact). If circumstances require that the electrodes be placed on the torso, be sure to position them as close to the appropriate limb as possible.

TABLE 2.3	Augmented Limb Leads	
Lead	**Positive Electrode**	**Heart Surface Viewed**
aVR	Right arm	None
aVL	Left arm	Lateral
aVF	Left leg	Inferior

HORIZONTAL PLANE LEADS

Six chest (i.e., precordial or "V") leads view the heart in the horizontal plane (see Fig. 2.16). This allows a view of the front and left side of the heart.

Chest Leads

The chest leads are identified as V_1, V_2, V_3, V_4, V_5, and V_6 (Fig. 2.17). Each electrode placed in a "V" position is a positive electrode, measuring electrical potential with respect to the WCT.

Lead V_1 is recorded with the positive electrode in the fourth intercostal space, just to the right of the sternum. Remember, the electrode positions refer to the location of the gel. For example, the gel of the V_1 electrode, not the entire adhesive patch, is positioned in the fourth intercostal space, just to the right of the sternum. Lead V_2 is recorded with the positive electrode in the fourth intercostal space, just to the left of the sternum. Lead V_3 is recorded with the positive electrode on a line midway between V_2 and V_4. Lead V_4 is recorded with the positive electrode in the left midclavicular line in the fifth intercostal space. To evaluate the right ventricle, lead V_4 may be moved to the same anatomic location but on the right side of the chest. The lead is then called V_4R, and it is viewed for ECG changes consistent with acute myocardial infarction. Lead V_5 is recorded with the positive electrode in the left anterior axillary line at the same level as V_4. Lead V_6 is recorded with the positive electrode in the left midaxillary line at the same level as V_4. Table 2.4 summarizes the chest leads.

 Did You Know? _____

Because their location varies, the nipples shouldn't be used as landmarks for chest electrode placement. If your patient is a woman, place the electrodes for leads V_3 through V_6 *under* the breast rather than *on* the breast.

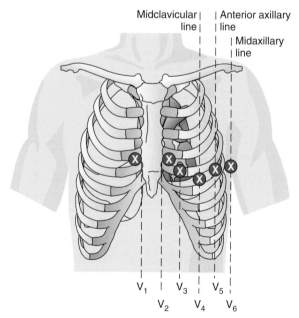

Fig. 2.17 Chest (precordial) leads V_1 through V_6. (From Copstead-Kirkhorn LE, Banasik JL: *Pathophysiology,* ed 5, St. Louis, 2013, Saunders.)

TABLE 2.4	Chest Leads	
Lead	Positive Electrode Position	Heart Area Viewed
V_1	Right side of sternum, fourth intercostal space	Interventricular septum
V_2	Left side of sternum, fourth intercostal space	Interventricular septum
V_3	Midway between V_2 and V_4	Anterior surface
V_4	Left midclavicular line, fifth intercostal space	Anterior surface
V_5	Left anterior axillary line; same level as V_4	Lateral surface
V_6	Left midaxillary line, fifth intercostal space	Lateral surface

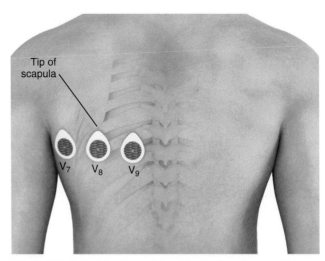

Fig. 2.19 Electrode locations for left posterior chest lead placement. (From Hedges JR: *Roberts and Hedges' clinical procedures in emergency medicine,* ed 6, Philadelphia, 2014, Saunders.)

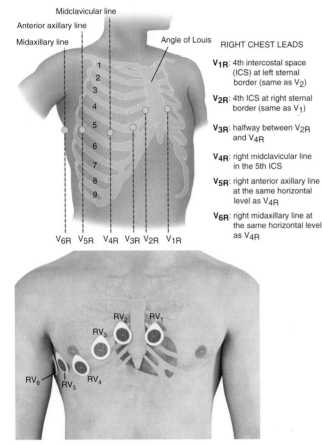

RIGHT CHEST LEADS

V_{1R}: 4th intercostal space (ICS) at left sternal border (same as V_2)

V_{2R}: 4th ICS at right sternal border (same as V_1)

V_{3R}: halfway between V_{2R} and V_{4R}

V_{4R}: right midclavicular line in the 5th ICS

V_{5R}: right anterior axillary line at the same horizontal level as V_{4R}

V_{6R}: right midaxillary line at the same horizontal level as V_{4R}

Fig. 2.18 Electrode locations for recording a right chest electrocardiogram (ECG). Right chest leads are not part of a standard 12-lead ECG but are used when a right ventricular infarction is suspected. (From Drew BJ, Ide B: Right ventricular infarction, *Prog Cardiovascular Nurs 10*:46, 1195; and Hedges JR: *Roberts and Hedges' clinical procedures in emergency medicine,* ed 6, Philadelphia, 2014, Saunders.)

Right Chest Leads

Other chest leads that are not part of a standard 12-lead ECG reveal specific surfaces of the heart. Right chest leads are used to evaluate the right ventricle (Fig. 2.18). The placement of right chest leads is identical to the placement of the standard chest leads except that it is done on the right side of the chest. Obtain a standard 12-lead ECG first; then

reposition the electrodes on the right side of the chest and attach the cables for the standard chest leads to the repositioned electrodes to obtain the additional leads. If time does not permit obtaining all of the right chest leads, the lead of choice is V_4R.

Posterior Chest Leads

On a standard 12-lead ECG, no leads look directly at the posterior surface of the heart. Additional chest leads may be used for this purpose. These leads are placed farther left and toward the back. All of the leads are placed on the same horizontal line as V_4 to V_6. Lead V_7 is placed at the posterior axillary line. Lead V_8 is placed at the angle of the scapula (i.e., the posterior scapular line), and lead V_9 is placed over the left border of the spine (Fig. 2.19).

→ *Lead In* _____

Multiple-Lead ECGs

Multiple-lead ECGs are being used with increasing frequency to help spot infarctions of the right ventricle and the posterior wall of the left ventricle. The 15-lead ECG uses all of the leads of a standard 12-lead ECG plus leads V_4R, V_8, and V_9. An 18-lead ECG uses all of the leads of the 15-lead ECG plus leads V_5R, V_6R, and V_7. A 16-lead ECG machine allows recording of two ECGs: (1) a standard 12-lead plus leads V_3R, V_4R, V_5R, and V_6R and (2) a standard 12-lead plus posterior leads V_7, V_8, and V_9.

ALTERNATIVE LEADS

Alternative lead configurations are sometimes useful in differentiating among types of dysrhythmias. For example, the Lewis lead is used to enhance viewing of atrial activity (Fig. 2.20). The right arm (negative) electrode is applied to the right of the sternum at the second intercostal space, the left arm (positive) electrode is placed at the right fourth

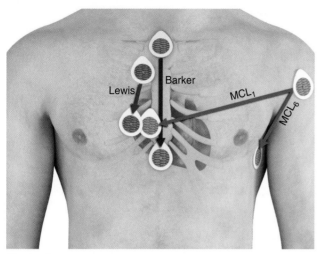

Fig. 2.20 Electrode locations for alternative electrocardiogram leads. *MCL,* Modified chest lead. (From Hedges JR: *Roberts and Hedges' clinical procedures in emergency medicine,* ed 6, Philadelphia, 2014, Saunders.)

intercostal space, and the ECG machine is set to record lead I (Bakker et al, 2009).

The vertical sternal leads, also known as *Barker leads,* have been reported to record P waves that are larger than those seen with other leads, including the Lewis lead (Harrigan et al, 2014). When this lead is used, the positive electrode is placed at the xiphoid process and the negative electrode is placed just below the suprasternal notch (see Fig. 2.20).

The modified chest leads (MCLs) are bipolar chest leads that are variations of the chest leads. Each MCL consists of a positive and negative electrode applied to a specific location on the chest. Lead MCL_1 views the interventricular septum. The negative electrode is placed just below the left clavicle toward the left shoulder, and the positive electrode is placed to the right of the sternum in the fourth intercostal space (see Fig. 2.20). Leads MCL_1 and V_1 are similar but not identical. In V_1, the negative electrode is calculated by the ECG machine at the center of the heart. In MCL_1, the negative electrode is located just below the left clavicle.

Lead MCL_6 is a variation of the chest lead V_6 and views the low lateral wall of the left ventricle. The negative electrode is placed below the left clavicle toward the left shoulder, and the positive electrode is placed at the fifth intercostal space, left midaxillary line.

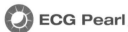 **ECG Pearl** _____

Lead MCL_1 was once used to help differentiate between right and left bundle blocks and distinguish ventricular tachycardia from supraventricular tachycardia with abnormal (i.e., aberrant) ventricular conduction. Because the shape (morphology) of the QRS complex in MCL_1 has been shown to differ in 40% of patients with ventricular tachycardia, chest lead V_1 should be used instead (Drew et al, 2004).

Ambulatory Cardiac Monitoring

External ambulatory cardiac monitoring, also known as *ambulatory electrocardiographic* (AECG) *monitoring,* is a noninvasive diagnostic tool used to monitor the patient's cardiac rhythm as he or she performs daily activities. Examples of indications for AECG monitoring include the following (Crawford et al, 1999; Mittal et al, 2011):

- To determine the association between a patient's symptoms (e.g., dizziness, palpitations, near syncope, shortness of breath, chest pain, fatigue) and cardiac rhythm disturbances
- To detect myocardial ischemia and to evaluate the efficacy of anti-ischemic medications in patients with coronary artery disease
- To assess the patient's risk of dysrhythmias after a myocardial infarction; for patients with heart failure, hypertrophic cardiomyopathy, diabetic neuropathy, systemic hypertension, or valvular heart disease; for patients receiving hemodialysis; and for the preoperative evaluation of patients and after cardiac operations
- To assess the efficacy of medications on the cardiac conduction system, the patient's cardiac rhythm, or both
- To aid in correlating patient symptoms with dysrhythmias and evaluating symptomatic patients for pacemaker implantation
- To assess the function of implanted devices, such as a pacemaker or an implantable cardioverter-defibrillator
- To assess the efficacy of ablation procedures

TYPES OF AMBULATORY MONITORS

A conventional Holter monitor is a battery-powered continuous AECG recorder that is used for 24 hours to a maximum of 72 hours to document ECG events that are likely to occur within this period. Electrodes and lead wires are connected to a portable, lightweight recorder that is attached to the patient and carried with a belt or shoulder strap (Fig. 2.21). Patients are asked to keep a log or diary while the device is in use. A typical diary consists of entries reflecting the time of day, activity being performed, and patient symptoms. When the monitoring period is complete, the patient returns the monitor and events that have been stored on a digital flash memory device is then scanned by a technician and interpreted by a physician. This information is then compared with the ECG events captured by the AECG recorder to determine if a relationship exists among the patient's symptoms, activities, and ECG.

Newer Holter monitors permit extended ECG monitoring, typically for 7 to 14 days, using a patch-based system (Fig. 2.22). During extended Holter monitoring, data are recorded continuously and transmitted to a central monitoring station. This approach is useful because involvement of a monitoring center enhances responsiveness to changes observed during ECG monitoring (Krahn et al, 2014).

Event recorders, also called *intermittent recorders,* may be used for longer periods (generally up to 30 days) to

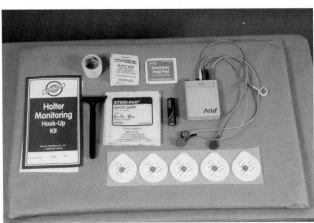

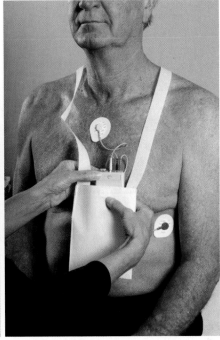

Fig. 2.21 A Holter monitor is an example of an ambulatory electrocardiographic monitor. (From Bonewit-West K: *Clinical procedures for medical assistants,* ed 9, St. Louis, 2015, Saunders.)

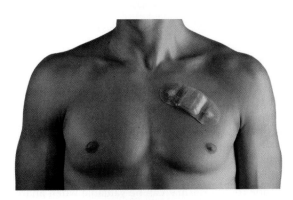

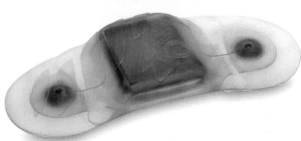

Fig. 2.22 Sample patch-based recording system that allows both acquisition and storage of a single-lead electrocardiogram for 7 to 14 days. (From Krahn AD, Yee R, Skanes AC, Klein GJ: Cardiac monitoring: Short and long-term recording. In DP Zipes & J Jalife (Eds.): *Cardiac electrophysiology: from cell to bedside,* ed 6, Philadelphia, 2014, Saunders.)

document events that are brief, that occur infrequently, or that are unlikely to be captured during a 24- to 72-hour period. Events may be captured by the patient or automatically captured by the recorder. For example, when the device

is attached to the patient, he or she is instructed to press a button on the recorder when experiencing symptoms, such as palpitations, to capture and store the ECG event for analysis when the monitoring interval is complete. Some event recorders automatically detect and store cardiac events (e.g., bradycardia, tachycardia, pauses, atrial fibrillation), and others automatically detect, store, and then transmit the ECG event by telephone for analysis.

ELECTROCARDIOGRAPHY PAPER

[Objectives 16, 17]

Remember that an ECG is a graphical representation of the heart's electrical activity. When you place electrodes on the patient's body and connect them to an electrocardiograph, the machine records the voltage (i.e., the potential difference) between the electrodes. The needle, or pen, of the ECG moves a specific distance depending on the voltage measured. This recording is made on ECG paper.

ECG paper is graph paper made up of small and large boxes measured in millimeters. The smallest boxes are 1 mm wide and 1 mm high (Fig. 2.23). The horizontal axis of the paper corresponds to time. Time is used to measure the interval between or duration of specific cardiac events, which is stated in seconds. Measuring how quickly or slowly an electrical impulse spreads through the heart provides important information about the condition of the heart's conduction system and the muscle itself.

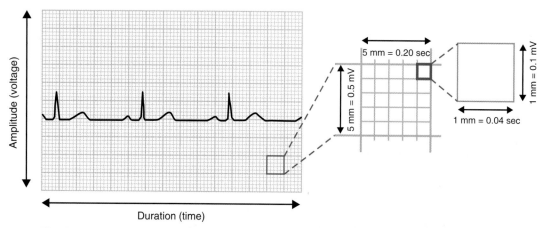

Fig. 2.23 Electrocardiographic strip showing the markings for measuring amplitude and duration of waveforms, using a standard recording speed of 25 mm/sec. (From Copstead-Kirkhorn LE, Banasik JL: *Pathophysiology,* ed 5, St. Louis, 2013, Saunders.)

ECG paper normally records at a constant speed of 25 mm/sec. Thus, each horizontal unit (i.e., each 1-mm box) represents 0.04 second (25 mm/sec × 0.04 second = 1 mm). The rate at which ECG paper goes through the printer is adjustable. A slower paper speed makes the rhythm appear faster. Increasing the paper speed to 50 mm/sec has the effect of making the rhythm appear slower. This technique is sometimes used by clinicians when evaluating rapid atrial or ventricular rhythms, making it easier to see the waveforms and analyze the tachycardia. Increasing the paper speed also exaggerates any existing irregularity and makes it possible to more accurately measure intervals on the ECG (Harrigan et al, 2014).

Look closely at the boxes in Fig. 2.23. You can see that the lines after every five small boxes on the paper are heavier. The heavier lines indicate one large box. Because each large box is the width of five small boxes, a large box represents 0.20 second. Five large boxes, each consisting of five small boxes, represent 1 second; 15 large boxes equal an interval of 3 seconds; and 30 large boxes represent 6 seconds.

The vertical axis of the graph paper represents the voltage or amplitude of the ECG waveforms or deflections. Voltage is measured in millivolts (mV). Voltage may appear as a positive or negative value because voltage is a force with direction as well as amplitude. Amplitude is measured in millimeters (mm). The default value for ECG machine calibration is 10 mm/mV. This means that when the ECG machine is properly calibrated, a 1-mV electrical signal produces a deflection that measures exactly 10 mm tall (i.e., the height of 10 small boxes) (Fig. 2.24). When a calibration marker is present, it appears at the extreme left side of the ECG tracing, before the first waveform. Clinically, the height of a waveform is usually stated in mm rather than in mV. Calibration, also called *standardization*, can be adjusted manually, by the clinician, or automatically, by the ECG machine's computer. Decreasing

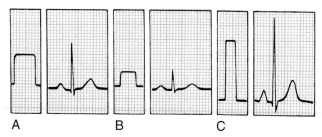

Fig. 2.24 A, When an electrocardiograph is properly calibrated, a 1-mV electrical signal will produce a deflection measuring exactly 10 mm tall (i.e., normal standardization). B, One-half standardization. C, Two times normal standardization. (From Goldberger AL: *Clinical electrocardiography: a simplified approach,* ed 8, Philadelphia, 2013, Saunders.)

the calibration to 5 mm/mV can be helpful when the QRS amplitude is so large that it encroaches on those of neighboring leads (Harrigan et al, 2014). Increasing the amplitude to 20 mm/mV can be valuable when analyzing waveforms.

Waveforms

[Objective 18]

A **waveform** (i.e., a deflection) is movement away from the baseline in a positive (i.e., upward) or negative (i.e., downward) direction (Box 2.1). Each waveform that you see on an ECG is related to a specific electrical event in

Box 2.1	Terminology

Baseline (isoelectric line): A straight line recorded when electrical activity is not detected
Waveform: Movement away from the baseline in either a positive or negative direction
Segment: A line between waveforms; named by the waveform that precedes or follows it
Complex: Several waveforms
Interval: A waveform and a segment

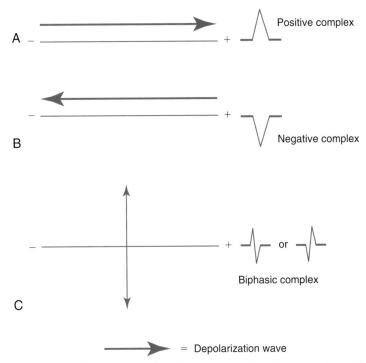

Fig. 2.25 Electrocardiographic waveforms may be positive or negative. A, A positive waveform is seen if the wave of depolarization spreads toward the positive pole of the lead. B, A negative waveform is seen if the depolarization wave spreads toward the negative pole (away from the positive pole) of the lead. C, A biphasic (partly positive, partly negative) waveform or a straight line is seen if the mean direction of the wave of depolarization moves perpendicularly (at a right angle) to the positive electrode. (From Sole ML, Klein DG, Moseley MJ: *Introduction to critical care nursing,* ed 6, St. Louis, 2013, Saunders.)

the heart. Waveforms are named alphabetically, beginning with P, QRS, T, and occasionally U. When electrical activity is not detected, a straight line is recorded. This line is called the **baseline** or **isoelectric line**. If the wave of depolarization (i.e., the electrical impulse) moves toward the positive electrode, the waveform recorded on ECG graph paper will be upright (i.e., a positive deflection) (Fig. 2.25). If the wave of depolarization moves away from the positive electrode, the waveform recorded will be inverted (i.e., a downward or negative deflection). A **biphasic** (i.e., partly positive, partly negative) waveform or a straight line is recorded when the wave of depolarization moves perpendicularly to the positive electrode. The term *equiphasic* may be used instead of *biphasic* to describe a waveform that has no net positive or negative deflection.

P WAVE

The first waveform in the cardiac cycle is the *P wave* (Fig. 2.26). Activation of the SA node occurs before the onset of the P wave. This event is not recorded on the ECG. However, the spread of that impulse throughout the right and left atrial muscle (atrial depolarization) is observed. The beginning of the P wave is recognized as the first abrupt or gradual movement away from the baseline; its end is the point at which the waveform returns to the baseline. The first half of the P wave is recorded when the

---

Box 2.2	Normal P-Wave Characteristics

- Smooth and rounded
- No more than 2.5 mm in height (Goldberger et al, 2013)
- No more than 0.12 second in duration
- Positive in leads I, II, aVF, and V_2 through V_6

electrical impulse that originated in the SA node stimulates the right atrium. The middle portion of the P wave represents completion of right atrial activation and the start of activation of the left atrium (Wagner, 2012). The downslope of the P wave reflects completion of left atrial activation; thus, the P wave represents the spread of the electrical impulse throughout the right and left atria (i.e., atrial depolarization). A P wave normally precedes each QRS complex. Normal P wave characteristics are shown in Box 2.2.

The atria contract a fraction of a second after the P wave begins. The atria begin to repolarize at the same time as the ventricles depolarize. A waveform representing atrial repolarization is usually not seen on the ECG because it is small and buried in the QRS complex.

Tall and pointed (i.e., peaked) or wide and notched P waves may be seen in conditions such as chronic obstructive pulmonary disease, heart failure, or valvular disease and may be indicative of atrial enlargement (Fig. 2.27).

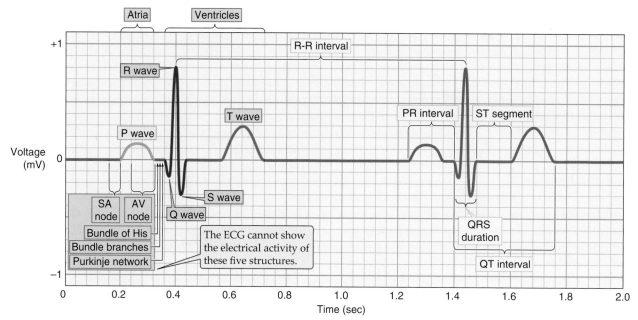

Fig. 2.26   Components of the electrocardiogram (ECG) recording. *AV,* Atrioventricular; *SA,* sinoatrial. (From Boron WF, Boulpaep EL: *Medical physiology,* ed 3, Philadelphia, 2017, Saunders.)

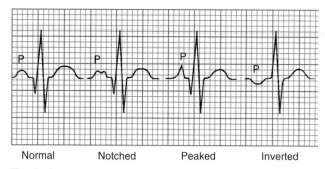

Fig. 2.27   Abnormal P waves may be notched, tall and pointed (peaked), or inverted (negative).

Enlargement of the right atrium produces an abnormally tall initial part of the P wave. The latter part of the P wave is prominent in left atrial enlargement (see Chapter 9).

P waves that begin at a site other than the SA node (i.e., ectopic P waves) may be positive or negative in lead II. If the ectopic pacemaker is in the atria, the P wave will be upright. If the ectopic pacemaker is in the AV bundle, the P wave will be negative (i.e., inverted) in lead II.

QRS COMPLEX

[Objective 19]

A **complex** consists of several waveforms. The QRS complex consists of the Q wave, R wave, and S wave (see Fig. 2.26) and represents the spread of the electrical impulse through the ventricles (i.e., ventricular depolarization) and the sum of all ventricular muscle cell depolarizations. Because the left ventricle is much larger than the right, in a normally conducted beat, the QRS complex represents the electrical activity occurring in the left ventricle. Ventricular depolarization normally triggers contraction of ventricular tissue. Thus, shortly after the QRS complex begins, the ventricles contract. The QRS complex is significantly larger than the P wave because depolarization of the ventricles involves a considerably greater muscle mass than depolarization of the atria. Remember that atrial repolarization takes place during ventricular depolarization, but the QRS complex overshadows it on the ECG.

A QRS complex normally follows each P wave. One or even two of the three waveforms that make up the QRS complex may be absent. When it is present, the Q wave is the first downward deflection following the P wave, and it represents depolarization of the interventricular septum, which normally occurs from left to right and posteriorly to anteriorly. A Q wave is *always* a negative waveform. The Q wave begins when the ECG leaves the isoelectric line in a downward direction and continues until it returns to the isoelectric line.

It is important to differentiate normal (i.e., a physiologic) Q waves from pathologic Q waves (Fig. 2.28). With the exception of leads III and aVR, a normal Q wave in the limb leads is less than 0.03 second in duration (Surawicz & Knilans, 2008). An abnormal (i.e., pathologic) Q wave is more than 0.03 second in duration or more than 30% of the height of the following R wave in that lead, or both (Anderson, 2012). Myocardial infarction is one possible cause of abnormal Q waves.

The QRS complex continues as a large, upright, triangular waveform known as the *R wave* (see Fig. 2.26). The R wave is the first positive (i.e., upright) waveform following the P

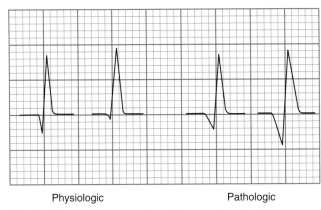

Physiologic   Pathologic

Fig. 2.28 Physiologic and pathologic Q waves. (From Phalen T, Aehlert BJ: *The 12-lead ECG in acute coronary syndromes*, ed 3, St. Louis, 2012, Mosby.)

wave. The S wave is the negative waveform following the R wave. An R wave is *always* positive, and an S wave is *always* negative. The R and S waves represent depolarization of the right and left ventricles.

Because of its greater muscle mass, the QRS complex generally represents the electrical activity occurring in the left ventricle. Factors other than the size or mass of the left ventricle affect QRS amplitude. For example, the sites of electrode placement, age, gender, and race influence QRS voltage (Hancock et al, 2009).

The QRS complex may appear predominantly positive, negative, or biphasic, depending on the lead. It is predominantly positive in leads that view the heart from the left (e.g., I, aVL, V_5, V_6) and in leads that look at the heart's inferior surface (e.g., II, III, aVF). In leads that view the heart from the right side, the QRS complex is predominantly negative (e.g., aVR, V_1, V_2). The QRS is normally biphasic in leads V_3, V_4, and sometimes III.

QRS Measurement

The QRS duration is a measurement of the time required for ventricular depolarization. The width of a QRS complex is most accurately determined when it is viewed and measured in more than one lead. The measurement should be taken from the QRS complex with the longest duration and clearest onset and end. The beginning of the QRS complex is measured from the point where the first wave of the complex begins to deviate from the baseline. The point at which the last wave of the complex begins to level out or distinctly changes direction at, above, or below the baseline marks the end of the QRS complex. In adults, the normal duration of the QRS complex is 0.11 second or less (Surawicz et al, 2009). In general, the QRS duration in women is shorter than that in men by about 5 to 8 milliseconds (msec) (Mirvis & Goldberger, 2015).

If an electrical impulse does not follow the normal ventricular conduction pathway, it will take longer to depolarize the myocardium. This delay in conduction through the ventricles produces a wider QRS complex. Normal characteristics of the QRS complex appear in Box 2.3.

 Box 2.3   Normal QRS Complex Characteristics

- Normal duration of 0.075 to 0.11 second in adults (Ganz, 2012)
- QRS amplitude varies among leads

Lead In _____

Applying Principles to Practice

Einthoven expressed the relationship among leads I, II, and III as the sum of any complex in leads I and III equals that of lead II. Thus, lead I + III = II. Stated another way, the voltage of a waveform in lead I plus the voltage of the same waveform in lead III equals the voltage of the same waveform in lead II. For example, when you look at leads I, II, and III, if the R wave in lead II does not appear to be the sum of the voltage of the R waves in leads I and III, the leads may have been incorrectly applied.

Abnormal QRS Complexes

- In adults, the duration of an abnormal QRS complex is greater than 0.11 second.
- The duration of a QRS caused by an impulse originating in an ectopic pacemaker in the Purkinje network or ventricular myocardium is usually greater than 0.12 second and often 0.16 second or greater.
- If the impulse originates in a bundle branch, a QRS duration between 0.11 and 0.12 second in adults is called an *incomplete* bundle branch block (Surawicz et al, 2009). In adults, a QRS measuring 0.12 second or more is called a *complete* bundle branch block (Surawicz et al, 2009). This is discussed in more detail in Chapter 9.
- Low-amplitude QRS complexes measure less than 5 mm or 0.5 mV (Ganz, 2012).
- Enlargement of the right ventricle produces an abnormally tall R wave; left ventricular enlargement produces an abnormally deep S wave.

QRS Variations

Although the term *QRS complex* is used, not every QRS complex contains a Q wave, R wave, and S wave. If the QRS complex consists entirely of a positive waveform, it is called an *R wave*. If the complex consists entirely of a negative waveform, it is called a *QS wave*. QS waves may be pathologic. If there are two positive deflections in the same complex, the second is called *R prime* and is written R'. If there are two negative deflections following an R wave, the second is called *S prime* and is written S'. Capital (i.e., upper case) letters are used to designate waveforms of relatively large amplitude, and small (i.e., lower case) letters are used to label relatively small waveforms (Fig. 2.29).

T WAVE

The T wave represents repolarization of both ventricles (Lederer, 2012) (Fig. 2.30). The ARP is still present during the beginning of the T wave. At the peak of the T wave, the

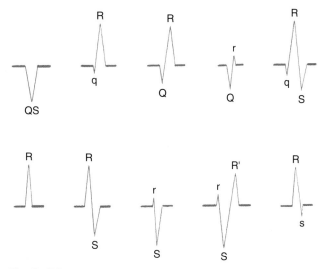

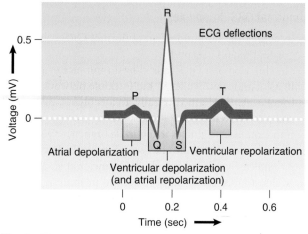

Fig. 2.29 Various QRS morphologies. (From Goldberger A: *Clinical electrocardiography: a simplified approach,* ed 6, St. Louis, 1999, Mosby.)

Fig. 2.30 The T wave reflects ventricular repolarization. (From Patton KT, Thibodeau GA: *Anatomy & physiology,* ed 9, St. Louis, 2016, Mosby.)

Box **2.4**	**Normal T Wave Characteristics**

- Slightly asymmetric
- Negative in aVR; may be positive or negative in leads III, aVL, and V_1
- Normally upright in leads I, II, and V_3 through V_6 (Rautaharju et al, 2009)
- Usually 0.5 mm or more in height in leads I and II
- Usually 5 mm or less in height in any limb lead or 10 mm or less in any chest lead

RRP has begun. It is during the RRP that a stronger than normal stimulus may produce ventricular dysrhythmias.

In the limb leads, lead II most commonly reveals the tallest T wave. The normal T wave is slightly asymmetric: The peak of the waveform is closer to its end than to the beginning, and the first half has a more gradual slope than the second half (Box 2.4). The beginning of the T wave is identified as the point where the slope of the ST segment appears to become abruptly or gradually steeper. The T wave ends when it returns to the baseline. It may be difficult to clearly determine the onset and end of the T wave. Examples of T waves are shown in Fig. 2.31.

The direction of the T wave is normally the same as the QRS complex that precedes it. This is because depolarization begins at the endocardial surface and spreads to the epicardium. Repolarization begins at the epicardium and spreads to the endocardium.

Abnormal T Waves

- A T wave following an abnormal QRS complex usually moves in a direction opposite that of the QRS. In other words, when the QRS complex points down, the T wave points up and vice versa. This pattern may be seen with ventricular beats or rhythms and in bundle branch block.
- In a patient experiencing an acute coronary syndrome (ACS), T-wave inversion suggests the presence of myocardial ischemia.
- Tall, pointed (i.e., peaked) T waves are commonly seen in hyperkalemia.
- Low-amplitude T waves may be seen in hypokalemia or hypomagnesemia.
- Tall, broad T waves may be seen with internal pacemakers.
- Deeply inverted T waves may be seen with acute central nervous system events (e.g., intracranial hemorrhage, massive stroke) and therapy with tricyclic antidepressants or phenothiazines (Amsterdam et al, 2014).
- The T wave in leads I, II, aVL, and V_2 to V_6 should be described as *inverted* when the T-wave amplitude is from −1 mm to −5 mm, as *deep negative* when the amplitude is from −5 mm to −10 mm, and as *giant negative* when the amplitude is more than −10 mm. The T wave is described as *low* when its amplitude is less than 10% of the R wave amplitude in the same lead and as *flat* when the peak T-wave amplitude is between 1 mm and −1 mm in leads I, II, aVL (with an R wave taller than 3 mm), and V_4 to V_6 (Rautaharju et al, 2009).

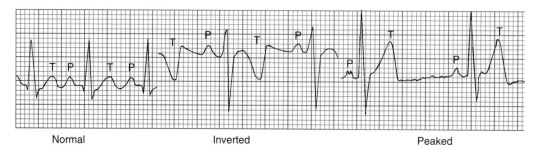

Normal   Inverted   Peaked

Fig. 2.31 Examples of T waves.

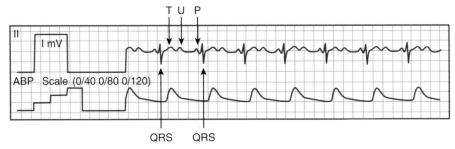

Fig. 2.32 Electrocardiogram tracing from a patient with a serum potassium of 2 to 6 mEq/L shows a prominent U wave. (From Urden L, Stacy K, Lough M: *Thelan's critical care nursing: diagnosis and management,* ed 5, St. Louis, 2006, Mosby.)

U WAVE

A U wave is a small waveform that, when seen, follows the T wave. The U wave is thought to represent late repolarization of the Purkinje fibers (Lederer, 2012). However, some cardiologists believe that U waves represent delayed repolarization in areas of the ventricle that undergo late mechanical relaxation (Mirvis & Goldberger, 2015) or they are simply two-part T waves resulting from a longer action potential duration in some ventricular myocardial cells (Patton & Thibodeau, 2013).

U waves are most easily seen when the heart rate is slow and are difficult to identify when the rate exceeds 95 beats/min (Rautaharju et al, 2009). When seen, they are generally tallest in leads V_2 and V_3 (Rautaharju et al, 2009). The amplitude of the normal U wave is usually less than 0.1 mV (Mirvis & Goldberger, 2015). Possible causes of prominent U waves include central nervous system disease, electrolyte imbalance (e.g., hypokalemia) (Fig. 2.32), hyperthyroidism, long QT syndrome, and medications (e.g., amiodarone, digitalis, disopyramide, phenothiazines, procainamide, quinidine).

U waves usually appear in the same direction as the T waves that precede them. Inverted U waves seen in leads V_2 through V_5 are abnormal and may appear during episodes of acute ischemia or in the presence of hypertension (Rautaharju et al, 2009).

Segments

[Objectives 18, 19]

A **segment** is a line between waveforms. It is named by the waveform that precedes or follows it.

PR SEGMENT

The PR segment is part of the PR interval, specifically, the horizontal line between the end of the P wave and the beginning of the QRS complex (Fig. 2.33). The PR segment is normally isoelectric and represents the spread of the electrical impulse from the AV node, through the AV bundle, the right and left bundle branches, and the Purkinje fibers to activate ventricular muscle. The PR segment ends when enough ventricular myocardium has been activated

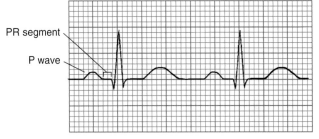

Fig. 2.33 The PR segment.

to initiate the recording of the QRS complex (Mirvis & Goldberger, 2015). Most of the conduction delay during the PR segment is a result of slow conduction within the AV node (Wagner, 2012).

TP SEGMENT

The TP segment is the portion of the ECG tracing between the end of the T wave and the beginning of the next P wave during which there is no electrical activity (Fig. 2.34). When the heart rate is within normal limits, the TP segment is usually isoelectric and used as the reference point from which to estimate the position of the isoelectric line and determine ST-segment displacement. With rapid heart rates, the TP segment is often unrecognizable because the P wave encroaches on the preceding T wave. When the TP segment is unrecognizable, the PR segment is typically used as the reference point from which to estimate the position of the isoelectric line.

ST SEGMENT

The portion of the ECG tracing between the QRS complex and the T wave is the ST segment. The term *ST segment* is used regardless of whether the final wave of the QRS complex is an R or an S wave. The ST segment represents the early part of repolarization of the right and left ventricles. The normal ST segment begins at the isoelectric line, extends from the end of the S wave, and curves gradually upward to the beginning of the T wave.

The point where the QRS complex and the ST segment meet is called the *ST junction* or the *J point* (Fig. 2.35). The ST segment is considered elevated if the segment is deviated above the baseline and is considered depressed if the segment deviates below it. When looking for ST-segment elevation or depression, first locate the J point. Next use the TP segment to estimate the position of the isoelectric line. Then compare the level of the ST segment with the isoelectric line. Deviation is measured as the number of mm of vertical ST segment displacement

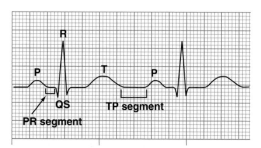

Fig. 2.34 When the heart rate is within normal limits, the TP segment is used as the reference point from which to estimate the position of the isoelectric line and determine ST-segment displacement.

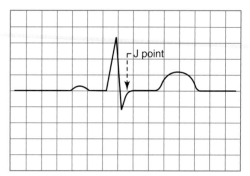

Fig. 2.35 The location of the J point.

from the isoelectric line or from the patient's baseline at the J point (Thygesen et al, 2012). It may be difficult to clearly determine the J point in patients with rapid heart rates or hyperkalemia. Some displacement of the ST segment from the isoelectric line is normal and dependent on age, gender, race, and ECG lead.

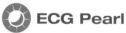 **ECG Pearl** _____

Proper machine calibration is critical when analyzing ST segments. The ST segment criteria described here apply *only* when the monitor is adjusted to standard calibration.

Various conditions may displace the ST segment from the isoelectric line in either a positive or a negative direction. Myocardial ischemia, injury, and infarction are among the causes of ST-segment deviation (Fig. 2.36). Other causes of ST-segment changes include a normal variant, pericarditis, myocarditis, left ventricular aneurysm, and bundle branch block, among other causes (Amsterdam et al, 2014). Pericarditis causes ST-segment elevation in all or virtually all leads.

When ECG changes of myocardial ischemia, injury, or infarction occur, they are not found in every lead of the ECG. Findings are considered significant if viewed in two or more leads looking at the same or adjacent area of the heart. If these findings are seen in leads that look directly at the affected area, they are called **indicative changes**. If findings are seen in leads opposite the affected area, they are called **reciprocal changes** (also called *mirror image* changes). Indicative changes are significant when they are seen in two *anatomically contiguous* leads. Two leads are contiguous if they look at the same or adjacent areas of the heart or if they are numerically consecutive chest leads (see Chapter 9).

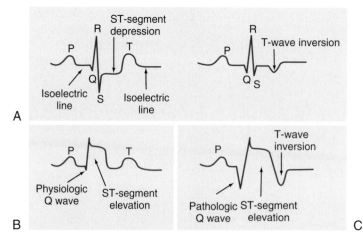

Fig. 2.36 ST segment, T wave, and Q wave changes associated with myocardial ischemia A, injury B, and infarction C. (From Lewis, SL, Bucher L, Heitkemper MM, Harding MM: *Medical-surgical nursing: assessment and management of clinical problems,* ed 10, St. Louis, 2017, Elsevier.)

Abnormal ST Segments

- ST-segment depression of 0.5 mm or more in a patient who is experiencing an ACS is suggestive of myocardial ischemia when it is seen in two or more anatomically contiguous leads (Thygesen et al, 2012).
- New or presumed new ST-segment elevation of 1 mm or more at the J-point in all leads other than V_2 and V_3 in a patient who is experiencing an ACS is suggestive of myocardial injury when observed in two or more anatomically contiguous leads (O'Gara et al, 2013). For leads V_2 and V_3, ST elevation is considered significant if it is elevated 2 mm or more in men older than 40 years or elevated 1.5 mm or more in women (O'Gara et al, 2013).
- A horizontal ST segment (i.e., forming a sharp angle with the T wave) is suggestive of ischemia.
- Digitalis causes a depression or scoop of the ST segment that is sometimes referred to as a "dig dip" (Fig. 2.37).

Intervals

PR INTERVAL

[Objective 18]

An **interval** is made up of a waveform and a segment. The P wave plus the PR segment equals the PR interval (PRI); thus, the PRI reflects total supraventricular activity.

The PRI is measured from the point where the P wave leaves the baseline to the beginning of the QRS complex (Fig. 2.38). The term *PQ interval* is preferred by some because it is the period that is actually measured unless a Q wave is absent. The PRI changes with heart rate but normally measures 0.12 to 0.20 second in adults (Box 2.5). As the heart rate increases, the duration of the PRI shortens. A PRI is considered *short* if it is less than 0.12 second and *long* if it is more than 0.20 second.

Abnormal PR Intervals

Delays in impulse conduction through the atria, AV node, or AV bundle can result in prolongation (greater than 0.20 second) of the PRI. Conditions causing such disturbances may be inflammatory, circulatory, nervous, endocrine, or pharmacologic in origin. The P wave associated with a prolonged PRI may be normal or abnormal.

A PRI of less than 0.12 second may be seen when the impulse originates in an ectopic pacemaker in the atria close to the AV node or in the AV bundle. A shortened PRI may also occur if the electrical impulse progresses from the atria to the ventricles through an abnormal conduction pathway that bypasses the AV node and depolarizes the ventricles earlier than usual.

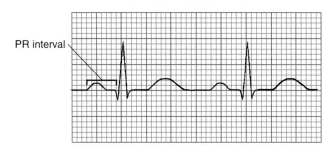

Fig. 2.38 The PR interval is measured from the onset of the P wave to the onset of the QRS complex.

Box 2.5	Normal PR Interval Characteristics

- Normally measures 0.12 to 0.20 second in adults; may be shorter in children and longer in older adults
- Normally shortens as heart rate increases

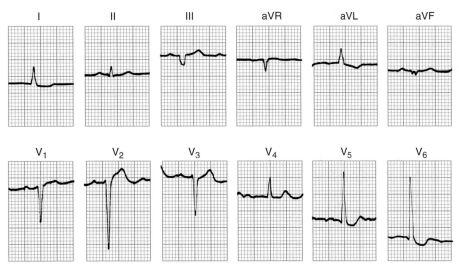

Fig. 2.37 Digitalis may produce a characteristic scooping of the ST segment, as seen here in leads V_5 and V_6. (From Goldberger A: *Clinical electrocardiography: a simplified approach,* ed 6, St. Louis, 1999, Mosby.)

QT INTERVAL

[Objective 18]

The **QT interval** is the period from the beginning of the QRS complex to the end of the T wave. It represents total ventricular activity; this is the time from ventricular depolarization (i.e., activation) to repolarization (i.e., recovery) (see Fig. 2.26). When measuring the QT interval, first select a lead with the most clearly defined T-wave end. To ensure meaningful comparisons of later tracings, use the same lead for subsequent measurements. The QT interval is usually longest in chest leads V_2 or V_3 (Rautaharju et al, 2009). In the absence of a Q wave, the QT interval is measured from the beginning of the R wave to the end of the T wave. The term *QT interval* is used regardless of whether the QRS complex begins with a Q wave or an R wave.

The duration of the QT interval varies in accordance with age, gender, and heart rate. As the heart rate increases, the QT interval shortens (i.e., decreases). As the heart rate decreases, the QT interval lengthens (i.e., increases). Because of the variability of the QT interval with the heart rate, it can be measured more accurately if it is corrected (i.e., adjusted) for the patient's heart rate. Several formulas have been used to calculate the corrected QT interval, which is noted as QT_c, and enable comparison of this measurement at differing heart rates. Bazett's formula, in which the corrected QT interval is calculated as the QT interval divided by the square root of the R-R interval, has been widely used for many years. This formula works well with heart rates within the normal range but overcorrects at rapid heart rates and undercorrects at slow rates (Anderson, 2012).

The QT interval is considered short if it is 0.39 second or less and prolonged if it is 0.46 second or longer in women or 0.45 second or longer in men (Rautaharju et al, 2009). A prolonged QT interval indicates a lengthened RRP. A QT_c of more than 0.50 second in either gender has been correlated with a higher risk for ventricular dysrhythmias (e.g., torsades de pointes [TdP]). A prolonged QT interval may be congenital or acquired. Myocardial ischemia or infarction, electrolyte disorders (e.g., hypokalemia, hypocalcemia), sudden decreases in heart rate, acute neurologic events, and medications (e.g., amiodarone, sotalol) can prolong the QT interval. Digitalis and hypercalcemia shorten the QT interval.

R-R AND P-P INTERVALS

The R-R (R wave-to-R wave) and P-P (P wave-to-P wave) intervals are used to determine the rate and regularity of a cardiac rhythm. To evaluate the regularity of the ventricular rhythm on a rhythm strip, the interval between two consecutive R waves is measured (see Fig. 2.26). The distance between succeeding R-R intervals is measured and compared. If the ventricular rhythm is regular, the R-R intervals will measure the same. To evaluate the regularity of the atrial rhythm, the same procedure is used but the interval between two consecutive P waves is measured and compared with succeeding P-P intervals.

Artifact

[Objective 20]

Accurate ECG rhythm recognition requires a tracing in which the waveforms and intervals are free of distortion. Distortion of an ECG tracing by electrical activity that is noncardiac in origin is called **artifact** (Fig. 2.39). Because artifact can mimic various cardiac dysrhythmias, including ventricular fibrillation, it is essential to evaluate the patient before initiating any medical intervention.

Proper preparation of the patient's skin and evaluation of the monitoring equipment (e.g., electrodes, wires) before use can minimize the problems associated with artifact. Electrodes may adhere poorly if the patient's skin is especially hairy, because the gel comes into contact with hair instead of skin. Skin contact is necessary for adequate signal penetration. If necessary, remove excessive chest hair from the areas where the electrodes will be applied.

Artifact may result from external or internal sources. Possible causes of external artifact include loose electrodes, broken ECG cables or broken lead wires, external chest compressions, and 60-cycle interference (Fig. 2.40). If 60-cycle interference is observed, check for crossing of cable wires with other electrical wires (e.g., a bed control) or frayed and broken wires. Verify that all electrical

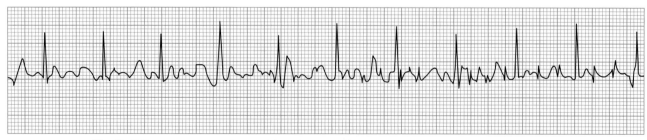

Fig. 2.39 A rhythm strip with artifact. (From Lynn-McHale Wiegand DM: *AACN procedure manual for critical care*, ed 6, St. Louis, 2011, Saunders.)

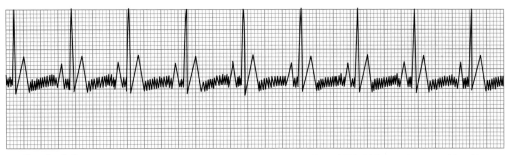

Fig. 2.40 Artifact caused by 60-cycle interference. (From Lynn-McHale Wiegand DM: *AACN procedure manual for critical care,* ed 6, St. Louis, 2011, Saunders.)

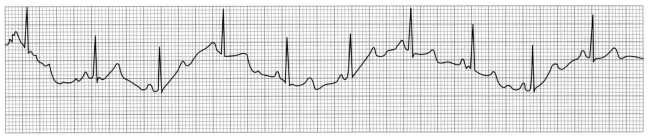

Fig. 2.41 Wandering baseline. (From Lynn-McHale Wiegand DM: *AACN procedure manual for critical care,* ed 6, St. Louis, 2011, Saunders.)

equipment is properly grounded and that the cable electrode connections are clean.

Internal artifact may result from patient movement, shivering, muscle tremors (e.g., seizures, Parkinson disease), or hiccups (McKinley, 2011). A wandering baseline may occur because of normal respiratory movement (particularly when electrodes have been applied directly over the ribs) or because of poor electrode contact with the patient's skin (Fig. 2.41). Consider clipping the ECG cable to the patient's clothing to minimize excessive movement.

SYSTEMATIC RHYTHM INTERPRETATION

[Objective 21]

A systematic approach to rhythm analysis that is consistently applied when analyzing a rhythm strip is essential (Box 2.6). If you do not develop such an approach, you are more likely to miss something important. Begin analyzing the rhythm strip from left to right.

Assess Regularity

The waveforms on an ECG strip are evaluated for regularity by measuring the distance between the P waves and QRS complexes.

Box 2.6	Systematic Rhythm Interpretation

1. Assess regularity (atrial and ventricular).
2. Assess rate (atrial and ventricular).
3. Identify and examine waveforms.
4. Assess intervals (e.g., PR, QRS, QT), and examine ST segments.
5. Interpret the rhythm, and assess its clinical significance.

 ECG Pearl

Conflicting information with regard to regularity exists among textbooks related to electrocardiography. Some texts indicate that a rhythm is irregular if the R-R or P-P intervals vary by more than 0.04 second, 0.06 second, 0.08 second, 0.12 second, or even 0.16 second, depending on the author. Because most texts indicate that *any* deviation in regularity is, by definition, an irregular rhythm, that is the criterion that is used with regard to regularity throughout this text.

VENTRICULAR REGULARITY

To determine if the ventricular rhythm is regular or irregular, measure the distance between two consecutive R-R intervals. Place one point of a pair of calipers or make a mark on a piece of paper on an R wave (Fig. 2.42). Place the other point of the calipers or make a second mark on the paper at an identical point on the R wave of the next QRS complex. Without adjusting the calipers, evaluate

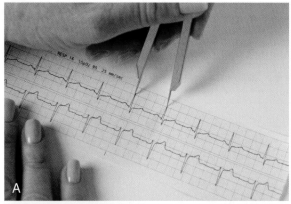

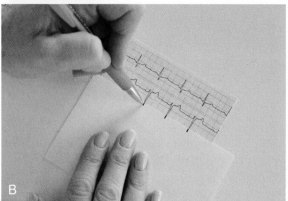

Fig. 2.42 A, Establishing ventricular regularity with calipers. B, Establishing ventricular regularity with paper and pencil. (From Sole, ML, Goldenberg Klein D, Moseley MJ: *Introduction to critical care nursing,* ed 5, Philadelphia, 2008, Saunders.)

each succeeding R-R interval. If paper is used, lift the paper and move it across the rhythm strip. Compare the distance measured with the other R-R intervals. If the ventricular rhythm is regular, the R-R intervals will be equal (measure the same). If the intervals are unequal, the ventricular rhythm is considered irregular.

You can also determine regularity by counting the small squares between intervals and comparing the intervals. Some ECG monitoring systems are equipped with electronic calipers that are used in the same way as physical calipers or paper and pencil.

ATRIAL REGULARITY

To determine if the atrial rhythm is regular or irregular, follow the same procedure previously described for evaluation of ventricular regularity but measure the distance between two consecutive P-P intervals (instead of R-R intervals) and compare that distance with the other P-P intervals. If the atrial rhythm is regular, the P-P intervals will be equal. If the intervals are unequal, the atrial rhythm is considered irregular. For accuracy, the R-R or P-P intervals should be evaluated across an entire 6-second rhythm strip.

Assess Rate

Calculating the heart rate is important because deviations from normal can affect the patient's ability to maintain an adequate blood pressure and cardiac output. Although the atrial rate and ventricular rate are normally the same, they differ in some dysrhythmias; you must therefore calculate both rates.

In adults, a **tachycardia** (*tachy* means "fast") exists if the rate is more than 100 beats/min. Some dysrhythmias with very rapid ventricular rates (faster than 150 beats/min) require the delivery of medications or a shock to stop the rhythm. A **bradycardia** exists if the rate is less than 60 beats/min (*brady* means "slow"). Many patients tolerate a heart rate of 50 to 60 beats/min but become symptomatic when the rate drops below 50 beats/min.

Several methods are used for calculating heart rate. A discussion of each method follows.

METHOD 1: SIX-SECOND METHOD

Most ECG paper is printed with 1-second or 3-second markers on the top or bottom of the paper. On ECG paper, 5 large boxes = 1 second, 15 large boxes = 3 seconds, and 30 large boxes = 6 seconds. To determine the ventricular rate, count the number of complete QRS complexes within a period of 6 seconds and multiply that number by 10 to find the number of complexes in 1 minute (Fig. 2.43). The 6-second method, also called *the rule of 10*, can be used for regular and irregular rhythms. This is the simplest, quickest, and most commonly used method of rate measurement, but it also is the most inaccurate.

METHOD 2: LARGE BOXES

The large box method of rate determination is also called the *rule of 300*. To determine the ventricular rate, count the number of large boxes between an R-R interval and divide into 300 (see Fig. 2.43). To determine the atrial rate, count the number of large boxes between a P-P interval and divide into 300 (Table 2.5). This method is best used if the rhythm is regular; however, it may be used if the rhythm is irregular and a rate range (slowest [longest R-R interval] and fastest [shortest R-R interval] rate) is given.

A variation of the large box method is called the *sequence method*. To determine the ventricular rate, select an R wave that falls on a dark vertical line. Number the next six consecutive dark vertical lines as follows: 300, 150, 100, 75, 60, and 50 (Fig. 2.44). Note where the next R wave falls in relation to the six dark vertical lines already marked. This is the heart rate.

METHOD 3: SMALL BOXES

The small box method of rate determination is also called *the rule of 1500*. Each 1-mm box on the graph paper represents 0.04 second. A total of 1500 boxes represents 1 minute (60 sec/min divided by 0.04 sec/box = 1500 boxes/min). To calculate the ventricular rate, count the number of small boxes between the R-R interval and divide into 1500 (see Fig. 2.43). To determine the atrial rate, count the number of small boxes between the P-P interval and divide into 1500 (Table 2.6). This method is time consuming but accurate.

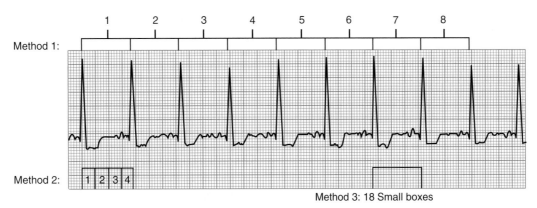

Method 1:

Method 2:

Method 3: 18 Small boxes

Fig. 2.43 Calculating heart rate. Method 1: Number of R-R intervals in 6 seconds × 10 (e.g., 8 × 10 = 80/min). Method 2: Number of large boxes between QRS complexes divided into 300 (e.g., 300 ÷ 4 = 75/min). Method 3: Number of small boxes between QRS complexes divided into 1500 (e.g., 1500 ÷ 18 = 84/min). (From Clochesy J: *Critical care nursing,* ed 2, Philadelphia, 1996, Saunders.)

TABLE 2.5	Heart Rate Determination Based on the Number of Large Boxes
Number of Large Boxes	Heart Rate (beats/min)
1	300
2	150
3	100
4	75
5	60
6	50
7	43
8	38
9	33
10	30

TABLE 2.6 Heart Rate Determination Based on the Number of Small Boxes			
Number of Small Boxes	Heart Rate (beats/min)	Number of Small Boxes	Heart Rate (beats/min)
5	300	28	54
6	250	29	52
7	214	30	50
8	188	31	48
9	167	32	47
10	150	33	45
11	136	34	44
12	125	35	43
13	115	36	42
14	107	37	41
15	100	38	40
16	94	39	39
17	88	40	38
18	83	41	37
19	79	42	36
20	75	43	35
21	71	44	34
22	68	45	33
23	65	46	33
24	62	47	32
25	60	48	31
26	58	49	31
27	56	50	30

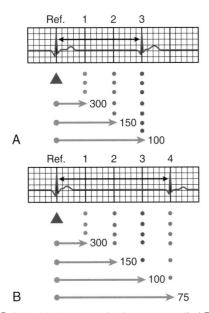

Fig. 2.44 Determining heart rate using the sequence method. To measure the ventricular rate, find a QRS complex that falls on a heavy dark line. Count 300, 150, 100, 75, 60, and 50 until a second QRS complex occurs. This will be the heart rate. A, Heart rate = 100 beats/min. B, Heart rate = 75 beats/min. (From Crawford MV, Spence MI: *Commonsense approach to coronary care,* rev ed 6, St. Louis, 1994, Mosby.)

Throughout this text, the 6-second method is used to calculate rate when the rhythm is irregular. The small box method of rate determination (i.e., the rule of 1500) is used when the rhythm is regular.

 ECG Pearl

During printing, distortion of ECGs can occur. This can result in slight variations in the measurements provided in this book when compared with the measurements that you obtain.

Identify and Examine Waveforms

Look to see if the normal waveforms (P, Q, R, S, and T) are present. To locate P waves, look to the left of each QRS complex. Normally, one P wave precedes each QRS complex (i.e., there is a 1:1 relationship); they occur regularly (P-P intervals are equal); and they look similar in size, shape, and position.

Next, evaluate the QRS complex. Are QRS complexes present? If so, does a QRS follow each P wave? Do the QRS complexes look alike? Assess the T waves. Does a T wave follow each QRS complex? Does a P wave follow the T wave? Are the T waves upright and of normal height? Look to see if a U wave is present. If so, note its height and direction (positive or negative).

Assess Intervals and Examine Segments
PR INTERVAL

Intervals are measured to evaluate conduction. Is a PRI present? If so, measure the PRIs and determine if they are equal. The PRI is measured from the point where the P wave leaves the baseline to the beginning of the QRS complex. Are the PRIs within normal limits? Remember that a normal PRI measures 0.12 to 0.20 seconds. If the PRIs are the same, they are said to be constant. If the PRIs are different, is a pattern present? In some dysrhythmias, the duration of the PRI will increase until a P wave appears with no QRS after it. This is referred to as lengthening of the PRI. PRIs that vary in duration and have no pattern are said to be variable.

QRS DURATION

Identify the QRS complexes and measure their duration. The beginning of the QRS is measured from the point where the first wave of the complex begins to deviate from the baseline. The point at which the last wave of the complex begins to level out at, above, or below the baseline marks the end of the QRS complex. The QRS is considered narrow (i.e., normal) if it measures 0.11 second or less and wide if it measures more than 0.11 second. A narrow QRS complex is presumed to be supraventricular in origin.

QT INTERVAL

To determine the QT interval, count the number of small boxes between the beginning of the QRS complex and the end of the T wave. Then multiply that number by 0.04 second. If no Q wave is present, measure the QT interval from the beginning of the R wave to the end of the T wave. The QT interval is prolonged if it is 0.46 second or longer in women or 0.45 second or longer in men (Rautaharju et al, 2009).

EXAMINE ST SEGMENTS

Determine the presence of ST segment elevation or depression. Remember that the TP segment is used as the baseline from which to evaluate the degree of displacement of the ST segment from the isoelectric line. If ST segment displacement is present, note the number of millimeters of deviation from the J point.

Interpret the Rhythm

Interpret the rhythm, specifying the site of origin (pacemaker site) of the rhythm (sinus), the mechanism (bradycardia), and the ventricular rate (for example, "Sinus bradycardia at 38 beats/min"). Assess the patient to find out how he or she is tolerating the rate and rhythm.

STOP & REVIEW

True/False

Indicate whether the statement is true or false.

____ **1.** The cardiac action potential is a reflection of the difference in the concentration of charged particles across a cell membrane at any given time.

____ **2.** If the wave of depolarization (electrical impulse) moves toward the positive electrode, the waveform recorded on ECG graph paper will be inverted (negative deflection).

____ **3.** Ventricular depolarization is reflected on the ECG as the T wave.

____ **4.** Leads V_1 and V_2 view the interventricular septum.

____ **5.** Abnormal automaticity is a disorder of impulse conduction.

____ **6.** The ERP is the period of the cardiac action potential that includes the ARP and the first half of the RRP.

Multiple Choice

Identify the choice that best completes the statement or answers the question.

____ **7.** The ST segment is measured from
- **a.** the end of the QRS complex to the end of the T wave.
- **b.** the beginning of the QRS complex to the end of the T wave.
- **c.** the end of the QRS complex to the beginning of the T wave.
- **d.** the beginning of the QRS complex to the beginning of the T wave.

____ **8.** Five large boxes, each consisting of five small boxes, represent _____ on ECG paper.
- **a.** 1 second
- **b.** 3 seconds
- **c.** 6 seconds
- **d.** 10 seconds

____ **9.** Which part of the conduction system receives an impulse from the SA node but delays relaying that impulse to the bundle of His, allowing time for the atria to empty their contents into the ventricles before the onset of ventricular contraction?
- **a.** AV node
- **b.** Right atrium
- **c.** Left bundle branch
- **d.** Right bundle branch

____ **10.** On the ECG, total supraventricular activity is reflected by the
- **a.** TP segment.
- **b.** PR interval.
- **c.** QT interval.
- **d.** QRS duration.

____ **11.** In an adult, the normal duration of the QRS complex is
- **a.** 0.06 second or less.
- **b.** 0.11 second or less.
- **c.** 0.04 to 0.14 second.
- **d.** 0.20 to 0.38 second.

____ **12.** The main electrolytes that affect cardiac function are
- **a.** sodium, potassium, calcium, and chloride.
- **b.** phosphate, sodium, sulfate, and potassium.
- **c.** chloride, sulfate, phosphate, and bicarbonate.
- **d.** bicarbonate, calcium, magnesium, and chloride.

____ **13.** The portion of the ECG tracing used to determine the degree of ST segment displacement is the
- **a.** PR interval.
- **b.** QT interval.
- **c.** TP segment.
- **d.** QRS complex.

____ **14.** In the normal heart, the primary pacemaker is the
- **a.** AV node.
- **b.** SA node.
- **c.** AV bundle.
- **d.** Purkinje fibers.

____ **15.** Which of the following surfaces of the heart are not directly viewed when using a standard 12-lead ECG?
- **a.** Anterior and lateral surfaces of the left ventricle
- **b.** Lateral and inferior surfaces of the left ventricle
- **c.** Inferior and posterior surfaces of the left ventricle
- **d.** Right ventricle and posterior surface of the left ventricle

____ **16.** U waves represent
  a. atrial repolarization.
  b. ventricular depolarization.
  c. depolarization of the bundle of His.
  d. repolarization of the Purkinje fibers.

____ **17.** _____ cells are specialized cells of the electrical conduction system responsible for the spontaneous generation and conduction of electrical impulses.
  a. Working
  b. Pacemaker
  c. Mechanical
  d. Contractile

____ **18.** Where is the positive electrode placed in lead III?
  a. Left arm
  b. Right arm
  c. Left leg or foot
  d. Right leg or foot

____ **19.** When an ECG machine is properly calibrated, a 1-mV electrical signal will produce a deflection measuring exactly _____ tall.
  a. 1 mm
  b. 5 mm
  c. 10 mm
  d. 20 mm

____ **20.** Which of the following are horizontal plane leads?
  a. Leads I and aVL
  b. Leads I, II, and III
  c. Leads V_1, V_2, V_3, V_4, V_5, and V_6
  d. Leads I, II, III, aVR, aVL, and aVF

Questions 21 through 26 pertain to the following scenario.
You are caring for a 64-year-old man complaining of chest pain that he rates a 9 on a 0 to 10 scale. He states his symptoms began 20 minutes ago while he was moving boxes in his garage.

____ **21.** You are applying ECG leads to this patient and will be using lead II for continuous monitoring. Lead II is an example of a(n)
  a. chest lead.
  b. horizontal lead.
  c. standard limb lead.
  d. augmented limb lead.

____ **22.** In lead II, the positive electrode is placed on the
  a. left leg.
  b. right leg.
  c. right arm.
  d. left wrist.

____ **23.** When analyzing this patient's ECG rhythm, the first areas of the rhythm strip that you should assess are
  a. regularity and rate.
  b. intervals and segments.
  c. P waves and QRS complexes.
  d. rate and waveform identification.

____ **24.** The patient's ECG shows four large squares between two consecutive R waves. Based on this information, you calculate the patient's heart rate to be _____ beats/min.
  a. 50
  b. 75
  c. 100
  d. 150

____ **25.** When analyzing the leads facing the affected area of the heart, ECG evidence of myocardial injury is displayed as
  a. inverted P waves.
  b. pathologic Q waves.
  c. ST-segment elevation.
  d. ST-segment depression.

____ **26.** Which of the following statements is true regarding analysis of the ST segment on this patient's ECG?
  a. ST-segment displacement should be measured at a point 0.12 sec after the J-point.
  b. ST-segment elevation viewed in lead II would be considered clinically significant if also seen in lead III or aVF.
  c. Based on this patient's age, ST-segment elevation seen in lead II would be considered clinically significant if elevated more than 0.5 mm.
  d. Use the PR interval as the baseline from which to evaluate the degree of ST-segment displacement from the isoelectric line.

Completion

Complete each statement.

27. _____ is the spread of an impulse through tissue already stimulated by that same impulse.

28. Distortion of an ECG tracing by electrical activity that is noncardiac in origin is called _____.

29. _____ refers to the ability of cardiac muscle cells to respond to an external stimulus, such as that from a chemical, mechanical, or electrical source.

Matching
Waveforms, Segments, and Intervals

Match the terms below with their descriptions by placing the letter of each correct answer in the space provided.

a. Waveform
b. Segment
c. J point
d. Interval
e. 0.12 to 0.20 sec
f. Q wave

g. 0.11 sec or less
h. Complex
i. 0.04 sec
j. Millimeters
k. 3 sec
l. R wave

_____ **30.** A waveform and a segment

_____ **31.** In adults, the normal duration of the QRS complex

_____ **32.** The amplitude of a waveform is measured in __.

_____ **33.** This waveform is always negative.

_____ **34.** Movement away from the baseline in either a positive or negative direction

_____ **35.** Normal duration of the PR interval

_____ **36.** This waveform is always positive.

_____ **37.** On ECG paper, each horizontal 1-mm box represents __.

_____ **38.** A line between waveforms

_____ **39.** On ECG paper, 15 large boxes represent __.

_____ **40.** The area where the QRS complex and the ST segment meet

_____ **41.** Several waveforms

The Cardiac Action Potential

Match the terms below with their descriptions by placing the letter of each correct answer in the space provided.

a. Procainamide and lidocaine
b. Fast response
c. Depolarization
d. Verapamil and diltiazem

e. Action potential
f. Wave of depolarization
g. Slow response
h. Repolarization

_____ **42.** This type of action potential occurs in the SA and AV nodes.

_____ **43.** A chain reaction that occurs from cell to cell in the heart's electrical conduction system until all the cells have been stimulated

_____ **44.** The movement of charged particles across a cell membrane in which the inside of the cell is restored to its negative charge

_____ **45.** Examples of antiarrhythmics that block sodium channels

_____ **46.** The rapid sequence of voltage changes that occur across the cell membrane during the electrical cardiac cycle

_____ **47.** This type of action potential occurs in normal atrial and ventricular myocardial cells and in the Purkinje fibers.

_____ **48.** The movement of ions across a cell membrane causing the inside of the cell to become more positive

_____ **49.** Examples of antiarrhythmics that slow the rate at which calcium passes through the cells

Short Answer

50. List three uses for ECG monitoring.
   1.
   2.
   3.

51. List four properties of cardiac cells.
   1.
   2.
   3.
   4.

52. Indicate the inherent rates for each of the following pacemaker sites:

    SA node: _____

    AV bundle: _____

    Purkinje fibers: _____

53. What are the R-R and P-P intervals used for in ECG monitoring?

    _____

    _____

    _____

54. Complete the following chart:

Lead	Positive Electrode	Negative Electrode	Heart Surface Viewed
Lead I	_____	_____	_____
Lead II	_____	_____	_____
Lead III	_____	_____	_____

55. List five steps used in ECG rhythm analysis.

    1. _____
    2. _____
    3. _____
    4. _____
    5. _____

56. List three possible causes of a poor ECG tracing.

    1. _____
    2. _____
    3. _____

Practice Rhythm Strips

For each of the following rhythm strips determine regularity and rate. Next, assess the relationship between P waves and QRS complexes, labeling the P wave, QRS complex, and T wave. Finally, measure the PR interval, QRS duration, and QT interval. *Not all waveforms will be present in each of the following rhythm strips.*

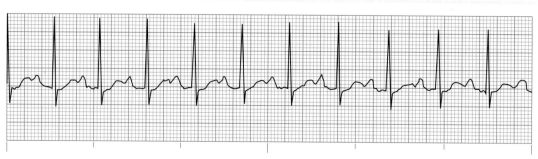

Fig. 2.45

57. **Fig. 2.45**

    Rhythm _____ Rate _____

    P waves _____ PR interval _____

    QRS duration _____ QT interval _____

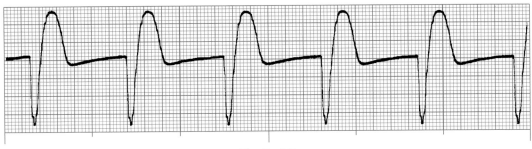

Fig. 2.46

58. Fig. 2.46

Rhythm _____ Rate _____

P waves _____ PR interval _____

QRS duration _____ QT interval _____

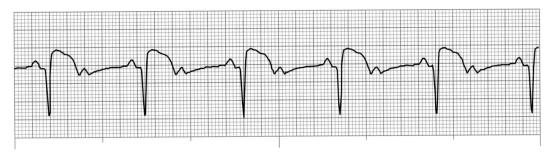

Fig. 2.47 (From Aehlert B: *ECG study cards,* St. Louis, 2004, Mosby.)

61. Fig. 2.47

Rhythm _____ Rate _____

P waves _____ PR interval _____

QRS duration _____ QT interval _____

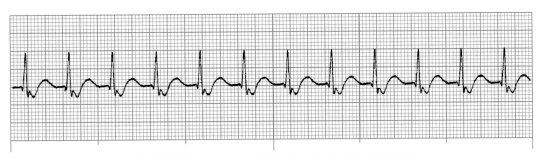

Fig. 2.48 (From Aehlert B: *ECG study cards,* St. Louis, 2004, Mosby.)

62. Fig. 2.48

Rhythm _____ Rate _____

P waves _____ PR interval _____

QRS duration _____ QT interval _____

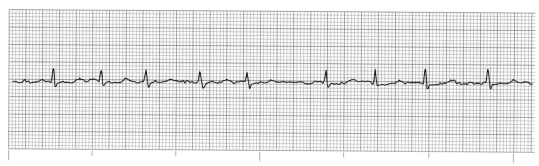

Fig. 2.49

63. **Fig. 2.49**

Rhythm _____ Rate _____

P waves _____ PR interval _____

QRS duration _____ QT interval _____

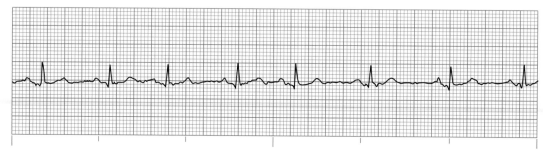

Fig. 2.50 (From Aehlert B: *ECG study cards*, St. Louis, 2004, Mosby.)

64. **Fig. 2.50**

Rhythm _____ Rate _____

P waves _____ PR interval _____

QRS duration _____ QT interval _____

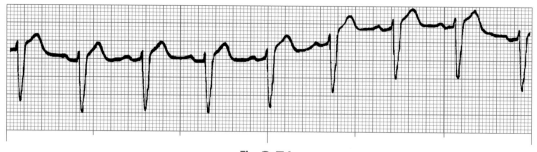

Fig. 2.51

65. **Fig. 2.51**

Rhythm _____ Rate _____

P waves _____ PR interval _____

QRS duration _____ QT interval _____

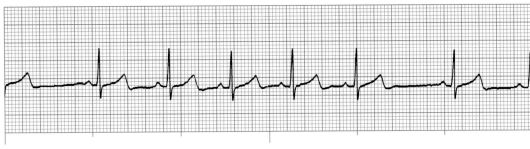

Fig. **2.52**

66. **Fig. 2.52**

Rhythm _____ Rate _____

P waves _____ PR interval _____

QRS duration _____ QT interval _____

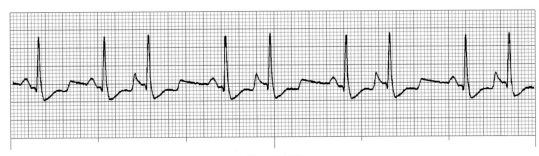

Fig. **2.53**

67. **Fig. 2.53**

Rhythm _____ Rate _____

P waves _____ PR interval _____

QRS duration _____ QT interval _____

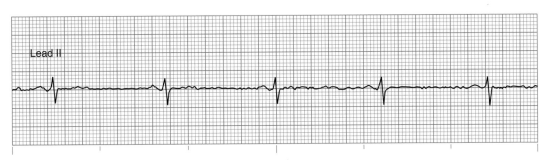

Lead II

Fig. **2.54**

68. **Fig. 2.54**

Rhythm _____ Rate _____

P waves _____ PR interval _____

QRS duration _____ QT interval _____

STOP & REVIEW / ANSWERS

1. T. The action potential of a cardiac cell reflects the rapid sequence of voltage changes that occur across the cell membrane during the electrical cardiac cycle. The configuration of the action potential varies depending on the location, size, and function of the cardiac cell.
OBJ: Define the *terms membrane potential, threshold potential, action potential, polarization, depolarization,* and *repolarization.*

2. F. If the wave of depolarization (electrical impulse) moves toward the positive electrode, the waveform recorded on ECG graph paper will be upright (positive deflection).
OBJ: Define the terms *membrane potential, threshold potential, action potential, polarization, depolarization,* and *repolarization.*

3. F. The QRS complex represents ventricular depolarization. Ventricular repolarization is recorded on the ECG as the ST segment and T wave.
OBJ: Define and describe the significance of each of the following as they relate to cardiac electrical activity: P wave, QRS complex, T wave, U wave, PR segment, TP segment, ST segment, PR interval, QRS duration, and QT interval.

4. T. Leads V_1 and V_2 are chest leads that view the interventricular septum.
OBJ: Relate the cardiac surfaces or areas represented by the ECG leads.

5. F. Abnormal automaticity is a condition in which one of the following occurs: (1) Cardiac cells that are not normally associated with a pacemaker function begin to depolarize spontaneously *or* (2) a pacemaker site other than the SA node increases its firing rate beyond that which is considered normal.
OBJ: Differentiate the primary mechanisms responsible for producing cardiac dysrhythmias.

6. T. The ERP is the period of the cardiac action potential that includes the ARP and the first half of the RRP.
OBJ: Define the absolute, effective, relative refractory, and supernormal periods and their locations in the cardiac cycle.

7. C. The portion of the ECG tracing between the QRS complex and the T wave is the ST segment. The term *ST segment* is used regardless of whether the final wave of the QRS complex is an R or an S wave. The ST segment represents the early part of repolarization of the right and left ventricles. The normal ST segment begins at the isoelectric line, extends from the end of the S wave, and curves gradually upward to the beginning of the T wave.
OBJ: Define and describe the significance of the following as they relate to cardiac electrical activity: P wave, QRS complex, T wave, U wave, PR segment, TP segment, ST segment, PR interval, QRS duration, and QT interval.

8. A. Five large boxes, each consisting of five small boxes, represent 1 second. Fifteen large boxes equal an interval of 3 seconds. Thirty large boxes represent 6 seconds.
OBJ: Identify the numeric values assigned to the small and large boxes on ECG paper.

9. A. As the electrical impulse enters the AV node through the internodal pathways, conduction is markedly slowed before the impulse reaches the ventricles. The delay in conduction allows both atrial chambers to contract and empty blood into the ventricles before the next ventricular contraction begins.
OBJ: Describe the normal sequence of electrical conduction through the heart.

10. B. The P wave plus the PR segment equals the PR interval (PRI); thus, the PRI reflects total supraventricular activity. The QT interval (which includes the QRS complex, ST segment, and T wave) represents total ventricular activity; this is the time from ventricular depolarization (i.e., activation) to repolarization (i.e., recovery).
OBJ: Define and describe the significance of each of the following as they relate to cardiac electrical activity: P wave, QRS complex, T wave, U wave, PR segment, TP segment, ST segment, PR interval, QRS duration, and QT interval.

11. B. In adults, the normal duration of the QRS complex is 0.11 sec or less. If an electrical impulse does not follow the normal ventricular conduction pathway, it will take longer to depolarize the myocardium. This delay in conduction through the ventricles produces a wider QRS complex.
OBJ: Define and describe the significance of each of the following as they relate to cardiac electrical activity: P wave, QRS complex, T wave, U wave, PR segment, TP segment, ST segment, PR interval, QRS duration, and QT interval.

12. A. The main electrolytes that affect the function of the heart are sodium, potassium, calcium, and chloride. Disorders that affect the concentration of these important electrolytes can have serious consequences. For example, an imbalance of potassium can cause life-threatening disturbances in the heart's rhythm.
OBJ: List the most important ions involved in the cardiac action potential and their primary function in this process.

13. C. When the heart rate is within normal limits, the TP segment is usually isoelectric and used as the reference point from which to estimate the position of the isoelectric line and determine ST segment displacement.
OBJ: Define and describe the significance of each of the following as they relate to cardiac electrical activity: P wave, QRS complex, T wave, U wave, PR segment, TP segment, ST segment, PR interval, QRS duration, and QT interval.

14. B. The SA node is normally the primary pacemaker of the heart because it has the fastest firing rate of all of the heart's normal pacemaker sites.
OBJ: Describe the normal sequence of electrical conduction through the heart.

15. D. The right ventricle and posterior surface of the left ventricle are not directly viewed when using a standard 12-lead ECG. Right chest leads and posterior chest leads, respectively, are used for this purpose.
OBJ: Relate the cardiac surfaces or areas represented by the ECG leads.

16. D. A U wave is a small waveform that, when seen, follows the T wave. The U wave is thought to represent late repolarization of the Purkinje fibers (Lederer, 2012). However, some cardiologists believe that U waves denote delayed repolarization in areas of the ventricle that undergo late mechanical relaxation (Mirvis & Goldberger, 2015) or they are simply two-part T waves resulting from a longer action potential duration in some ventricular myocardial cells (Patton & Thibodeau, 2013).
OBJ: Define and describe the significance of each of the following as they relate to cardiac electrical activity: P wave, QRS complex, T wave, U wave, PR segment, TP segment, ST segment, PR interval, QRS duration, and QT interval.

17. B. Pacemaker cells are specialized cells of the heart's electrical system. Pacemaker cells also may be referred to as *conducting cells* or *automatic cells*. They are responsible for spontaneously generating and conducting electrical impulses.
OBJ: Describe the two basic types of cardiac cells in the heart, where they are found, and their function.

18. C. Lead III records the difference in electrical potential between the left leg (+) and left arm (−) electrodes. In lead III, the positive electrode is placed on the left leg, and the negative electrode is placed on the left arm.
OBJ: Describe correct anatomic placement of the standard limb leads, augmented leads, and chest leads.

19. C. An ECG machine's sensitivity must be calibrated so that a 1-mV electrical signal will produce a deflection measuring exactly 10-mm tall. When properly calibrated, a small box is 1 mm high (0.1 mV), and a large box (equal to five small boxes) is 5 mm high (0.5 mV).
OBJ: Identify how heart rates, durations, and amplitudes can be determined from ECG recordings.

20. C. Six chest (precordial or "V") leads view the heart in the horizontal plane. The chest leads are identified as V_1, V_2, V_3, V_4, V_5, and V_6.
OBJ: Differentiate between the frontal plane and the horizontal plane leads.

21. C. Frontal plane leads view the heart from the front of the body as if it were flat. Directions in the frontal plane are superior, inferior, right, and left. Six leads view the heart in the frontal plane. Leads I, II, and III are called *standard limb leads*. Leads aVR, aVL, and aVF are called *augmented limb leads*.
OBJ: Differentiate between the frontal plane and the horizontal plane leads.

22. A. Lead II records the difference in electrical potential between the left leg (+) and right arm (−) electrodes. The positive electrode is placed on the left leg and the negative electrode is placed on the right arm.
OBJ: Describe correct anatomic placement of the standard limb leads, augmented leads, and chest leads.

23. A. When analyzing a rhythm strip, begin by assessing regularity (atrial and ventricular) and rate (atrial and ventricular).
OBJ: Describe a systematic approach to the analysis and interpretation of cardiac dysrhythmias.

24. B. Using the large box (rule of 300) method to calculate heart rate, four large boxes between two consecutive R waves equal a heart rate of 75 beats/min (300 divided by 4).
OBJ: Identify how heart rates, durations, and amplitudes can be determined from ECG recordings.

25. C. In a patient experiencing an acute coronary syndrome, ECG evidence of myocardial injury is displayed as ST segment elevation in the leads facing the affected area of the heart.
OBJ: Recognize the changes on the ECG that may indicate myocardial ischemia, injury, and infarction.

26. B. The TP segment is used as the baseline from which to evaluate the degree of displacement of the ST segment from the isoelectric line. If ST segment displacement is present, note the number of millimeters of deviation from the isoelectric line or from the patient's baseline at the J-point.

When ECG changes of myocardial ischemia, injury, or infarction occur, they are not found in every lead of the ECG. Findings are considered significant if viewed in two or more leads looking at the same or adjacent area of the heart. If these findings are seen in leads that look directly at the affected area, they are called *indicative changes*. Indicative changes are significant when they are seen in two *anatomically contiguous* leads. Two leads are contiguous if they look at the same or adjacent area of the heart or they are numerically consecutive chest leads. Remember that leads II, III, and aVF view the inferior wall of the left ventricle. Therefore, in this patient situation, ST segment changes viewed in lead II would be considered clinically significant if elevated more than 1 mm and also seen in lead III or aVF.
OBJ: Recognize the changes on the ECG that may indicate myocardial ischemia, injury, and infarction.

27. <u>Reentry</u> is the spread of an impulse through tissue already stimulated by that same impulse.
OBJ: Describe reentry.

28. Distortion of an ECG tracing by electrical activity that is noncardiac in origin is called <u>artifact</u>.
OBJ: Define the term *artifact*, and explain methods used to minimize its occurrence.

29. <u>Excitability</u> (or irritability) refers to the ability of cardiac muscle cells to respond to an external stimulus, such as that from a chemical, mechanical, or electrical source.
OBJ: Describe the primary characteristics of cardiac cells.

30. D
31. G
32. J
33. F
34. A
35. E
36. L
37. I
38. B
39. K
40. C
41. H
42. G
43. F
44. H
45. A
46. E
47. B
48. C
49. D

50. ECG monitoring can be used for the following purposes:
- To monitor a patient's heart rate
- To evaluate the effects of disease or injury on heart function
- To evaluate pacemaker function
- To evaluate the response to medications (e.g., antiarrhythmics)
- To obtain a baseline recording before, during, and after a medical procedure
- To evaluate for signs of myocardial ischemia, injury, and infarction
OBJ: Explain the purpose of ECG monitoring.

51. The four properties of cardiac cells are automaticity, excitability (or irritability), conductivity, and contractility.
OBJ: Describe the primary characteristics of cardiac cells.

52. SA node: 60 to 100 beats/min
AV bundle: 40 to 60 beats/min
Purkinje fibers: 20 to 40 beats/min
OBJ: Describe the location, function, and (when appropriate), the intrinsic rate of the following structures: sinoatrial node, atrioventricular bundle, and Purkinje fibers.

53. The R-R (R wave-to-R wave) and P-P (P wave-to-P wave) intervals are used to determine the rate and regularity of a cardiac rhythm.
OBJ: Describe a systematic approach to the analysis and interpretation of cardiac dysrhythmias.

54.

Lead	Positive Electrode	Negative Electrode	Heart Surface Viewed
Lead I	Left arm	Right arm	Lateral
Lead II	Left leg	Right arm	Inferior
Lead III	Left leg	Left arm	Inferior

OBJ: Relate the cardiac surfaces or areas represented by the ECG leads.

55.
1. Assess regularity (atrial and ventricular).
2. Assess rate (atrial and ventricular).
3. Identify and examine waveforms.
4. Assess intervals (e.g., PR, QRS, QT), and examine ST segments.
5. Interpret the rhythm, and assess its clinical significance.
OBJ: Describe a systematic approach to the analysis and interpretation of cardiac dysrhythmias.

56. Possible causes of a poor ECG tracing include excessive body hair, loose electrode, muscle tremor, dried electrode gel, improper lead placement, 60-cycle interference, broken ECG cables or wires, poor electrical contact (e.g., diaphoresis), and external chest compressions.
OBJ: Define the term *artifact*, and explain methods used to minimize its occurrence.

Practice Rhythm Strip Answers

Note: Because of the distortion of ECGs that can occur during printing, a range of acceptable measurements is provided in the rhythm strip answers throughout this textbook.

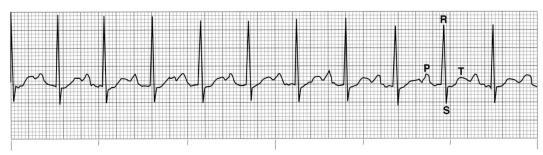

Fig. 2.55 (Answer to Fig. 2.45)

57. **Fig. 2.55 (Answer to Fig. 2.45)**
    Rhythm: Regular
    Rate: 107 beats/min
    P waves: Uniform; upright before each QRS
    PR interval: 0.24 second
    QRS duration: 0.06 to 0.08 second
    QT interval: 0.28 to 0.32 second

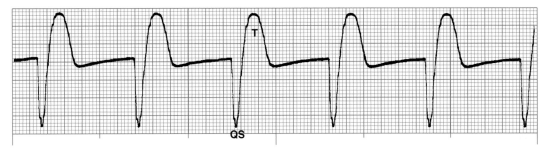

Fig. 2.56 (Answer to Fig. 2.46)

60. **Fig. 2.56 (Answer to Fig. 2.46)**
    Rhythm: Regular
    Rate: 56 beats/min
    P waves: No identifiable P waves
    PR interval: None
    QRS duration: 0.12 second
    QT interval: 0.44 second

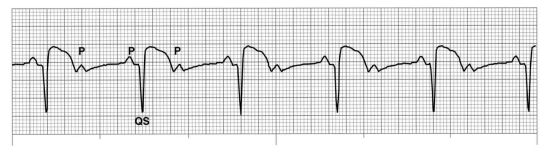

Fig. 2.57 (Answer to Fig. 2.47)

61. **Fig. 2.57 (Answer to Fig. 2.47)**
    Rhythm: Regular
    Rate: Atrial, 107 beats/min; ventricular, 56 beats/min
    P waves: Two upright Ps before each QRS
    PR interval: 0.16 second
    QRS duration: 0.04 to 0.06 second; elevated ST segments
    QT interval: 0.36 sec (estimated; difficult to determine because T wave is not clearly visible)

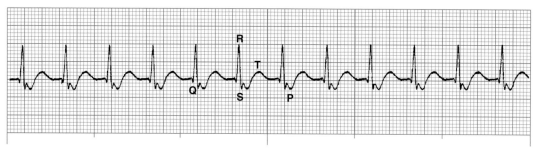

Fig. 2.58 (Answer to Fig. 2.48)

62. **Fig. 2.58 (Answer to Fig. 2.48)**
    Rhythm: Regular
    Rate: 115 beats/min
    P waves: One P appears after each QRS
    PR interval: None
    QRS duration: 0.08 to 0.10 second
    QT interval: 0.36 to 0.40 second

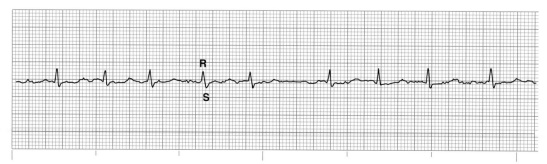

Fig. 2.59 (Answer to Fig. 2.49)

63. **Fig. 2.59 (Answer to Fig. 2.49)**
    Rhythm: Irregular
    Rate: 90 beats/min
    P waves: No identifiable P waves
    PR interval: None
    QRS duration: 0.06 to 0.08 second
    QT interval: Unable to determine; no consistently identifiable T waves

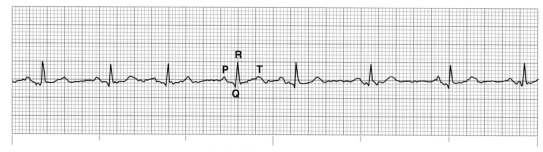

Fig. 2.60 (Answer to Fig. 2.50)

64. **Fig. 2.60 (Answer to Fig. 2.50)**
    Rhythm: Irregular
    Rate: 80 beats/min
    P waves: Upright before each QRS; some are smooth and rounded, others are pointed
    PR interval: 0.16 to 0.20 sec
    QRS duration: 0.08 second
    QT interval: 0.36 second

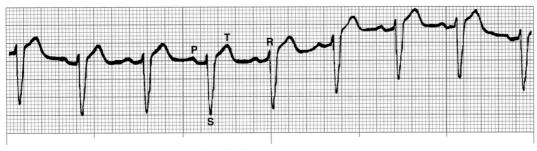

Fig. 2.61 (Answer to Fig. 2.51)

65. **Fig. 2.61 (Answer to Fig. 2.51)**
Rhythm: Regular
Rate: 83 beats/min
P waves: Uniform; upright before each QRS
PR interval: 0.16 to 0.20 second
QRS duration: 0.12 second; ST segment elevation
QT interval: 0.32 to 0.36 second

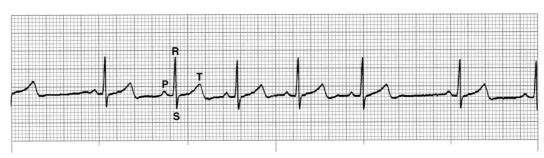

Fig. 2.62 (Answer to Fig. 2.52)

66. **Fig. 2.62 (Answer to Fig. 2.52)**
Rhythm: Irregular
Rate: 70 beats/min
P waves: Uniform; upright before each QRS
PR interval: 0.12 to 0.14 second
QRS duration: 0.06 to 0.08 second
QT interval: 0.36 second

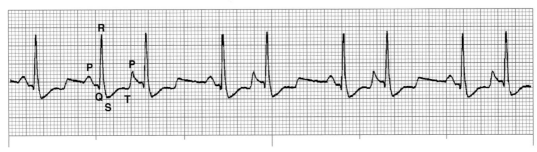

Fig. 2.63 (Answer to Fig. 2.53)

67. **Fig. 2.63 (Answer to Fig. 2.53)**
Rhythm: Irregular
Rate: 90 beats/min
P waves: Upright before each QRS; the P waves of beats 3, 5, 7, and 9 differ from the others
PR interval: 0.16 sec
QRS duration: 0.08 second; ST segment depression
QT interval: 0.40 second; inverted T waves

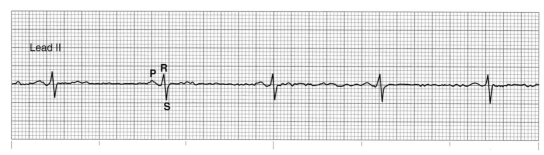

Fig. 2.64 (Answer to Fig. 2.54)

68. **Fig. 2.64 (Answer to Fig. 2.54)**

    Rhythm: Irregular

    Rate: 50 beats/min

    P waves: Upright before each QRS

    PR interval: 0.16 to 0.20 second

    QRS duration: 0.08 second

    QT interval: Unable to determine; no identifiable T waves

REFERENCES

Amsterdam, E. A., Wenger, N. K., Brindis, R. G., Casey, D. E., Jr., Ganiats, T. G., Holmes, D. R., Jr., & Zieman, S. J. (2014). 2014 AHA/ACC guideline for the management of patients with non-ST-elevation acute coronary syndromes. *J Am Coll Cardiol, 64*(24), 1–150.

Anderson, J. L. (2012). ST segment elevation acute myocardial infarction and complications of myocardial infarction. In L. Goldman & A. I. Schafer (Eds.), *Goldman's Cecil medicine* (24th ed.) (pp. 434–448). Philadelphia: Saunders.

Aronson, P. S., Boron, W. F., & Boulpaep, E. L. (2012). Transport of solutes and water. In W. F. Boron & E. L. Boulpaep (Eds.), *Medical physiology: A cellular and molecular approach* (2nd ed.) (pp. 106–146). Philadelphia: Saunders.

Bakker, A. L., Nijkerk, G., Groenemeijer, B. E., Waalewijn, R. A., Koomen, E. M., Braam, R. L., & Wellens, H. J. (2009). The Lewis lead: making recognition of P waves easy during wide QRS complex tachycardia. *Circulation, 119*(24), e592–e593.

Boulpaep, E. L. (2017). The heart as a pump. In W. F. Boron & E. L. Boulpaep (Eds.), *Medical physiology: A cellular and molecular approach* (3rd ed.) (pp. 507–532). Philadelphia: Saunders.

Brashers, V. L., & McCance, K. L. (2012). Structure and function of the cardiovascular and lymphatic systems. In S. E. Huether, K. L. McCance, V. L. Brashers, & N. S. Rote (Eds.), *Understanding pathophysiology* (5th ed.) (pp. 551–584). St. Louis: Mosby.

Costanzo, L. S. (2014). Cardiovascular physiology. In *Physiology* (5th ed.) (pp. 113–184). Philadelphia: Saunders.

Crawford, M. H., Bernstein, S. J., Deedwania, P. C., DiMarco, J. P., Ferrick, K. J., Garson, A., Jr., & Smith, S. C., Jr. (1999). ACC/AHA Guidelines for Ambulatory Electrocardiography. A report of the American College of Cardiology/American Heart Association Task Force on Practice Guidelines (Committee to Revise the Guidelines for Ambulatory Electrocardiography). *J Am Coll Cardiol, 34*(3), 912–948.

DeBeasi, L. C. (2003a). Anatomy of the cardiovascular system. In S. A. Price & L. M. Wilson (Eds.), *Pathophysiology: Clinical concepts of disease processes* (6th ed.) (pp. 405–415). St. Louis: Mosby.

DeBeasi, L. C. (2003b). Physiology of the cardiovascular system. In S. A. Price & L. M. Wilson (Eds.), *Pathophysiology: Clinical concepts of disease processes* (6th ed.) (pp. 416–428). St. Louis: Mosby.

Drew, B. J., Califf, R. M., Funk, M., Kaufman, E. S., Krucoff, M. W., Laks, M. M., & Van Hare, G. F. (2004). Practice standards for electrocardiographic monitoring in hospital settings: an American Heart Association scientific statement from the Councils on Cardiovascular Nursing, Clinical Cardiology, and Cardiovascular Disease in the Young. *Circulation, 110*(17), 2721–2746.

Ganz, L. (2012). Electrocardiography. In L. Goldman & A. I. Schafer (Eds.), *Goldman's Cecil medicine* (24th ed.) (pp. 272–278). Philadelphia: Saunders.

Goldberger, A. L., Goldberger, Z. D., & Shvilkin, A. (2013). Atrial and ventricular enlargement. In *Clinical electrocardiography: A simplified approach* (6th ed.) (pp. 45–74). Philadelphia: Saunders.

Gorgels, A. P., Engelen, D. J., & Wellens, H. J. (2001). Lead aVR, a mostly ignored but very valuable lead in clinical electrocardiography. *J Am Coll Cardiol, 38*(5), 1355–1356.

Hall, J. E. (2016). The heart. In *Guyton and Hall textbook of medical physiology* (13th ed.) (pp. 107–166). Philadelphia: Saunders.

Hancock, E. W., Deal, B. J., Mirvis, D. M., Okin, P., Kligfield, P., & Gettes, L. S. (2009). AHA/ACCF/HRS recommendations for the standardization and interpretation of the electrocardiogram: Part V: electrocardiogram changes associated with cardiac chamber hypertrophy. *J Am Coll Cardiol, 53*(11), 992–1002.

Harrigan, R. A., Chan, T. C., & Brady, W. J. (2014). Basic electrocardiographic techniques. In J. R. Roberts (Ed.), *Roberts and Hedges' clinical procedures in emergency medicine* (6th ed.) (pp. 263–276). Philadelphia: Saunders.

Hwang, H. J., Ng, F. S., & Efimov, I. R. (2014). Mechanisms of atrioventricular nodal excitability and propagation. In D. P. Zipes & J. Jalife (Eds.), *Cardiac electrophysiology: From cell to bedside* (6th ed.) (pp. 275–285). Philadelphia: Saunders.

Issa, Z. F., Miller, J. M., & Zipes, D. P. (2012). Atrioventricular nodal reentrant tachycardia. In *Clinical arrhythmology and electrophysiology: A companion to Braunwald's heart disease* (2nd ed.) (pp. 381–410). Philadelphia: Saunders.

Krahn, A. D., Yee, R., Skanes, A. C., & Klein, G. J. (2014). Cardiac monitoring: Short and long-term recording. In D. P. Zipes & J. Jalife (Eds.), *Cardiac electrophysiology: From cell to bedside* (pp. 621–627). Philadelphia: Saunders.

Lederer, W. J. (2012). Cardiac electrophysiology and the electrocardiogram. In W. F. Boron & E. L. Boulpaep (Eds.), *Medical physiology: A cellular and molecular approach* (2nd ed.) (pp. 504–528). Philadelphia: Saunders.

McKinley, M. G. (2011). Procedure 57: Electrocardiographic leads and cardiac monitoring. In D. J. Lynn-McHale Wiegand (Ed.), *AACN Procedure Manual for Critical Care* (6th ed.) (pp. 490–501). St. Louis: Saunders.

Mirvis, D. M., & Goldberger, A. L. (2015). Electrocardiography. In D. L. Mann, D. P. Zipes, P. Libby, R. O. Bonow, & E. Braunwald (Eds.), *Braunwald's heart disease: A textbook of cardiovascular medicine* (10th ed.) (pp. 114–154). Philadelphia: Saunders.

Mittal, S., Movsowitz, C., & Steinberg, J. S. (2011). Ambulatory external electrocardiographic monitoring: focus on atrial fibrillation. *J Am Coll Cardiol*, 58(17), 1741–1749.

O'Gara, P. T., Kushner, F. G., Ascheim, D. D., Casey, D. E., Jr., Chung, M. K., de Lemos, J. A., & Zhao, D. X. (2013). 2013 ACCF/AHA guideline for the management of ST-elevation myocardial infarction. *J Am Coll Cardiol*, 61(4), e78–e140.

Pappano, A. J. (2010). Elements of cardiac function. In B. M. Koeppen & B. A. Stanton (Eds.), *Berne & Levy physiology* (6th ed.) (pp. 292–329). Philadelphia: Mosby.

Patton, K. T., & Thibodeau, G. A. (2013). Physiology of the cardiovascular system. In *Anatomy & physiology* (8th ed.) (pp. 681–721). St. Louis: Mosby.

Peterson, K. J. (2009). Advanced dysrhythmias. In K. K. Carlson (Ed.), *AACN Advanced Critical Care Nursing* (1st ed.) (pp. 173–206). St. Louis: Saunders.

Phalen, T., & Aehlert, B. (2012). Introduction to the 12-lead ECG. In *The 12-lead in acute coronary syndromes* (3rd ed.) (pp. 21–50). Maryland Heights, Missouri: Mosby.

Rautaharju, P. M., Surawicz, B., & Gettes, L. S. (2009). AHA/ACCF/HRS Recommendations for the standardization and interpretation of the electrocardiogram: Part IV: The ST segment, T and U waves, and the QT interval: a scientific statement from the American Heart Association Electrocardiography and Arrhythmias. *J Am Coll Cardiol*, 53(11), 982–991.

Rubart, M., & Zipes, D. P. (2015). Genesis of cardiac arrhythmias: Electrophysiologic considerations. In D. L. Mann, D. P. Zipes, P. Libby, R. O. Bonow, & E. Braunwald (Eds.), *Braunwald's heart disease: A textbook of cardiovascular medicine* (10th ed.) (pp. 629–661). Philadelphia: Saunders.

Saksena, S., Bharati, S., Lindsay, B. D., & Levy, S. (2012). Paroxysmal supraventricular tachycardia and pre-excitation syndromes. In S. Saksena & A. J. Camm (Eds.), *Electrophysiological disorders of the heart* (2nd ed.) (pp. 531–558). Philadelphia: Saunders.

Surawicz, B., & Knilans, T. K. (2008). Normal electrocardiogram: origin and description. In *Chou's electrocardiography in clinical practice* (6th ed.) (pp. 1–28). Philadelphia: Saunders.

Surawicz, B., Childers, R., Deal, B. J., & Gettes, L. S. (2009). AHA/ACCF/HRS Recommendations for the standardization and interpretation of the electrocardiogram: Part III: Intraventricular conduction disturbances: a scientific statement from the American Heart Association Electrocardiography and Arrhythmias Committee. *J Am Coll Cardiol*, 53(11), 976–981.

Thygesen, K., Alpert, J. S., Jaffe, A. S., Simoons, M. L., Chaitman, B. R., & White, H. D. (2012). Third universal definition of myocardial infarction. *Circulation*, 126(16), 2020–2035.

Vorobiof, G., & Ellestad, M. H. (2011). Lead aVR: dead or simply forgotten? *JACC Cardiovasc Imaging*, 4(2), 187–190.

Wagner, G. (2012). Basic electrocardiography. In S. Saksena & A. J. Camm (Eds.), *Electrophysiological disorders of the heart* (2nd ed.) (pp. 125–158). Philadelphia: Saunders.

Wagner, G. S., Macfarlane, P., Wellens, H., Josephson, M., Gorgels, A., Mirvis, D. M., & Gettes, L. S. (2009). AHA/ACCF/HRS recommendations for the standardization and interpretation of the electrocardiogram: Part VI: acute ischemia/infarction; a scientific statement from the American Heart Association Electrocardiography and Arrhythmias Committee. *J Am Coll Cardiol*, 53(11), 1003–1011.

Zimetbaum, P. (2016). Cardiac arrhythmias with supraventricular origin. In L. Goldman & A. I. Schafer (Eds.), *Goldman's Cecil medicine* (25th ed.) (pp. 356–366). Philadelphia: Saunders.

Sinus Mechanisms

3

INTRODUCTION

In this chapter, you will begin learning the characteristics of specific cardiac rhythms. Study these characteristics carefully and commit them to memory. Throughout this text, all ECG characteristics pertain to adult patients unless otherwise noted.

The normal heartbeat is the result of an electrical impulse that starts in the sinoatrial (SA) node (Fig. 3.1). Normally, pacemaker cells within the SA node spontaneously depolarize more rapidly than other cardiac cells. As a result, the SA node usually dominates other areas that are depolarizing at a slightly slower rate. The impulse is sent to cells at the outside edge of the SA node and then to the myocardial cells of the surrounding atrium.

A rhythm that begins in the SA node has the following characteristics:

- A positive (i.e., upright) P wave before each QRS complex
- P waves that look alike
- A constant PR interval
- A regular atrial and ventricular rhythm (usually)

An electrical impulse that begins in the SA node may be affected by the following:

- Medications
- Diseases or conditions that cause the heart rate to speed up, slow down, or beat irregularly
- Diseases or conditions that delay or block the impulse from leaving the SA node
- Diseases or conditions that prevent an impulse from being generated in the SA node

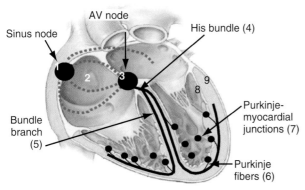

Fig. 3.1 The cardiac action potential originates in the sinoatrial (SA) node (1), continues in the atrial wall (2), and is delayed in the atrioventricular (AV) node (3). Conduction within the ventricles is initially rapid within the rapid conduction system: His bundle (4), right and left bundle branches (5), and Purkinje fibers (6). The impulse is transferred from the rapid conduction system to the working myocardium in the Purkinje-myocardial junctions (7), which are located in the endocardium. Within the slowly conducting working myocardium, the impulse is conducted from endocardium to epicardium. The SA node normally depolarizes faster than any other part of the heart's conduction system. As a result, the SA node is normally the heart's primary pacemaker. (From Ellenbogen KA, Kay GN, Lau CP, Wilkoff BL: *Clinical cardiac pacing, defibrillation and resynchronization therapy,* ed 4, Philadelphia, 2011, Saunders.)

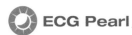 **ECG Pearl**

Most, but not all, rhythms that begin in the SA node are regular.

SINUS RHYTHM

[Objective 1]

Sinus rhythm is the name given to a normal heart rhythm. Sinus rhythm is sometimes called a *regular sinus rhythm* (RSR) or *normal sinus rhythm* (NSR). Sinus rhythm reflects normal electrical activity—that is, the rhythm starts in the SA node and then heads down the normal conduction pathway through the atria, atrioventricular (AV) node and bundle, right and left bundle branches, and Purkinje fibers.

A person's heart rate varies with age (Table 3.1). In adults and adolescents, the SA node normally fires at a regular rate of 60 to 100 beats/min.

How Do I Recognize It?

Fig. 3.2 shows an example of a sinus rhythm recorded simultaneously in three leads: V_1, II, and V_5. As you look as this figure from left to right, note the 10-mm calibration marker that appears at the far left of each lead. Although we will focus on lead II as we examine this rhythm strip, you will find that it is helpful to view waveforms, segments, and intervals in more than one lead.

A sinus rhythm has a regular atrial and ventricular rhythm. Find the QRS complexes on the rhythm strip. Place one point of your calipers or make a mark on a piece of paper on the beginning of an R wave. Place the other point of the

TABLE 3.1	Normal Resting Heart Rates by Age
Age	Heart Rate (beats/min)
Infant (1 to 12 months)	100 to 160
Toddler (1 to 3 years)	90 to 150
Preschooler (4 to 5 years)	80 to 140
School age (6 to 12 years)	70 to 120
Adolescent (13 to 18 years)	60 to 100
Adult	60 to 100

calipers or make a second mark on the paper on the beginning of the R wave of the next QRS complex. Without adjusting the calipers, evaluate each succeeding R-R interval. If you are using paper, lift the paper and move it across the rhythm strip. The R-R intervals in this example are regular. Because you have already identified the R waves, determine the ventricular rate. Because the rhythm is regular, calculate the rate using the small box method. There are 19 small boxes between R waves; therefore, the ventricular rate is about 79 beats/min. Remember, the built-in (i.e., intrinsic) rate for a rhythm that begins in the SA node is 60 to 100 beats/min; therefore, the rate of the rhythm in our example fits within the criteria for a sinus rhythm.

Now look to the left of the QRS complexes to find the P waves on the rhythm strip. A rhythm that begins in the SA node should have a positive (i.e., upright) P wave in lead II before each QRS complex (i.e., there should be a 1:1 relationship between P waves and QRS complexes). When you look at this rhythm strip, you can see one upright P wave before each QRS complex. Every P wave looks alike. Measure the P-P interval to see if the P waves occur regularly, and then determine the atrial rate. You will find that the P waves occur regularly at a rate of 79 beats/min.

Now measure the PR interval and QRS duration. In a sinus rhythm, the PR interval measures 0.12 to 0.20 second and is constant from beat to beat. In this example, the PR interval is 0.16 second. The QRS complex normally measures 0.11 second or less. If there is a delay in conduction through the bundle branches, the QRS may be wide (i.e., greater than 0.11 second). In our example, the QRS measures between 0.04 and 0.08 second depending on the lead and complex selected for the measurement. Next, determine the QT interval by counting the number of small boxes between the beginning of the QRS complex and the end of the T wave and multiplying that number by 0.04 second. In our example, the QT interval measures about 8.5 boxes (0.34 second). This value is within normal limits.

Next, locate the TP segment and then the J point. Remember that deviation is measured as the number of millimeters of vertical ST-segment displacement from the J point (O'Gara et al, 2013). You will see that the ST segments in leads II and III of this rhythm strip are elevated. Now interpret the rhythm, specifying the site of origin (pacemaker site) of the rhythm and the ventricular rate. Because the rhythm shown in Fig. 3.2 fits the ECG criteria for a sinus rhythm,

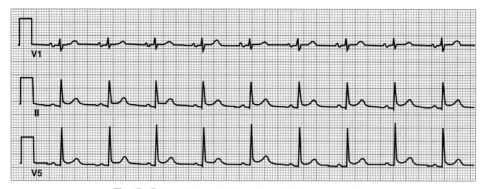

Fig. 3.2 Sinus rhythm at 79 beats/min with ST-segment elevation.

TABLE **3.2**	Characteristics of Sinus Rhythm
Rhythm	R-R and P-P intervals are regular
Rate	60 to 100 beats/min
P waves	Positive (upright) in lead II; one precedes each QRS complex; P waves look alike
PR interval	0.12 to 0.20 sec and constant from beat to beat
QRS duration	0.11 sec or less unless abnormally conducted

TABLE **3.3**	Characteristics of Sinus Bradycardia
Rhythm	R-R and P-P intervals are regular
Rate	Less than 60 beats/min
P waves	Positive (upright) in lead II; one precedes each QRS complex; P waves look alike
PR interval	0.12 to 0.20 sec and constant from beat to beat
QRS duration	0.11 sec or less unless abnormally conducted

your interpretation should be sinus rhythm at 79 beats/min with ST-segment elevation (STE). A summary of the ECG characteristics of a sinus rhythm are shown in Table 3.2.

SINUS BRADYCARDIA

[Objective 2]

If the SA node fires at a rate slower than normal for the patient's age, the rhythm is called **sinus bradycardia**. The rhythm starts in the SA node and then travels the normal conduction pathway, resulting in atrial and ventricular depolarization. In adults and adolescents, a sinus bradycardia has a heart rate of less than 60 beats/min. The term *severe sinus bradycardia* is sometimes used to describe a sinus bradycardia with a rate of less than 40 beats/min.

How Do I Recognize It?

Fig. 3.3 is an example of sinus bradycardia. Table 3.3 lists the ECG characteristics of sinus bradycardia. You will note they are the same as the characteristics of a sinus rhythm with one exception—the rate. The rate of a sinus rhythm is 60 to 100 beats/min. The rate of a sinus bradycardia is less than 60 beats/min.

Examine this rhythm strip with the use of the same systematic format that you previously used. Begin by locating the QRS complexes on the rhythm strip. Evaluate each succeeding R-R interval. The R-R intervals in this example are regular. Now determine the ventricular rate. In this rhythm strip, the ventricular rate is 40 beats/min. Next, find the P waves on the rhythm strip. Remember that a rhythm that

begins in the SA node should have a positive P wave (in lead II) before each QRS complex. In our example, you can see that there is a 1:1 relationship between P waves and QRS complexes, and every P wave looks alike. Now measure the P-to-P interval to see if the P waves occur regularly and determine the atrial rate. The P waves occur regularly at a rate of 40 beats/min. Next, measure the PR interval, QRS duration, and QT interval. In this example, the PR interval is 0.16 second, the QRS complex measures 0.08 second, and the QT interval is 0.40 second. ST-segment depression is present, and negative (i.e., inverted) T waves appear after each QRS complex. These findings must be noted in your final description of the rhythm. Therefore, correct interpretation of this rhythm would be sinus bradycardia at 40 beats/min with ST-segment depression and inverted T waves.

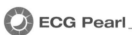 **ECG Pearl**

In sinus bradycardia, the QT interval may be longer than normal because of the slower heart rate.

What Causes It?

Sinus bradycardia occurs in adults during sleep and in well-conditioned athletes. It is also present in up to 35% of people younger than 25 years of age while at rest. Sinus bradycardia is common in some myocardial infarctions (MIs). Prolonged standing and stimulation of the vagus nerve can also result in slowing of the heart rate. For example, coughing, vomiting, straining to have a bowel movement, or sudden exposure of

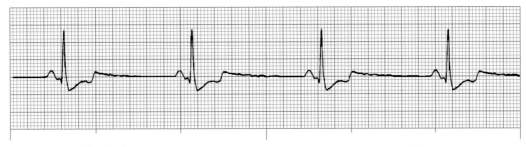

Fig. 3.3 Sinus bradycardia at 40 beats/min with ST-segment depression and inverted T waves.

Box **3.1**	**Causes of Sinus Bradycardia**

- Disease of the sinoatrial node
- Hyperkalemia
- Hypokalemia
- Hypothermia
- Hypothyroidism
- Hypoxia
- Increased intracranial pressure
- Inferior myocardial infarction (MI)
- Medications such as calcium channel blockers, digitalis, beta-blockers, amiodarone, and sotalol
- Obstructive sleep apnea
- Post heart transplant
- Posterior MI
- Vagal stimulation

Box **3.2**	**Signs and Symptoms of Hemodynamic Compromise**

- Acute changes in mental status
- Chest pain or discomfort
- Cold, clammy skin
- Fall in urine output
- Heart failure
- Hypotension
- Pulmonary congestion
- Shock
- Shortness of breath

the face to cold water can result in slowing of the heart rate. In people who have a sensitive carotid sinus, slowing of the heart rate can occur when a tight collar is worn or with the impact of the stream of water on the neck while in the shower. Other causes of sinus bradycardia are shown in Box 3.1.

What Do I Do About It?

Remember that cardiac output equals stroke volume × heart rate. Therefore, a decrease in either stroke volume or heart rate may result in a decrease in cardiac output. Many patients tolerate a heart rate of 50 to 60 beats/min but become symptomatic when the rate drops below 50 beats/min. A patient with an unusually slow heart rate may complain of light-headedness, dizziness, or weakness, and fainting (i.e., syncope) can occur. Decreasing cardiac output will eventually produce hemodynamic compromise (Box 3.2).

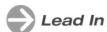 **Lead In** _____

Policy and Protocol

Interventions and treatments discussed in this text assume that an assessment has been performed, the patient's clinical problem identified, and a physician order has been obtained when indicated. In the out-of-hospital setting, paramedics and nurses typically operate under standing physician orders, local protocols, or both. In the hospital setting, agency policy may permit the use of standing orders to direct patient care when a patient's condition changes rapidly and requires immediate intervention. These orders, when performed by a clinician with appropriate training per that institution's policy, may include routine therapies, monitoring guidelines, diagnostic procedures, and medication administration. Physician contact is necessary when standing orders or local protocols are not available.

If a patient presents with a bradycardia, assess how she or he is tolerating the rhythm at rest and with activity. If the patient has no symptoms, no treatment is necessary. The term *symptomatic bradycardia* refers to signs and symptoms of hemodynamic compromise related to a slow heart rate. Treatment of a symptomatic bradycardia should include assessment of the patient's oxygen saturation level and determining if signs of increased work of breathing are present (e.g., retractions, tachypnea, paradoxic abdominal breathing). Give supplemental oxygen if oxygenation is inadequate and assist breathing if ventilation is inadequate. Establish intravenous (IV) access and obtain a 12-lead ECG. Atropine, administered intravenously, is the drug of choice for symptomatic bradycardia. Reassess the patient's response and continue monitoring the patient.

In the setting of an MI, sinus bradycardia is often transient. A slow heart rate can be beneficial in a patient who has had an MI and who has no symptoms because of the slow rate. This is because the heart's demand for oxygen is less when the heart rate is slow.

 Drug Pearl _____

Atropine is a drug used to increase the heart rate. It works by blocking acetylcholine at the endings of the vagus nerves. The vagus nerves innervate the heart at the SA and AV nodes. Thus, atropine is most effective for narrow-QRS bradycardias. By blocking the effects of acetylcholine, atropine allows more activity from the sympathetic division of the autonomic nervous system. As a result, the rate at which the SA node can fire is increased. Atropine also increases the rate at which an impulse is conducted through the AV node. Areas of the heart that are not innervated or that are minimally innervated by the vagus nerves (e.g., the ventricles) will not respond to atropine. Transplanted hearts do not usually respond to atropine because they lack vagal nerve innervation.

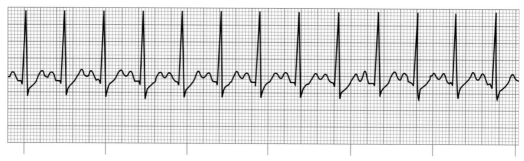

Fig. 3.4 Sinus tachycardia at 125 beats/min with ST-segment depression.

SINUS TACHYCARDIA

[Objective 3]

If the SA node fires at a rate faster than normal for the patient's age, the rhythm is called **sinus tachycardia**. Sinus tachycardia begins and ends gradually. The rhythm starts in the SA node and travels the normal pathway of conduction through the heart, resulting in atrial and ventricular depolarization.

How Do I Recognize It?

A sinus tachycardia looks much like a sinus rhythm except that it is faster. At very fast rates, it may be hard to tell the difference between a P wave and T wave. Keep in mind that the QT interval normally shortens as heart rate increases.

Normal heart rates vary with age. In adults, the rate associated with sinus tachycardia is usually between 101 and 180 beats/min, although faster rates have been documented. Some experts consider the upper rate of sinus tachycardia to be about 220 beats/min, minus the patient's age in years (Link et al, 2015).

Because an infant or child's heart rate can transiently increase during episodes of crying, pain, or fever, the term *tachycardia* describes a significant and persistent increase in heart rate. With a sinus tachycardia, the heart rate is faster than normal for age, but it is usually less than 220 beats/min in infants or 180 beats/min in children.

Fig. 3.4 is an example of sinus tachycardia. Table 3.4 lists the ECG characteristics of sinus tachycardia. Let us examine this rhythm strip more closely. By glancing at the strip from left to right, you can see that the rate is faster than that of a sinus rhythm. Locate the QRS complexes, evaluate the R-R intervals, and then determine the ventricular rate. The R-R intervals in this example are regular, and the ventricular rate is 125 beats/min. The ventricular rate fits within the parameters of a sinus tachycardia.

Look at the P waves on the rhythm strip, evaluate the P-P intervals for regularity, and then determine the atrial rate. One upright P wave appears before each QRS complex, every P wave looks alike, and the P waves occur regularly at a rate of 125 beats/min. Now measure the PR interval, QRS duration, and QT interval. In this example, the PR interval is 0.16 second, the QRS complex measures 0.06 second, and the QT interval is 0.32 second. Now interpret the rhythm, noting the ST-segment

TABLE 3.4	Characteristics of Sinus Tachycardia
Rhythm	R-R and P-P intervals are regular
Rate	Usually between 101 and 180 beats/min; alternatively, the upper ventricular rate limit may be calculated as 220 beats/min minus the patient's age in years
P waves	Positive (upright) in lead II; one precedes each QRS complex; P waves look alike
PR interval	0.12 to 0.20 sec and constant from beat to beat
QRS duration	0.11 sec or less unless abnormally conducted

Box 3.3	Causes of Sinus Tachycardia
• Acute myocardial infarction • Caffeine-containing beverages • Dehydration, hypovolemia • Drugs such as cocaine, amphetamines, ecstasy, and cannabis • Exercise • Fear and anxiety • Fever • Heart failure • Hyperthyroidism	• Hypoxia • Infection • Medications (e.g., epinephrine, atropine, dopamine) • Nicotine • Pain • Pulmonary embolism • Shock • Sympathetic stimulation

depression that is present. The correct interpretation is sinus tachycardia at 125 beats/min with ST-segment depression.

What Causes It?

Sinus tachycardia is a normal response to the body's demand for increased oxygen, which results from many conditions (Box 3.3). The patient is often aware of an increase in heart rate. Some patients complain of palpitations, a racing heart, or a feeling of pounding in their chests. Sinus tachycardia is seen in some patients with acute MI, especially in those with an anterior infarction.

In a patient with coronary artery disease (CAD), sinus tachycardia can cause problems. The heart's demand for oxygen increases as the heart rate increases. As the heart rate increases, there is less time for the ventricles to fill and less blood for the ventricles to pump out with each contraction, which can lead to decreased cardiac output. Because the coronary arteries fill when the ventricles are at rest, rapid heart rates decrease the time available for coronary artery filling. This decreases the heart's blood supply. Chest discomfort can result if the supplies of blood and oxygen to the heart are inadequate. Sinus tachycardia in a patient who is having an acute MI may be an early warning signal for heart failure, cardiogenic shock, and more serious dysrhythmias.

What Do I Do About It?

Treatment for sinus tachycardia is directed at correcting the underlying cause (i.e., fluid replacement, relief of pain, removal of offending medications or substances, reducing fever or anxiety). Sinus tachycardia in a patient experiencing an acute MI may be treated with medications to slow the heart rate and decrease myocardial oxygen demand (e.g., beta-blockers), provided there are no signs of heart failure or other contraindications.

Some dysrhythmias with very rapid ventricular rates (i.e., above 150 beats/min) require the delivery of medications or a shock to stop the rhythm. However, it is important to remember that shocking a sinus tachycardia is inappropriate; rather, treat the cause of the tachycardia.

SINUS ARRHYTHMIA

As you have seen so far, the SA node fires quite regularly most of the time. When it fires irregularly, the resulting rhythm is called **sinus arrhythmia**. Sinus arrhythmia begins in the SA node and follows the normal conduction pathway in the heart, resulting in atrial and ventricular depolarization. A sinus arrhythmia usually occurs at a rate of 60 to 100 beats/min. Sinus arrhythmia associated with the phases of breathing and changes in intrathoracic pressure is called *respiratory sinus arrhythmia*. Sinus arrhythmia unrelated to the ventilatory cycle is called *nonrespiratory sinus arrhythmia*.

How Do I Recognize It?

Let's look at the rhythm strip in Fig. 3.5. How does this rhythm differ from the others we have discussed so far? Without using calipers or a piece of paper, you can see that

it is irregular. Recognizing that, the rhythm cannot be a sinus rhythm because a sinus rhythm is regular. Because the rhythm is irregular, we will use the 6-second method to calculate the rate, which is 70 beats/min. Alternately, the rate could be calculated by finding the slowest and fastest parts of the rhythm and giving a rate range. Looking closely at the rest of the rhythm strip, you can see one upright P wave before each QRS complex. Upon measuring the PR interval, the QRS duration, and the QT interval, you will find that they are within normal limits.

This rhythm strip was obtained from a 39-year-old man who was complaining of "feeling faint." If we were able to see the patient and watch his ventilatory rate and ECG at the same time, you would see a pattern. The patient's heart rate increases gradually during inspiration (i.e., the R-R intervals shorten) and decreases with expiration (i.e., the R-R intervals lengthen). To identify this rhythm, we will call it a sinus arrhythmia at 70 beats/min. Table 3.5 lists the characteristics of sinus arrhythmia.

What Causes It?

Respiratory sinus arrhythmia, which is the most common type of sinus arrhythmia, is a normal phenomenon that occurs with phases of breathing and changes in intrathoracic pressure. The heart rate increases with inspiration (i.e., the R-R intervals shorten) and decreases with expiration (i.e., the R-R intervals lengthen). The changes in rhythm disappear when patients hold their breath. Sinus arrhythmia is most commonly observed in children and young adults.

TABLE 3.5	Characteristics of Sinus Arrhythmia
Rhythm	Irregular and often phasic with breathing; heart rate increases gradually during inspiration (R-R intervals shorten) and decreases with expiration (R-R intervals lengthen)
Rate	Usually 60 to 100 beats/min
P waves	Positive (upright) in lead II; one precedes each QRS complex; P waves look alike
PR interval	0.12 to 0.20 sec and constant from beat to beat
QRS duration	0.11 sec or less unless abnormally conducted

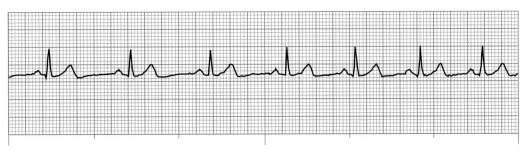

Fig. 3.5 Sinus arrhythmia at 70 beats/min.

Nonrespiratory sinus arrhythmia can be seen in people with normal hearts, but it is more likely to be found in older individuals and in those with heart disease. It is common after acute inferior wall MI, and it may be seen with increased intracranial pressure. Nonrespiratory sinus arrhythmia may be the result of the effects of medications (e.g., digitalis, morphine) or carotid sinus pressure.

What Do I Do About It?

Sinus arrhythmia usually does not require treatment unless it is accompanied by a slow heart rate that causes hemodynamic compromise. If hemodynamic compromise is present because of the slow rate, IV atropine may be indicated to treat the bradycardia.

SINOATRIAL BLOCK

With SA block, also called *sinus exit block*, the pacemaker cells within the SA node initiate an impulse, but it is blocked as it exits the SA node. This results in periodically absent PQRST complexes. SA block is thought to occur because of failure of the transitional cells in the SA node to conduct the impulse from the pacemaker cells to the surrounding atrium. Thus, SA block is a disorder of impulse conduction.

How Do I Recognize It?

When an impulse is blocked as it exits the SA node, the atria are not activated. This appears on the ECG as a single missed beat (i.e., a P wave, QRS complex, and T wave are missing). The pause caused by the missed beat is the same as, or an exact multiple of, the distance between two P-P intervals of the underlying rhythm.

Look at the example of SA block in Fig. 3.6. As you quickly scan the rhythm strip from left to right, the pause between the third and fourth beats should be obvious. The atrial and ventricular rhythm is irregular because of the pause. The rate is about 60 beats/min using the 6-second method of rate calculation. You can see a positive P wave in front of each QRS complex. The P waves look alike. The PR interval is 0.16 second and constant from beat to beat. The QRS complex measures 0.06 to 0.08 second, and the QT interval measures 0.32

to 0.36 second, which is within normal limits. Because the P waves are upright and each P wave is associated with a QRS complex, we know that the underlying rhythm came from the SA node. So far, we can identify this rhythm as a sinus rhythm with a ventricular rate of 60 beats/min.

Now we need to figure out what caused the pause between beats 3 and 4. First, look to the left of the pause and examine the waveforms of the beat that comes before the pause. Compare these waveforms with the others in the rhythm strip. It is important to do this because sometimes waveforms hide on top of other waveforms, distorting their shape. In our example, nothing seems to be amiss. Now use your calipers or paper and plot P waves and R waves from left to right across the strip. When you do this, make a mark on the rhythm strip where the next PQRST cycle should have occurred. You will find that exactly one PQRST cycle is missing. The P-P interval is an exact multiple of the distance between two P-P intervals of the underlying sinus rhythm. This occurred because impulses were generated regularly but failed to exit the SA node between beats 3 and 4. To complete our interpretation of this rhythm, we will explain the pause as an SA block. Putting it all together, we have a sinus rhythm at a rate of 60 beats/min with an episode of SA block. Table 3.6 lists the ECG characteristics of SA block.

What Causes It?

SA block is rather uncommon. Possible causes of SA block include hypoxia, damage or disease to the SA node from CAD, myocarditis, or acute MI; carotid sinus sensitivity;

TABLE 3.6	Characteristics of Sinoatrial (SA) Block
Rhythm	Irregular as a result of the pause(s) caused by the sinoatrial block—the pause is the same as, or an exact multiple of, the distance between two other P-P intervals
Rate	Usually normal but varies because of the pause
P waves	Positive (upright) in lead II; P waves look alike; when present, one precedes each QRS complex.
PR interval	0.12 to 0.20 sec and constant from beat to beat
QRS duration	0.11 sec or less unless abnormally conducted

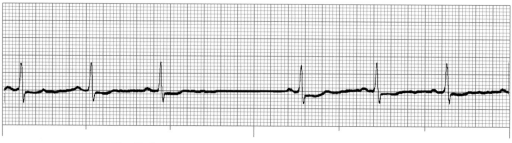

Fig. 3.6 Sinus rhythm at 60 beats/min with an episode of sinoatrial block.

increased vagal tone on the SA node; and medications (e.g., digitalis, quinidine, procainamide, salicylates). If episodes of SA block are frequent and accompanied by a slow heart rate, the patient may show signs and symptoms of hemodynamic compromise.

What Do I Do About It?

Signs and symptoms associated with SA block depend on the number of sinus beats blocked. If the episodes of SA block are transient and there are no significant signs or symptoms, the patient is observed. If signs of hemodynamic compromise are present and are the result of medication toxicity, the offending agents should be withheld. If the episodes of SA block are frequent, IV atropine, temporary pacing, or insertion of a permanent pacemaker may be needed.

SINUS ARREST

[Objective 6]

Sinus arrest, also called *sinus pause* or *sinoatrial arrest*, is a disorder of impulse formation. With sinus arrest, the pacemaker cells of the SA node fail to initiate an electrical impulse for one or more beats resulting in absent PQRST complexes on the ECG.

When the SA node fails to initiate an impulse, an escape pacemaker site (e.g., the AV junction or the Purkinje fibers) should kick in and assume responsibility for pacing the heart. The term *junctional* denotes a beat or rhythm originating at the AV junction. Therefore, when the SA node fails to fire and an escape pacemaker kicks in, the pause associated with a sinus arrest may be terminated by a junctional or ventricular escape beat. If an escape pacemaker site does not fire, you will see absent PQRST complexes on the ECG.

How Do I Recognize It?

An example of sinus arrest is shown in Fig. 3.7. Looking at the rhythm strip from left to right, you can see a period of no electrical activity between the third and fourth beats. Begin analyzing the rhythm strip by determining the atrial and ventricular rhythmicity and rate. The rate is about 60 beats/min using the 6-second method of rate calculation because the rhythm is irregular.

You can see a positive P wave in front of each QRS complex. The P waves look alike. The PR interval is 0.20 second and constant from beat to beat. The QRS complex is 0.10 second, and the QT interval is 0.36 second. Because the P waves are upright and each P wave is associated with a QRS complex, we know that the underlying rhythm came from the SA node.

Now let's try to explain what caused the pause between beats 3 and 4. Look to the left of the pause and examine the waveforms of the beat that comes before the pause. Compare these waveforms with the others in the rhythm strip. There does not appear to be any distortion of the waveforms. With the use of your calipers or paper, plot P waves and R waves from left to right across the strip. When you do this, make a mark on the rhythm strip where the next PQRST cycles should have occurred. You will find that more than one PQRST cycle is missing. Because the SA node periodically failed to produce impulses, the P-P intervals are not exact multiples of other P-P intervals. This is characteristic of a sinus arrest. To complete our interpretation of this rhythm strip, we must add this explanation for the pause we saw; therefore, our final interpretation is a sinus rhythm at a rate of 60 beats/min with an episode of sinus arrest. Table 3.7 lists the ECG characteristics of sinus arrest.

What Causes It?

Causes of sinus arrest include damage to or disease of the SA node from CAD, acute MI, or rheumatic disease; carotid sinus pressure, a sudden increase in parasympathetic activity

TABLE 3.7	Characteristics of Sinus Arrest
Rhythm	Irregular; the pause is of undetermined length, more than one PQRST complex is missing, and it is not the same distance as other P-P intervals
Rate	Usually normal but varies because of the pause
P waves	Positive (upright) in lead II; P waves look alike; when present, one precedes each QRS complex
PR interval	0.12 to 0.20 sec and constant from beat to beat
QRS duration	0.11 sec or less unless abnormally conducted

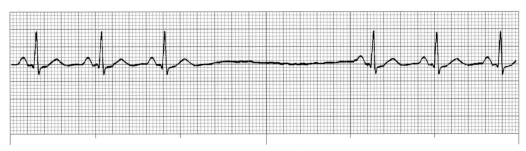

Fig. 3.7 Sinus rhythm at a rate of 60 beats/min with an episode of sinus arrest.

on the SA node, stimulation of the pharynx, obstructive sleep apnea, hypothermia, and reactions to medications such as beta-blockers and calcium channel blockers.

What Do I Do About It?

Signs and symptoms associated with sinus arrest depend on the number of absent sinus beats and the length of the sinus arrest because there is no cardiac output during the period of arrest. Signs of hemodynamic compromise such as weakness, lightheadedness, dizziness, or syncope may be associated with this dysrhythmia. If the episodes of sinus arrest are transient and there are no significant signs or symptoms, observe the patient. If signs and symptoms are a result of carotid sinus sensitivity and resultant vagal stimulation, remove tight clothing, if applicable. If hemodynamic compromise is present, IV atropine, temporary pacing, or both may be indicated. If the episodes of sinus arrest are frequent and prolonged (i.e., more than 3 seconds) or a result of disease of the SA node, insertion of a permanent pacemaker is generally warranted.

A summary of the characteristics of sinus mechanisms can be found in Table 3.8.

TABLE 3.8 **Sinus Mechanisms: Summary of Characteristics**

Characteristic	Sinus Rhythm	Sinus Bradycardia	Sinus Tachycardia	Sinus Arrhythmia	Sinoatrial Block	Sinus Arrest
Rhythm	Regular	Regular	Regular	Irregular, typically phasic with breathing	Regular except for the event; pause is the same (or an exact multiple of) as the distance between two P-P intervals of underlying rhythm	Regular except for the event; pause of undetermined length; not a multiple of other P-P intervals
Rate (beats/min)	60 to 100	Less than 60	Usually between 101 and 180; alternatively, the upper ventricular rate limit may be calculated as 220 beats/min minus the patient's age in years	Usually 60 to 100	Varies	Varies
P waves (lead II)	Positive; one precedes each QRS	Positive; one precedes each QRS	Positive; one precedes each QRS	Positive; one precedes each QRS	When present, positive; one precedes each QRS	When present, positive; one precedes each QRS
PR interval	0.12 to 0.20 sec	0.12 to 0.20 sec	0.12 to 0.20 sec	0.12 to 0.20 sec	When present, 0.12 to 0.20 sec	When present, 0.12 to 0.20 sec
QRS duration	0.11 sec or less unless abnormally conducted	0.11 sec or less unless abnormally conducted	0.11 sec or less unless abnormally conducted	0.11 sec or less unless abnormally conducted	0.11 sec or less unless abnormally conducted	0.11 sec or less unless abnormally conducted

STOP & REVIEW

Multiple Choice

Identify the choice that best completes the statement or answers the question.

_____ 1. A lead II rhythm strip obtained from a 38-year-old woman with difficulty breathing reveals a regular atrial and ventricular rhythm, a ventricular rate of 120 beats/min, an upright P wave before each QRS complex, and a normal PR interval and QRS duration. This rhythm is
   a. sinus rhythm.
   b. SA block.
   c. sinus arrhythmia.
   d. sinus tachycardia.

_____ 2. Which of the following rhythms originates in the SA node and is commonly phasic with breathing?
   a. Sinus arrest
   b. Sinus arrhythmia
   c. Sinus tachycardia
   d. Sinus bradycardia

_____ 3. Sinus arrest is a disorder of
   a. reentry.
   b. conductivity.
   c. impulse formation.
   d. impulse conduction.

_____ 4. SA block is a disorder of
   a. reentry.
   b. contractility.
   c. impulse formation.
   d. impulse conduction.

Questions 5 through 11 pertain to the following scenario.
A 75-year-old man presents with weakness and "feeling lightheaded." His symptoms began about 30 minutes ago.

_____ 5. The patient's blood pressure is 75/40 mm Hg, pulse is 44 beats/min, and ventilations are 16 breaths/min. A bradycardia is present when the heart rate is less than
   a. 60 beats/min.
   b. 75 beats/min.
   c. 85 beats/min.
   d. 100 beats/min.

_____ 6. You prepare to apply electrodes and lead wires to the patient for continuous ECG monitoring in lead II. Lead II views the
   a. lateral surface of the left ventricle.
   b. inferior surface of the left ventricle.
   c. anterior surface of the left ventricle.
   d. posterior surface of the right ventricle.

_____ 7. You are examining the waveforms on this patient's ECG. What is the name given to the first negative deflection observed after the P wave?
   a. Q wave
   b. R wave
   c. S wave
   d. T wave

_____ 8. As you measure the intervals on this patient's rhythm strip, you recall that the normal duration of the PR interval is _____ second.
   a. 0.04 to 0.10
   b. 0.06 to 0.14
   c. 0.12 to 0.20
   d. 0.16 to 0.24

_____ 9. Analysis of the patient's ECG reveals ST-segment depression in lead II. Although this ECG finding must be noted in additional leads viewing the same area of the heart to be considered clinically significant, the presence of ST-segment depression suggests
   a. myocardial injury.
   b. myocardial ischemia.
   c. death of a portion of the left ventricular tissue.
   d. death of a portion of the cardiac conduction system.

_____ 10. You interpret the patient's cardiac rhythm to be a sinus bradycardia. A coworker applied a pulse oximeter, which revealed an oxygen saturation level of 89% on room air. Supplemental oxygen is now being administered. The patient reports that he continues to feel weak and lightheaded. A second set of vital signs have been obtained and are essentially unchanged. Which of the following statements is true with regard to this patient situation?
   a. The patient is asymptomatic. No treatment is necessary.
   b. The patient is showing signs of hemodynamic compromise. An IV line should be established and a 12-lead ECG obtained.
   c. The patient's complaints of weakness and lightheadedness warrant an IV line start but no further interventions.
   d. The patient is not complaining of chest pain or discomfort; therefore, no additional interventions are necessary at this time.

_____ 11. The patient's symptoms persist, and his vital signs are essentially unchanged. The cardiac monitor shows a sinus bradycardia with ST-segment depression. You should prepare to administer
   a. atropine.
   b. atenolol.
   c. adenosine.
   d. amiodarone.

Matching

Match the terms below with their descriptions by placing the letter of each correct answer in the space provided.

a. Inferior MI, prolonged standing
b. AV junction
c. Symptomatic bradycardia
d. Sinus tachycardia
e. Palpitations, racing heart
f. SA block

g. Exercise, fever, pain, dehydration
h. Sinus arrhythmia
i. Smooth, rounded, upright
j. Sinus arrest
k. Atropine
l. Damage or disease to the SA node from acute MI

_____ **12.** Possible causes of sinus tachycardia
_____ **13.** Appearance of P waves that originate from the SA node
_____ **14.** Dysrhythmia with a pause that is the same as (or an exact multiple of) the distance between two other P-P intervals
_____ **15.** If the SA node fails to generate an impulse, the next (escape) pacemaker that should generate an impulse.
_____ **16.** Common dysrhythmia associated with changes in intrathoracic pressure
_____ **17.** Possible causes of SA block
_____ **18.** Dysrhythmia with a pause of undetermined length that is not the same distance as other P-P intervals
_____ **19.** Examples of symptoms that may be associated with a sinus tachycardia
_____ **20.** Vagolytic medication used to increase heart rate
_____ **21.** Signs and symptoms of hemodynamic compromise related to a slow heart rate
_____ **22.** Possible causes of sinus bradycardia
_____ **23.** Dysrhythmia that originates from the SA node and has a ventricular rate faster than 100 beats/min

Short Answer

24. Fill in the blank areas in the table below to help you recall the primary differences among sinus bradycardia, sinus tachycardia, and sinus arrhythmia.

ECG Finding	Sinus Bradycardia	Sinus Tachycardia	Sinus Arrhythmia
Rhythm	_____	_____	_____
Rate (beats/min)	_____		
P waves (lead II)	Positive; one precedes each QRS	Positive; one precedes each QRS	Positive; one precedes each QRS
PR interval	0.12 to 0.20 sec	0.12 to 0.20 sec	0.12 to 0.20 sec
QRS duration	0.11 sec or less unless abnormally conducted	0.11 sec or less unless abnormally conducted	0.11 sec or less unless abnormally conducted

25. Fill in the blank areas in the table below to help you recall the differences among sinus rhythm, SA block, and sinus arrest.

ECG Finding	Sinus Rhythm	Sinoatrial Block	Sinus Arrest
Rhythm	_____	_____	_____
Rate (beats/min)	_____		
P waves (lead II)	Positive; one precedes each QRS	When present, positive; one precedes each QRS	When present, positive; one precedes each QRS
PR interval	0.12 to 0.20 sec	When present, 0.12 to 0.20 sec	When present, 0.12 to 0.20 sec
QRS duration	0.11 sec or less unless abnormally conducted	0.11 sec or less unless abnormally conducted	0.11 sec or less unless abnormally conducted

Sinus Mechanisms—Practice Rhythm Strips

Use the five steps of rhythm interpretation discussed in Chapter 2 to interpret each of the following rhythm strips. All rhythms were recorded in lead II unless otherwise noted.

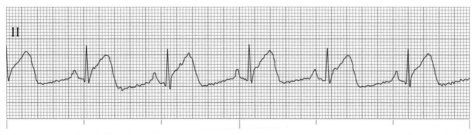

Fig. 3.8

26. **Fig. 3.8**

Rhythm: _____ Rate: _____ P waves: _____

PR interval: _____ QRS duration: _____ QT interval: _____

Interpretation: _____

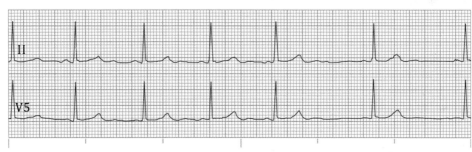

Fig. 3.9

27. **Fig. 3.9**

Rhythm: _____ Rate: _____ P waves: _____

PR interval: _____ QRS duration: _____ QT interval: _____

Interpretation: _____

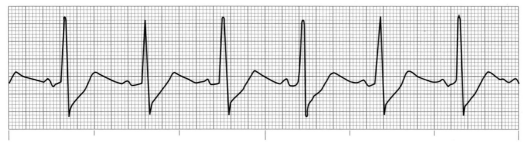

Fig. 3.10 (From Aehlert B: *ECG study cards,* St. Louis, 2004, Mosby.)

28. **Fig. 3.10**. This rhythm strip is from a 61-year-old woman with an altered level of responsiveness. Her blood pressure is 112/62 mm Hg, and her blood sugar is 42 mg/dL.

Rhythm: _____ Rate: _____ P waves: _____

PR interval: _____ QRS duration: _____ QT interval: _____

Interpretation: _____

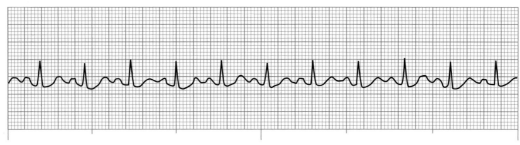

Fig. 3.11 (From Aehlert B: *ECG study cards,* St. Louis, 2004, Mosby.)

29. **Fig. 3.11**. This rhythm strip is from a 90-year-old woman with difficulty breathing.

Rhythm: _____ Rate: _____ P waves: _____

PR interval: _____ QRS duration: _____ QT interval: _____

Interpretation: _____

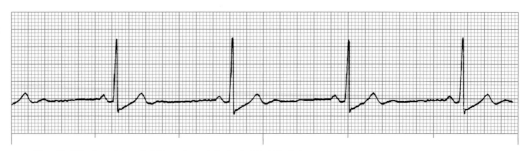

Fig. 3.12 (From Aehlert B: *ECG study cards,* St. Louis, 2004, Mosby.)

30. **Fig. 3.12**. This rhythm strip is from a 73-year-old man complaining of chest pain. He has a history of hypertension and lung disease. Medications include aspirin, albuterol, and Lotensin.

Rhythm: _____ Rate: _____ P waves: _____

PR interval: _____ QRS duration: _____ QT interval: _____

Interpretation: _____

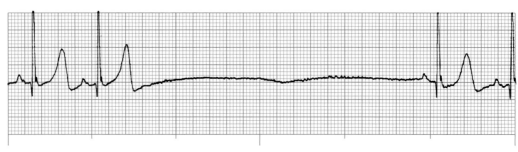

Fig. 3.13

31. **Fig. 3.13**

Rhythm: _____ Rate: _____ P waves: _____

PR interval: _____ QRS duration: _____ QT interval: _____

Interpretation: _____

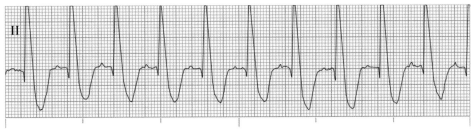

Fig. 3.14

32. **Fig. 3.14**. This rhythm strip is from a 57-year-old man with chest pain.

Rhythm: _____ Rate: _____ P waves: _____

PR interval: _____ QRS duration: _____ QT interval: _____

Interpretation: _____

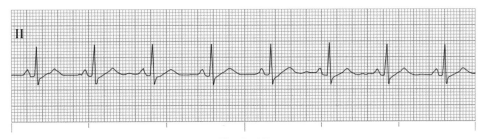

Fig. 3.15

33. **Fig. 3.15**.

Rhythm: _____ Rate: _____ P waves: _____

PR interval: _____ QRS duration: _____ QT interval: _____

Interpretation: _____

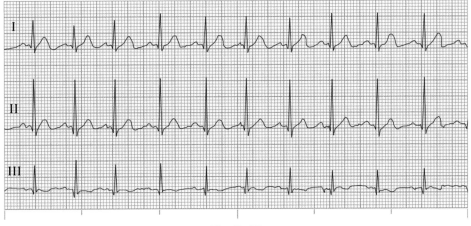

Fig. 3.16

34. **Fig. 3.16**. This rhythm strip is from a 4-month-old infant who reportedly ingested an oral pain reliever.

Rhythm: _____ Rate: _____ P waves: _____

PR interval: _____ QRS duration: _____ QT interval: _____

Interpretation: _____

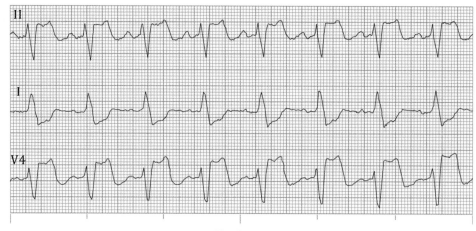

Fig. 3.17

35. **Fig. 3.17**

 Rhythm: _____ Rate: _____ P waves: _____

 PR interval: _____ QRS duration: _____ QT interval: _____

 Interpretation: _____

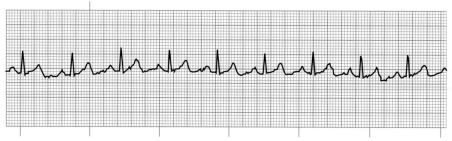

Fig. 3.18

36. **Fig. 3.18**. This rhythm strip is from a 40-year-old man complaining of back pain after jumping from a burning second floor balcony.

 Rhythm: _____ Rate: _____ P waves: _____

 PR interval: _____ QRS duration: _____ QT interval: _____

 Interpretation: _____

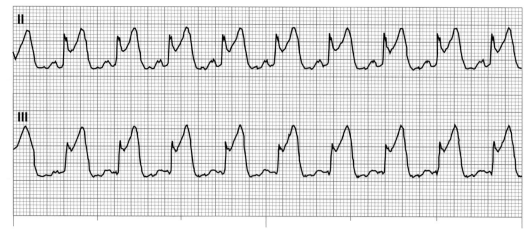

Fig. 3.19 (From Aehlert B: *ECG study cards,* St. Louis, 2004, Mosby.)

37. **Fig. 3.19**. These rhythm strips are from a 44-year-old woman with chest pain.

 Rhythm: _____ Rate: _____ P waves: _____

 PR interval: _____ QRS duration: _____ QT interval: _____

 Interpretation: _____

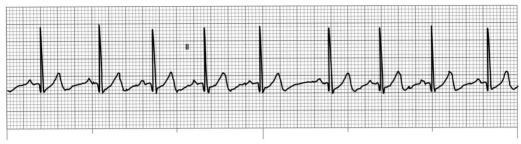

Fig. 3.20 (From Aehlert B: *ECG study cards,* St. Louis, 2004, Mosby.)

38. **Fig. 3.20.** This rhythm strip is from a 6-year-old girl complaining of abdominal pain. Her blood pressure is 100/60 mm Hg.

Rhythm: _____ Rate: _____ P waves: _____

PR interval: _____ QRS duration: _____ QT interval: _____

Interpretation: _____

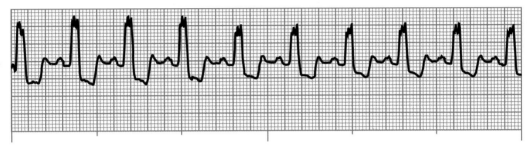

Fig. 3.21 (From Aehlert B: *ECG study cards,* St. Louis, 2004, Mosby.)

39. **Fig. 3.21**

Rhythm: _____ Rate: _____ P waves: _____

PR interval: _____ QRS duration: _____ QT interval: _____

Interpretation: _____

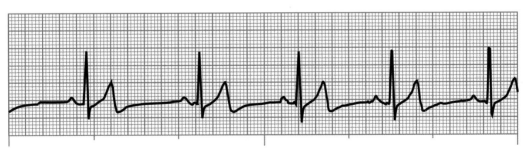

Fig. 3.22 (From Aehlert B: *ECG study cards,* St. Louis, 2004, Mosby.)

40. **Fig. 3.22.** This rhythm strip is from a 24-year-old woman complaining of weakness and fatigue.

Rhythm: _____ Rate: _____ P waves: _____

PR interval: _____ QRS duration: _____ QT interval: _____

Interpretation: _____

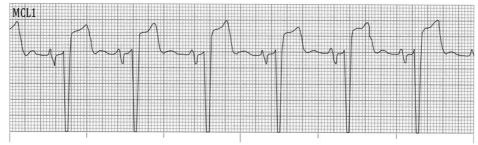

Fig. 3.23

41. **Fig. 3.23**

    Rhythm: _____ Rate: _____ P waves: _____

    PR interval: _____ QRS duration: _____ QT interval: _____

    Interpretation: _____

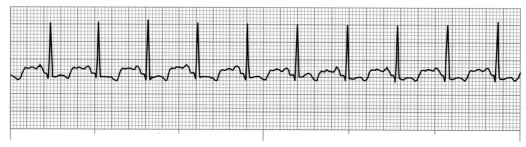

Fig. 3.24 (From Aehlert B: *ECG study cards,* St. Louis, 2004, Mosby.)

42. **Fig. 3.24**. This rhythm strip is from a 29-year-old woman with a kidney stone.

    Rhythm: _____ Rate: _____ P waves: _____

    PR interval: _____ QRS duration: _____ QT interval: _____

    Interpretation: _____

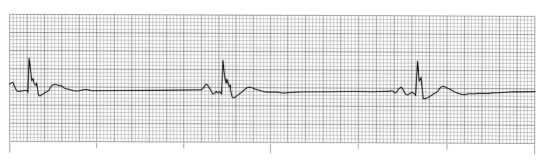

Fig. 3.25 (From Aehlert B: *ECG study cards,* St. Louis, 2004, Mosby.)

43. **Fig. 3.25**

    Rhythm: _____ Rate: _____ P waves: _____

    PR interval: _____ QRS duration: _____ QT interval: _____

    Interpretation: _____

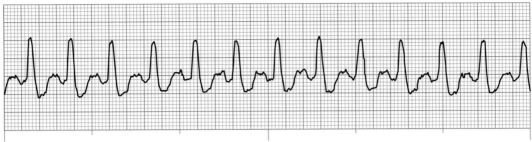

Fig. 3.26 (From Aehlert B: *ECG study cards,* St. Louis, 2004, Mosby.)

44. **Fig. 3.26.** This rhythm strip is from a 79-year-old woman with epistaxis. Her blood pressure is 222/118 mm Hg.

Rhythm: _____ Rate: _____ P waves: _____

PR interval: _____ QRS duration: _____ QT interval: _____

Interpretation: _____

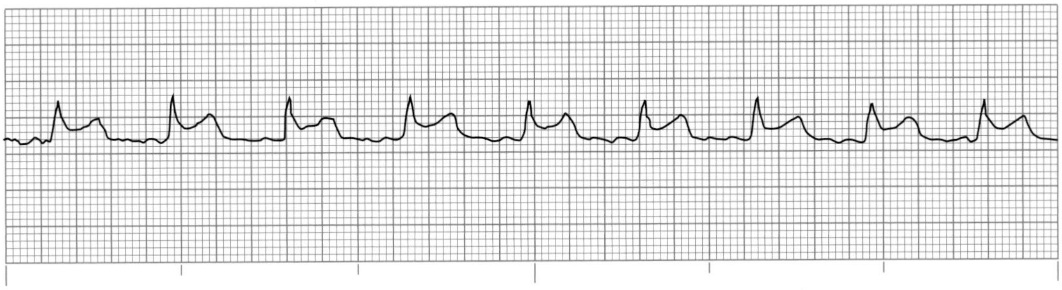

Fig. 3.27 (From Aehlert B: *ECG study cards,* St. Louis, 2004, Mosby.)

45. **Fig. 3.27.** This rhythm strip is from a 62-year-old man complaining of chest pain.

Rhythm: _____ Rate: _____ P waves: _____

PR interval: _____ QRS duration: _____ QT interval: _____

Interpretation: _____

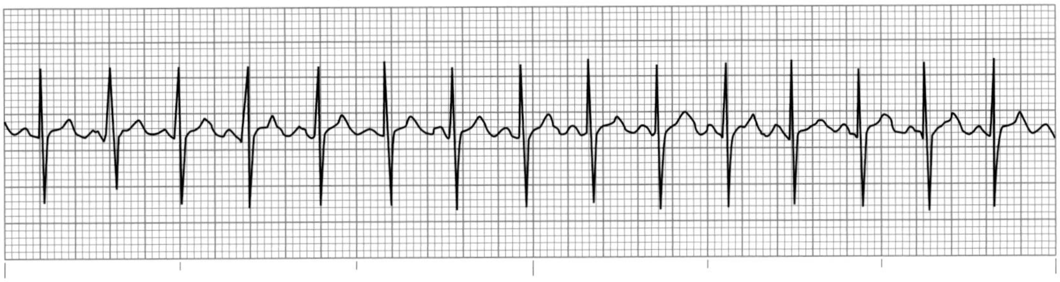

Fig. 3.28 (From Aehlert B: *ECG study cards,* St. Louis, 2004, Mosby.)

46. **Fig. 3.28.** This rhythm strip is from an 8-month-old infant after a seizure.

Rhythm: _____ Rate: _____ P waves: _____

PR interval: _____ QRS duration: _____ QT interval: _____

Interpretation: _____

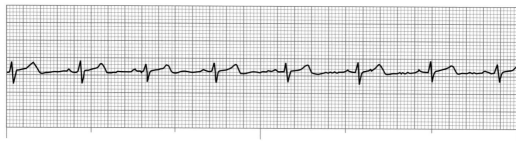

Fig. 3.29 (From Aehlert B: *ECG study cards,* St. Louis, 2004, Mosby.)

47. **Fig. 3.29**. This rhythm strip is from a 33-year-old woman complaining of abdominal pain.

Rhythm: _____ Rate: _____ P waves: _____

PR interval: _____ QRS duration: _____ QT interval: _____

Interpretation: _____

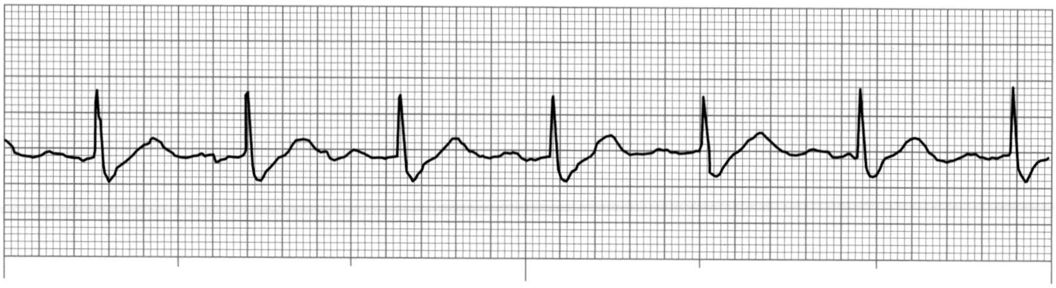

Fig. 3.30

48. **Fig. 3.30**

Rhythm: _____ Rate: _____ P waves: _____

PR interval: _____ QRS duration: _____ QT interval: _____

Interpretation: _____

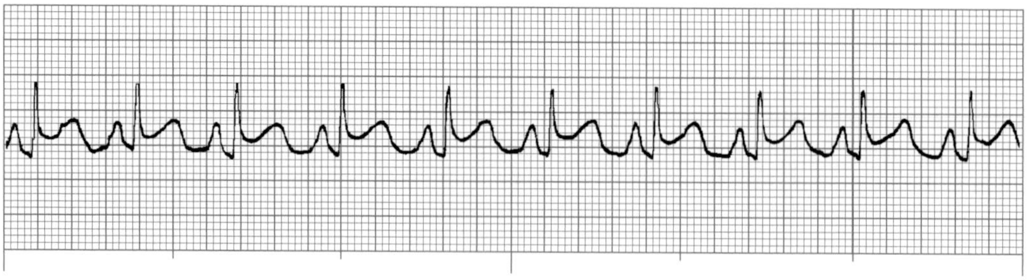

Fig. 3.31

49. **Fig. 3.31**

Rhythm: _____ Rate: _____ P waves: _____

PR interval: _____ QRS duration: _____ QT interval: _____

Interpretation: _____

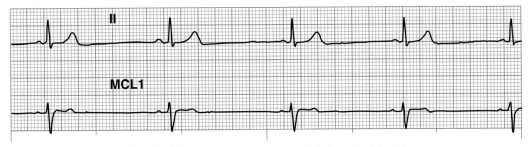

Fig. 3.32 (From Aehlert B: *ECG study cards,* St. Louis, 2004, Mosby.)

50. **Fig. 3.32.** This rhythm strip is from a 37-year-old asymptomatic man.

Rhythm: _____ Rate: _____ P waves: _____

PR interval: _____ QRS duration: _____ QT interval: _____

Interpretation: _____

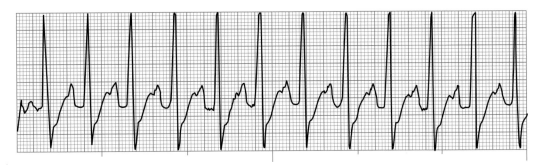

Fig. 3.33 (From Aehlert B: *ECG study cards,* St. Louis, 2004, Mosby.)

51. **Fig. 3.33**

Rhythm: _____ Rate: _____ P waves: _____

PR interval: _____ QRS duration: _____ QT interval: _____

Interpretation: _____

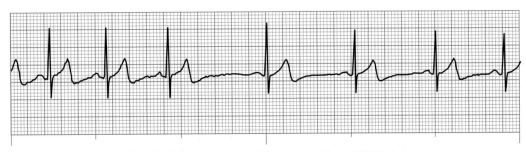

Fig. 3.34 (From Aehlert B: *ECG study cards,* St. Louis, 2004, Mosby.)

52. **Fig. 3.34.** This rhythm strip is from a 44-year-old construction worker with a sudden onset of chest pressure.

Rhythm: _____ Rate: _____ P waves: _____

PR interval: _____ QRS duration: _____ QT interval: _____

Interpretation: _____

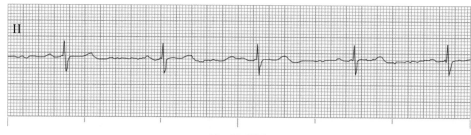

Fig. 3.35

53. **Fig. 3.35**

Rhythm: _____ Rate: _____ P waves: _____

PR interval: _____ QRS duration: _____ QT interval: _____

Interpretation: _____

1. D. A sinus tachycardia is differentiated from other rhythms that originate in the SA node by its rate (faster than 100 beats/min).
OBJ: Describe the ECG characteristics, possible causes, signs and symptoms, and emergency management of sinus tachycardia.

2. B. Respiratory sinus arrhythmia, which is the most common type of sinus arrhythmia, is a normal phenomenon that occurs with phases of breathing and changes in intrathoracic pressure. The heart rate increases with inspiration (i.e., the R-R intervals shorten) and decreases with expiration (i.e., the R-R intervals lengthen). Sinus arrhythmia is most commonly observed in children and young adults.
OBJ: Describe the ECG characteristics, possible causes, signs and symptoms, and emergency management of sinus arrhythmia.

3. C. Sinus arrest is a disorder of impulse formation. In sinus arrest, the pacemaker cells of the SA node fail to initiate an electrical impulse for one or more beats resulting in absent PQRST complexes on the ECG.
OBJ: Describe the ECG characteristics, possible causes, signs and symptoms, and emergency management of sinus arrest.

4. D. With SA block, the pacemaker cells within the SA node initiate an impulse but it is blocked as it exits the SA node. Thus, SA block is a disorder of impulse conduction. Blocking of the sinus impulses results in periodically absent PQRST complexes.
OBJ: Describe the ECG characteristics, possible causes, signs and symptoms, and emergency management of sinoatrial block.

5. A. In adults, a bradycardia exists if the rate is less than 60 beats/min (*brady* = slow).
OBJ: Describe the ECG characteristics, possible causes, signs and symptoms, and emergency management of sinus bradycardia.

6. B. Lead II views the inferior surface of the left ventricle.
OBJ: Relate the cardiac surfaces or areas represented by the ECG leads.

7. A. A QRS complex normally follows each P wave. The QRS complex begins as a downward deflection, the *Q wave*, and represents depolarization of the interventricular septum.
OBJ: Define and describe the significance of each of the following as they relate to cardiac electrical activity: P wave, QRS complex, T wave, U wave, PR segment, TP segment, ST segment, PR interval, QRS duration, and QT interval.

8. C. The PR interval changes with heart rate but normally measures 0.12 to 0.20 second in adults. As the heart rate increases, the duration of the PR interval shortens. A PR interval is considered *short* if it is less than 0.12 second and *long* if it is more than 0.20 second.
OBJ: Define and describe the significance of each of the following as they relate to cardiac electrical activity: P wave, QRS complex, T wave, U wave, PR segment, TP segment, ST segment, PR interval, QRS duration, and QT interval.

9. B. ST-segment depression of 0.5 mm or more in a patient who is experiencing an acute coronary syndrome is suggestive of myocardial ischemia when it is seen in two or more anatomically contiguous leads.
OBJ: Recognize the changes on the ECG that may reflect evidence of myocardial ischemia and injury.

10. B. The term *symptomatic bradycardia* describes signs and symptoms of hemodynamic compromise related to a slow heart rate. Because this patient is complaining of weakness and lightheadedness and he is hypotensive, he is clearly symptomatic with his slow heart rate. Treatment of a symptomatic bradycardia should include application of a pulse oximeter and administration of supplemental oxygen if indicated, which have already been done. Next, establish IV access and obtain a 12-lead ECG.
OBJ: Describe the ECG characteristics, possible causes, signs and symptoms, and emergency management of sinus bradycardia.

11. A. Atropine, administered intravenously, is the drug of choice for symptomatic bradycardia. Reassess the patient's response to the therapeutic interventions provided and continue monitoring the patient. Adenosine is used to slow the ventricular rate. Atenolol, a beta-blocker, would further slow the heart rate. Although amiodarone is an antiarrhythmic used to treat many atrial and ventricular dysrhythmias, it is not used to treat a sinus bradycardia.
OBJ: Describe the ECG characteristics, possible causes, signs and symptoms, and emergency management of sinus bradycardia.

12. G
13. I
14. F
15. B
16. H
17. L
18. J
19. E
20. K
21. C
22. A
23. D

24. ANS:

ECG Finding	Sinus Bradycardia	Sinus Tachycardia	Sinus Arrhythmia
Rhythm	Regular	Regular	Irregular, typically phasic with breathing
Rate (beats/min)	Slower than 60	101 to 180; alternatively, the upper ventricular rate limit may be calculated as 220 beats/min minus the patient's age in years	Usually 60 to 100
P waves (lead II)	Positive; one precedes each QRS	Positive; one precedes each QRS	Positive; one precedes each QRS
PR interval	0.12 to 0.20 sec	0.12 to 0.20 sec	0.12 to 0.20 sec
QRS duration	0.11 sec or less unless abnormally conducted	0.11 sec or less unless abnormally conducted	0.11 sec or less unless abnormally conducted

OBJ: Describe the ECG characteristics, possible causes, signs and symptoms, and emergency management of sinus bradycardia, sinus tachycardia, and sinus arrhythmia.

25. ANS:

ECG Finding	Sinus Rhythm	Sinoatrial Block	Sinus Arrest
Rhythm	Regular	Regular except for the event; pause is the same (or an exact multiple of) as the distance between two P-P intervals of underlying rhythm	Regular except for the event; pause of undetermined length; not a multiple of other P-P intervals
Rate (beats/min)	60 to 100	Varies	Varies
P waves (lead II)	Positive; one precedes each QRS	When present, positive; one precedes each QRS	When present, positive; one precedes each QRS
PR interval	0.12 to 0.20 sec	When present, 0.12 to 0.20 sec	When present, 0.12 to 0.20 sec
QRS duration	0.11 sec or less unless abnormally conducted	0.11 sec or less unless abnormally conducted	0.11 sec or less unless abnormally conducted

OBJ: Describe the ECG characteristics, possible causes, signs and symptoms, and emergency management of sinoatrial block and sinus arrest.

Practice Rhythm Strip Answers

Note: Because of the distortion of ECGs that can occur during printing, a range of acceptable measurements is provided in the rhythm strip answers throughout this textbook.

26. Fig. 3.8
Rhythm: Regular
Rate: 58 beats/min
P waves: Uniform and upright before each QRS complex
PR interval: 0.16 second
QRS duration: 0.08 second
QT interval: 0.40 to 0.44 second
Interpretation: Sinus bradycardia at 58 beats/min

27. Fig. 3.9
Rhythm: Irregular
Rate: 70 beats/min
P waves: Uniform and upright before each QRS complex
PR interval: 0.12 to 0.16 second
QRS duration: 0.04 to 0.06 second
QT interval: 0.36 second
Interpretation: Sinus arrhythmia at 70 beats/min

28. Fig. 3.10
Rhythm: Regular
Rate: 65 beats/min
P waves: Uniform and upright before each QRS complex
PR interval: 0.20 second
QRS duration: 0.10 to 0.12 second
QT interval: 0.60 to 0.64 second (prolonged)
Interpretation: Sinus rhythm at 65 beats/min with ST-segment depression; prolonged QT interval

29. Fig. 3.11
Rhythm: Regular
Rate: 111 beats/min
P waves: Uniform and upright before each QRS complex
PR interval: 0.16 second
QRS duration: 0.04 to 0.06 second
QT interval: 0.32 to 0.34 second
Interpretation: Sinus tachycardia at 111 beats/min with ST-segment depression

30. **Fig. 3.12**
Rhythm: Regular
Rate: 44 beats/min
P waves: Uniform and upright before each QRS complex
PR interval: 0.16 second
QRS duration: 0.06 second
QT interval: 0.40 second
Interpretation: Sinus bradycardia at 44 beats/min, ST-segment depression. Note the upright U waves after each T wave.

31. **Fig. 3.13**
Rhythm: Irregular
Rate: 75 beats/min
P waves: Uniform and upright before each QRS complex
PR interval: 0.16 second
QRS duration: 0.08 second
QT interval: 0.44 second
Interpretation: Sinus rhythm at 75 beats/min with an episode of sinus arrest; tall T waves

32. **Fig. 3.14**
Rhythm: Regular
Rate: 107 beats/min
P waves: Small but upright before each QRS
PR interval: 0.16 second
QRS duration: 0.16 second
QT interval: 0.32 to 0.40 second
Interpretation: Sinus tachycardia at 107 beats/min with a wide QRS and deeply inverted T waves

33. **Fig. 3.15**
Rhythm: Regular
Rate: 79 beats/min
P waves: Uniform and upright before each QRS complex
PR interval: 0.12 to 0.16 second
QRS duration: 0.06 to 0.08 second
QT interval: 0.32 second
Interpretation: Sinus rhythm at 79 beats/min, ST-segment depression

34. **Fig. 3.16**
Rhythm: Irregular
Rate: 100 beats/min (within normal limits for age)
P waves: Uniform and upright before each QRS
PR interval: 0.16 second
QRS duration: 0.08 second
QT interval: 0.28 second
Interpretation: Sinus arrhythmia at 100 beats/min

35. **Fig. 3.17**
Rhythm: Regular
Rate: 79 beats/min
P waves: Uniform and upright before each QRS
PR interval: 0.24 second

QRS duration: 0.12 to 0.14 second
QT interval: 0.36 second
Interpretation: Sinus rhythm at 79 beats/min with a prolonged PR interval, wide QRS, ST-segment elevation in leads II and V_4, and ST-segment depression in lead I

36. **Fig. 3.18**
Rhythm: Regular
Rate: 88 beats/min
P waves: Uniform and upright before each QRS
PR interval: 0.16 second
QRS duration: 0.06 second
QT interval: 0.32 second
Interpretation: Sinus rhythm at 88 beats/min

37. **Fig. 3.19**
Rhythm: Regular
Rate: 94 beats/min
P waves: Uniform and upright before each QRS
PR interval: 0.16 second
QRS duration: 0.08 second
QT interval: 0.28 second
Interpretation: Sinus rhythm at 94 beats/min with STE

38. **Fig. 3.20**
Rhythm: Irregular
Rate: 90 beats/min
P waves: Uniform and upright before each QRS
PR interval: 0.14 to 0.16 second
QRS duration: 0.08 second
QT interval: 0.32 second
Interpretation: Sinus arrhythmia at 90 beats/min

39. **Fig. 3.21**
Rhythm: Regular
Rate: 94 beats/min
P waves: Uniform and upright before each QRS
PR interval: 0.16 to 0.18 second
QRS duration: 0.12 second
QT interval: 0.36 to 0.40 second
Interpretation: Sinus rhythm at 94 beats/min with a wide QRS and ST-segment depression

40. **Fig. 3.22**
Rhythm: Irregular
Rate: 50 beats/min
P waves: Upright before each QRS
PR interval: 0.16 to 0.20 second
QRS duration: 0.08 second
QT interval: 0.40 second
Interpretation: Sinus bradyarrhythmia at 50 beats/min (the interpretation reflects that the rhythm is slow and irregular)

41. **Fig. 3.23**
Rhythm: Regular
Rate: 65 beats/min
P waves: Biphasic P waves before each QRS (a normal finding in leads MCL_1 and V_1)

PR interval: 0.20 second

QRS duration: 0.10 to 0.12 second

QT interval: 0.36 second

Interpretation: Sinus rhythm at 65 beats/min with biphasic P waves and STE

42. **Fig. 3.24**

Rhythm: Regular

Rate: 103 beats/min

P waves: Uniform and upright before each QRS

PR interval: 0.14 second

QRS duration: 0.08 second

QT interval: 0.28 to 0.32 second

Interpretation: Sinus tachycardia at 103 beats/min; inverted T waves

43. **Fig. 3.25**

Rhythm: Regular

Rate: 25 beats/min

P waves: Uniform and upright before each QRS

PR interval: 0.22 to 0.24 second

QRS duration: 0.10 to 0.12 second

QT interval: 0.40 second

Interpretation: Sinus bradycardia at 25 beats/min with a prolonged PR interval and ST-segment depression

44. **Fig. 3.26**

Rhythm: Regular

Rate: 125 beats/min

P waves: Upright before each QRS; some P waves are notched

PR interval: 0.16 second

QRS duration: 0.10 to 0.12 second

QT interval: Unable to determine because T waves are not clearly visible

Interpretation: Sinus tachycardia at 125 beats/min with a wide QRS and ST-segment depression

45. **Fig. 3.27**

Rhythm: Regular

Rate: 94 beats/min

P waves: Upright but low amplitude P waves before each QRS

PR interval: 0.12 to 0.14 second

QRS duration: 0.08 to 0.10 second

QT interval: 0.32 second

Interpretation: Sinus rhythm at 94 beats/min with STE

46. **Fig. 3.28**

Rhythm: Regular

Rate: 150 beats/min

P waves: Upright before each QRS

PR interval: 0.12 second

QRS duration: 0.06 to 0.08 second

QT interval: 0.20 to 0.24 second

Interpretation: Sinus rhythm at 150 beats/min (rate within normal limits for age)

47. **Fig. 3.29**

Rhythm: Slightly irregular

Rate: 80 beats/min

P waves: Uniform and upright before each QRS

PR interval: 0.12 to 0.14 second

QRS duration: 0.08 second

QT interval: 0.24 to 0.26 second

Interpretation: Sinus arrhythmia at 80 beats/min

48. **Fig. 3.30**

Rhythm: Regular

Rate: 68 beats/min

P waves: Uniform and upright before each QRS

PR interval: 0.28 to 0.32 second

QRS duration: 0.06 to 0.08 second

QT interval: 0.44 to 0.48 second

Interpretation: Sinus rhythm at 68 beats/min with a prolonged PR interval and ST-segment depression

49. **Fig. 3.31**

Rhythm: Regular

Rate: 97 beats/min

P waves: Uniform and upright before each QRS

PR interval: 0.16 second

QRS duration: 0.04 to 0.06 second

QT interval: 0.32 second

Interpretation: Sinus rhythm at 97 beats/min with STE

50. **Fig. 3.32**

Rhythm: Irregular

Rate: 50 beats/min

P waves: Uniform and upright before each QRS

PR interval: 0.12 to 0.16 second

QRS duration: 0.08 second

QT interval: 0.36 to 0.40 second

Interpretation: Sinus bradyarrhythmia at 50 beats/min

51. **Fig. 3.33**

Rhythm: Regular

Rate: 115 beats/min

P waves: Upright before each QRS

PR interval: 0.20 second

QRS duration: 0.10 to 0.12 second

QT interval: Unable to determine because T waves are not clearly visible

Interpretation: Sinus tachycardia at 115 beats/min with ST-segment depression

52. **Fig. 3.34**

Rhythm: Irregular

Rate: 70 beats/min

P waves: Upright before each QRS

PR interval: 0.12 to 0.16 second

QRS duration: 0.06 to 0.08 second

QT interval: 0.28 to 0.32 second

Interpretation: Sinus arrhythmia at 70 beats/min with STE

53. **Fig. 3.35**
Rhythm: Irregular
Rate: 50 beats/min
P waves: Uniform and upright before each QRS
PR interval: 0.20 to 0.22 second
QRS duration: 0.08 second
QT interval: 0.40 to 0.44 second
Interpretation: Sinus bradyarrhythmia at 50 beats/min with a prolonged PR interval

REFERENCES

Link, M. S., Berkow, L. C., Kudenchuk, P. J., Halperin, H. R., Hess, E. P., Moitra, V. K., Donnino, M. W. (2015, Oct). 2015 *American Heart Association Guidelines for CPR & ECC. Retrieved Oct 30, 2015, from American Heart Association.* Web-based Integrated Guidelines for Cardiopulmonary Resuscitation and Emergency Cardiovascular Care – Part 7: Adult Advanced Cardiovascular Life Support: Eccguidelines.heart.org

O'Gara, P. T., Kushner, F. G., Ascheim, D. D., Casey, D. E., Jr., Chung, M. K., de Lemos, J. A., & Zhao, D. X. (2013). 2013 ACCF/AHA guideline for the management of ST-elevation myocardial infarction. *J Am Coll Cardiol, 61*(4), e78–e140.

Atrial Rhythms

4

LEARNING OBJECTIVES

After reading this chapter, you should be able to:

1. Explain the concepts of abnormal automaticity, triggered activity, and reentry.
2. Explain the terms *bigeminy*, *trigeminy*, *quadrigeminy*, and *run* when used to describe premature complexes.
3. Describe the electrocardiogram (ECG) characteristics, possible causes, signs and symptoms, and initial emergency care for premature atrial complexes (PACs).
4. Explain the difference between a compensatory and noncompensatory pause.
5. Explain the terms *wandering atrial pacemaker* and *multifocal atrial tachycardia (MAT)*.
6. Describe the ECG characteristics, possible causes, signs and symptoms, and initial emergency care for wandering atrial pacemaker (multiform atrial rhythm).
7. Describe the ECG characteristics, possible causes, signs and symptoms, and initial emergency care for MAT.
8. Describe the ECG characteristics, possible causes, signs and symptoms, and initial emergency care for atrial tachycardia (AT).
9. Explain the terms *paroxysmal atrial tachycardia* and *paroxysmal supra-ventricular tachycardia* (PSVT).
10. List examples of vagal maneuvers.
11. Discuss the indications for synchronized cardioversion.
12. Describe the ECG characteristics, possible causes, signs and symptoms, and initial emergency care for atrioventricular nodal reentrant tachycardia (AVNRT).
13. Describe the ECG characteristics, possible causes, signs and symptoms, and initial emergency care for atrioventricular reentrant tachycardia (AVRT).
14. Describe the ECG characteristics, possible causes, signs and symptoms, and initial emergency care for atrial flutter.
15. Describe the ECG characteristics, possible causes, signs and symptoms, and initial emergency care for atrial fibrillation (AFib).

KEY TERMS

abnormal automaticity: A condition in which cardiac cells not normally associated with the property of automaticity begin to depolarize spontaneously or when escape pacemaker sites increase their firing rate beyond that considered normal

accessory pathway: An extra bundle of working myocardial tissue that forms a connection between the atria and ventricles outside the normal conduction system; also called a *bypass tract*

atrial kick: Blood pushed into the ventricles because of atrial contraction

atrial tachycardia (AT): A regular rhythm that arises from an ectopic focus in the atria at a rate faster than 100 beats/min and does not require the participation of the atrioventricular (AV) node to maintain the dysrhythmia

bigeminy: Dysrhythmia in which every other beat is a premature ectopic beat

blocked (nonconducted) PAC: PAC not followed by a QRS complex

bruit: Blowing or swishing sound

bursts: Three or more sequential ectopic beats; also referred to as a "salvo" or "run"

carotid sinus pressure: Type of vagal maneuver in which pressure is applied to the carotid sinus for a brief period to slow conduction through the AV node

compensatory pause: Pause for which the normal beat after a premature complex occurs when expected; also called a *complete pause*

couplet: Two consecutive premature complexes

delta wave: Slurring of the beginning portion of the QRS complex, caused by preexcitation

f waves: Fibrillatory waves; irregularly shaped atrial waves associated with AFib; occurring at a rate of 300 to 600 beats/min

F waves: Flutter waves; atrial waves associated with atrial flutter; usually shaped like the teeth of a saw or a picket fence

focal atrial tachycardia: AT that begins in a small area (focus) within the atria

multiform atrial rhythm: Dysrhythmia that occurs because of impulses originating from various sites, including the sinoatrial (SA) node, the atria, and/or the AV junction; requires at least three different P waves, seen in the same lead, for proper diagnosis

multifocal atrial tachycardia (MAT): An irregular rhythm at a rate faster than 100 beats/min with three or more P waves of differing shapes observed in the same lead

noncompensatory pause: A pause that often follows a PAC that represents the delay during which the SA node resets its rhythm for the next beat; the pause is noncompensatory if the normal beat after the premature complex occurs before it was expected (i.e., the period between the complex before and after the premature beat is less than two normal R-R intervals)

nonconducted (blocked) PAC: PAC that is not followed by a QRS complex

palpitations: An unpleasant awareness of one's heartbeat

paroxysmal atrial tachycardia: AT that starts or ends suddenly

paroxysmal supraventricular tachycardia (PSVT): A regular, narrow-QRS tachycardia that starts or ends suddenly; also called *paroxysmal atrial tachycardia*

preexcitation: Term used to describe a rhythm that originates above the ventricles and transmits an impulse along a pathway outside the AV node and bundle of His; this supraventricular impulse excites the ventricles earlier than normal.

premature complex: Early beat occurring before the next expected beat; can be atrial, junctional, or ventricular

quadrigeminy: Dysrhythmia in which every fourth beat is a premature ectopic beat

reentry: A disorder of impulse conduction that results from the spread of an impulse through tissue already stimulated by that same impulse

supraventricular: Originating from a site above the bifurcation of the bundle of His, such as the SA node, atria, or AV junction

synchronized cardioversion: The timed delivery of a shock to the heart by means of a defibrillator to terminate a rapid dysrhythmia

trigeminy: Dysrhythmia in which every third beat is a premature ectopic beat

triggered activity: A disorder of impulse formation that occurs when escape pacemaker and myocardial working cells fire more than once after stimulation by a single impulse

vagal maneuvers: Methods used to stimulate the vagus nerve in an attempt to slow conduction through the AV node, thereby slowing the heart rate

wandering atrial pacemaker (multiform atrial rhythm): Cardiac dysrhythmia that occurs because of impulses originating from various sites, including the SA node, the atria, and/or the AV junction; requires at least three different P waves, seen in the same lead, for proper diagnosis.

Wolff-Parkinson-White (WPW) pattern: Type of preexcitation pattern, characterized by a short PR interval, a slurred upstroke of the QRS complex (delta wave), and a wide QRS complex

INTRODUCTION

The atria are thin-walled, low-pressure chambers that receive blood from the systemic circulation and lungs. There is normally a continuous flow of blood from the superior and inferior vena cavae into the atria. About 70% of this blood flows directly through the atria and into the ventricles before the atria contract. When the atria contract, an additional 30% is added to filling of the ventricles. This additional contribution of blood because of atrial contraction is called **atrial kick**.

P waves reflect atrial depolarization. A rhythm that begins in the sinoatrial (SA) node has one positive (i.e., upright) P wave before each QRS complex. A rhythm that begins in the atria will have a positive P wave that is shaped differently than P waves that begin in the SA node. This difference in P wave configuration occurs because the impulse begins in the atria and follows a different conduction pathway to the atrioventricular (AV) node.

ATRIAL DYSRHYTHMIAS: MECHANISMS

[Objective 1]

Atrial dysrhythmias reflect abnormal electrical impulse formation and conduction in the atria. They result from abnormal automaticity, triggered activity, or reentry. Abnormal automaticity and triggered activity are disorders in impulse *formation*. Reentry is a disorder in impulse *conduction*. Dysrhythmias caused by disorders of impulse formation are often referred to as *automatic*. Dysrhythmias caused by a disorder in impulse conduction are referred to as *reentrant*.

Abnormal Automaticity

Abnormal automaticity occurs in normal pacemaker cells and in myocardial working cells that do not normally function as pacemaker sites. With abnormal automaticity, these cells fire and initiate impulses before a normal SA node impulse. If the rapid firing rate occurs for more than 50% of the day, it is said to be *incessant*. The rapid firing rate may also occur periodically. In these cases, it is said to be *episodic*. Atrial dysrhythmias associated with abnormal automaticity include PACs, multifocal atrial tachycardia (MAT), and atrial fibrillation (AFib).

 ECG Pearl _____

Causes of Abnormal Automaticity

- Chemical or toxic substance exposure
- Electrolyte disorders
- Hypoxia
- Ischemia

Triggered Activity

Triggered activity results from abnormal electrical impulses that sometimes occur during repolarization (i.e., afterdepolarizations), when cells are normally quiet. Triggered activity occurs when escape pacemaker and working cells fire more than once after stimulation by a single impulse. Triggered activity can result in atrial or ventricular beats that occur alone, in pairs, in runs of three or more beats, or as a sustained ectopic rhythm.

 ECG Pearl _____

Causes of Triggered Activity

- Catecholamine increase
- Digitalis toxicity
- Hypomagnesemia
- Hypoxia
- Medications that prolong repolarization (e.g., quinidine)
- Myocardial ischemia and injury

Reentry

Normally, an impulse spreads through the heart only once after it is initiated by pacemaker cells. With **reentry**, also called *reactivation*, an electrical impulse is delayed, blocked, or both in one or more areas of the conduction system while being conducted normally through the rest of the system (see Fig. 2.13). This results in the delayed electrical impulse entering cardiac cells that have just been depolarized by the normally conducted impulse. If the delayed impulse stimulates an area that is relatively refractory, the impulse can cause those cells to fire. This can produce a single early (i.e., premature) beat or repetitive electrical impulses, resulting in short periods of rapid rhythms (i.e., tachydysrhythmias). Atrial rhythms associated with reentry include atrial flutter, AVNRT, and AVRT. Common causes of reentry include hyperkalemia, myocardial ischemia, some antiarrhythmic medications, and the presence of an accessory pathway.

Most atrial dysrhythmias are not life threatening, but some may be associated with extremely fast ventricular rates. Increases in heart rate shorten all phases of the cardiac cycle, but the most important is a decrease in the length of time spent in diastole. Remember that as the heart rate increases, there is less time for the ventricles to fill and less blood for the ventricles to pump out with each contraction; therefore, an excessively fast heart rate can decrease cardiac output. Examples of factors that influence heart rate include hormone levels (e.g., thyroxin, epinephrine, norepinephrine), medications, stress, anxiety, fear, and body temperature.

PREMATURE ATRIAL COMPLEXES

[Objective 2]
Premature beats appear early, that is, they occur before the next expected beat. Premature beats are identified by their site of origin:
- Premature atrial complexes (PACs)
- Premature junctional complexes (PJCs)
- Premature ventricular complexes (PVCs)

The term *complex* is used instead of *contraction* to correctly identify an early beat because the electrocardiogram (ECG) depicts electrical activity, not mechanical function of the heart. Some practitioners prefer the term *conduction* instead of complex.

Premature beats may occur in patterns:
- Paired beats (**couplet**): Two premature beats in a row
- Runs or **bursts**: Three or more premature beats in a row
- **Bigeminy:** Every other beat is a premature beat
- **Trigeminy:** Every third beat is a premature beat
- **Quadrigeminy:** Every fourth beat is a premature beat

How Do I Recognize It?

[Objective 3]
A PAC occurs when an irritable site (i.e., focus) within the atria fires before the next SA node impulse is expected to fire. This interrupts the sinus rhythm. If the irritable site is close to the SA node, the atrial P wave will look very similar to the P waves initiated by the SA node. The P wave of a PAC may be biphasic (i.e., partly positive, partly negative), flattened, notched, pointed, or lost in the preceding T wave.

When compared with the P-P intervals of the underlying rhythm, a PAC is premature—occurring before the next expected sinus P wave. PACs are identified by the following:
- Early (premature) P waves
- Positive (upright) P waves (in lead II) that differ in shape from sinus P waves
- Early P waves that may or may not be followed by a QRS complex

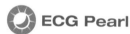 ECG Pearl

A PAC has a positive P wave before the QRS complex. Sometimes the P waves are clearly seen, and sometimes they are not. If the P wave of an early beat isn't obvious, look for it in the T wave of the preceding beat. The T wave of the preceding beat may be of higher amplitude than other T waves or have an extra "hump," which suggests the presence of a hidden P wave.

Look at the rhythm strip in Fig. 4.1. At a glance, you can see that the ventricular rhythm is irregular and that the rate is about 110 beats/min. Now let's look more

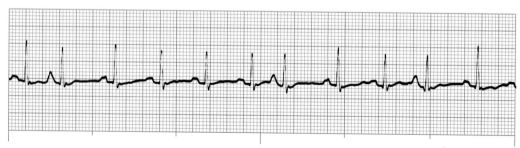

Fig. 4.1 Sinus tachycardia at 111 beats/min with three premature atrial complexes (PACs). From the left, beats 2, 7, and 10 are PACs.

closely. Begin by locating the QRS complexes on the rhythm strip. Evaluate each succeeding R-R interval. The R-R intervals in this example occur regularly except for three beats.

Now find the P waves on the rhythm strip. Remember that P waves that begin in the SA node are normally smooth and rounded. Atrial P waves will look different. Using a pen or pencil, mark an "S," for SA node, above each normal looking P wave. Mark an "A," for atrial, above those P waves that look different. When you are finished, you should have an "A" marked over the P waves in beats 2, 7, and 10. The rest of the P waves should be marked with an "S." Notice that the waveforms marked with an "S" above them occur regularly except when they are interrupted by the three atrial beats.

With the use of your calipers or a piece of paper, find two sinus beats that appear next to each other, such as beats 4 and 5. Using the sinus beats as your guide, determine the atrial rate. The distance between the sinus beats is about 13.5 boxes, or 111 beats/min, which is close to our initial estimated rate of 110 beats/min. Based on the rate (i.e., faster than 100 beats/min) and an upright P wave before each QRS, we know that the underlying rhythm is a sinus tachycardia. Now move your calipers or paper to the right. If beat 6 occurred on time, it will line up with your calipers or paper. It is on time. Now move your calipers to the right again. The right point of your calipers shows where the next sinus beat should have occurred. You can see that beat 7 occurred earlier than expected. This is a premature beat. When you continue this process, you will find that beat 10 is also early. Working backward and without adjusting your calipers, if you place the left point of your calipers on beat 1 in the rhythm strip, you will see that beat 2 is also early. So far, we can identify this rhythm as a sinus tachycardia at 111 beats/min with three premature beats.

Next, measure the PR interval, QRS duration, and QT interval. The PR interval is 0.16 second, and the QRS is 0.08 second in duration. Because it is difficult to clearly identify T waves in this rhythm strip, accurate determination of the QT interval is not possible.

We must identify where the premature beats came from because premature beats can start from more than one area of the heart. To do this, we must examine the premature beats more closely. Look carefully at beats 2, 7, and 10. The QRS complexes look the same as those of the underlying rhythm. This is because the impulse journeyed normally through the conduction system. Now look to the left of the QRS complex in each of these early beats and look at the P waves. Each P wave is positive (i.e., upright) but looks different from the P waves of the sinus beats. This is an important finding and one that tells you that the P waves came from the atria. The early beats are premature atrial complexes. A PAC is not an entire rhythm—it is a single beat; therefore, you must identify the underlying rhythm and the ectopic

beat(s). To complete our identification of this rhythm, we have a sinus tachycardia at 111 beats/min with three premature atrial complexes. The ECG characteristics of PACs are shown in Table 4.1.

Noncompensatory versus Compensatory Pause

[Objective 4]

A **noncompensatory** (i.e., incomplete) **pause** often follows a PAC. This represents the delay during which the SA node resets its rhythm for the next beat. A **compensatory** (i.e., complete) **pause** often follows PVCs (Fig. 4.2).

TABLE **4.1**	Characteristics of Premature Atrial Complexes
Rhythm	Irregular because of the early beat(s)
Rate	Usually within normal range but depends on underlying rhythm
P waves	Premature (occurring earlier than the next expected sinus P wave), positive (upright) in lead II, one before each QRS complex, often differ in shape from sinus P waves—may be flattened, notched, pointed, biphasic, or lost in the preceding T wave
PR interval	May be normal or prolonged depending on the prematurity of the beat
QRS duration	Usually 0.11 sec or less but may be wide (aberrant) or absent, depending on the prematurity of the beat; the QRS of the premature atrial complex (PAC) is similar in shape to those of the underlying rhythm unless the PAC is abnormally conducted

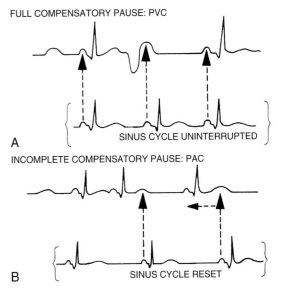

Fig. 4.2 A, A premature ventricular complex (PVC) is often followed by a full compensatory pause. B, A premature atrial complex (PAC) is often followed by a noncompensatory (incomplete) pause. (From Crawford MV, Spence MI: *Commonsense approach to coronary care,* rev ed 6, St. Louis, 1994, Mosby.)

To find out whether or not the pause after a **premature complex** is compensatory or noncompensatory, measure the distance between the R-R intervals of three normal beats. Then compare that measurement with the distance between the R-R intervals of three beats, one of which includes the premature complex. The pause is *noncompensatory* if the period between the complex before and after a premature beat is less than two normal R-R intervals (Fig. 4.3). The pause is *compensatory* if the period between the complex before and after a premature beat is the same as two normal R-R intervals.

Aberrantly Conducted Premature Atrial Complexes

If a PAC occurs very early, the right bundle branch can be slow to respond to the impulse (i.e., refractory). The impulse travels down the left bundle branch with no problem. Stimulation of the left bundle branch subsequently results in stimulation of the right bundle branch. The QRS will appear wide (i.e., greater than 0.11 second) because of this delay in ventricular depolarization. PACs associated with a wide QRS complex are called *aberrantly conducted PACs*. This indicates that conduction through the ventricles is abnormal. Fig. 4.4

shows a rhythm strip with two PACs. The first PAC (*arrow* in Fig. 4.4) was conducted abnormally, producing a wide QRS complex. The second PAC (*arrow* in Fig. 4.4) was conducted normally. Compare the T waves before each PAC with those of the underlying sinus bradycardia.

Nonconducted Premature Atrial Complexes

Sometimes when a PAC occurs very early and close to the T wave of the preceding beat, only a P wave may be seen with no QRS after it, appearing as a pause (Fig. 4.5). This type of PAC is called a **nonconducted** or **blocked PAC** because the P wave occurred too early to be conducted. Nonconducted PACs occur because the AV junction is still refractory to stimulation and unable to conduct the impulse to the ventricles (thus no QRS complex). Look for the early P wave in the T wave of the preceding beat.

WHAT CAUSES THEM?

[Objective 3]

PACs may be the result of abnormal automaticity or reentry. PACs are very common and can occur at any age. They are very frequent in older adults. Their presence does not

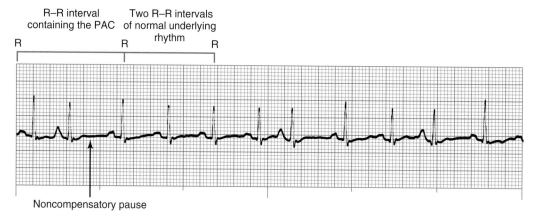

R—R interval
containing the PAC

Two R—R intervals
of normal underlying
rhythm

R   R   R

Noncompensatory pause

Fig. 4.3   A noncompensatory pause is present if the period between the complex before and after a premature beat is less than two normal R-R intervals. *PAC,* Premature atrial complex.

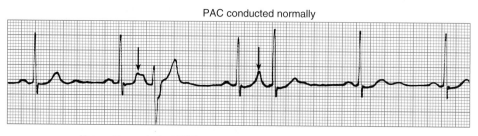

PAC conducted normally

Aberrantly conducted PAC

Fig. 4.4   Premature atrial complexes (PACs) with and without abnormal conduction (aberrancy). (From Kinney MP, Packa DR: *Andreoli's comprehensive cardiac care,* ed 8, St. Louis, 1996, Mosby.)

necessarily imply underlying cardiac disease. Possible causes of PACs include the following:

- Acute coronary syndromes
- Atrial enlargement
- Digitalis toxicity
- Electrolyte imbalance
- Emotional stress
- Heart failure
- Hyperthyroidism
- Mental and physical fatigue
- Stimulants: caffeine, tobacco, cocaine
- Sympathomimetic medications, such as epinephrine
- Valvular heart disease

What Do I Do About Them?
[Objective 3]

PACs usually do not require treatment if they are infrequent. If PACs are frequent, the patient may perceive a skipped beat or occasional **palpitations.** Some patients are unaware of their occurrence. In susceptible individuals, frequent PACs may induce episodes of AFib or PSVT. Frequent PACs are treated by correcting the underlying cause:

- Correcting electrolyte imbalances
- Reducing stress
- Reducing or eliminating stimulants
- Treating heart failure

If the patient is symptomatic, frequent PACs may be treated with beta-blockers, such as atenolol or metoprolol.

WANDERING ATRIAL PACEMAKER

How Do I Recognize It?
[Objectives 5, 6]

Multiform atrial rhythm is an updated term for the rhythm formerly known as **wandering atrial pacemaker**. With this rhythm, the size, shape, and direction of the P waves vary, sometimes from beat to beat. The difference in the look of the P waves is a result of the gradual shifting of the dominant pacemaker among the SA node, the atria, and/or the AV junction (Fig. 4.6). Wandering atrial pacemaker requires at least three different P waves, seen in the same lead, for proper diagnosis.

Wandering atrial pacemaker is associated with a normal or slow rate and irregular P-P, R-R, and PR intervals because of the different sites of impulse formation. The QRS duration is normally 0.11 second or less because conduction through the ventricles is usually normal. The ECG characteristics of wandering atrial pacemaker are shown in Table 4.2.

 ECG Pearl _____

At least three different P-wave configurations, seen in the same lead, are required for a diagnosis of wandering atrial pacemaker or multifocal atrial tachycardia.

What Causes It?

Wandering atrial pacemaker may be observed in normal, healthy hearts (particularly in athletes) and during sleep. It may also occur with some types of underlying heart disease and with digitalis toxicity. This dysrhythmia usually produces no signs and symptoms unless it is associated with a slow rate.

What Do I Do About It?

Wandering atrial pacemaker is usually a transient rhythm that resolves on its own when the firing rate of the SA node increases and the sinus resumes pacing responsibility. If the rhythm occurs because of digitalis toxicity, the drug should be withheld.

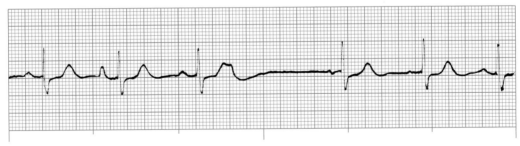

Fig. 4.5 Sinus rhythm with a nonconducted (blocked) premature atrial complex (PAC). Note the distorted T wave of the third QRS complex from the left.

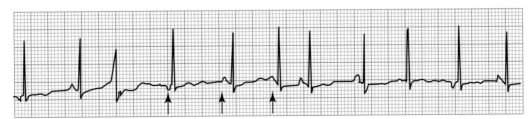

Fig. 4.6 Wandering atrial pacemaker. Note the differences in the shapes of the P waves. (From Paul S, Hebra JD: *The nurse's guide to cardiac rhythm interpretation: implications for patient care,* Philadelphia, 1998, Saunders.)

TABLE 4.2	Characteristics of Wandering Atrial Pacemaker
Rhythm	Usually irregular as the pacemaker site shifts from the SA node to ectopic atrial locations or AV junction
Rate	Usually 60 to 100 beats/min but may be slower; if the rate is faster than 100 beats/min, the rhythm is termed *multifocal atrial tachycardia*
P waves	Size, shape, and direction may change from beat to beat; may be upright, inverted, biphasic, rounded, flat, pointed, notched, or buried in the QRS complex
PR interval	Varies as the pacemaker site shifts from the SA node to ectopic atrial locations or AV junction
QRS duration	0.11 sec or less unless abnormally conducted

AV, Atrioventricular; *SA,* sinoatrial.

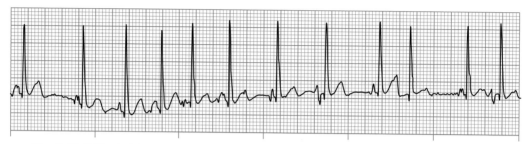

Fig. 4.7 Multifocal atrial tachycardia (MAT). (From Braunwald E, Libby P, Zipes DP, et al: *Heart disease: a textbook of cardiovascular medicine,* ed 6, St. Louis, 2001, Mosby.)

MULTIFOCAL ATRIAL TACHYCARDIA

How Do I Recognize It?

[Objective 7]

When the wandering atrial pacemaker rhythm is associated with a ventricular rate of more than 100 beats/min, the dysrhythmia is called **multifocal atrial tachycardia (MAT)** (Fig. 4.7). As evidenced by its name, MAT is the result of the random and chaotic firing of multiple ectopic sites in the atria. The ECG characteristics of MAT are shown in Table 4.3.

What Causes It?

MAT is most often seen in patients with severe chronic obstructive pulmonary disease (COPD), but it is also seen in the setting of acute coronary syndromes, valvular heart disease, or hypomagnesemia; and it may be a precursor of AFib (Hamdan, 2010).

What Do I Do About It?

The treatment of MAT is directed at the underlying cause. If the patient is symptomatic, it is best to consult a cardiologist before starting treatment.

SUPRAVENTRICULAR TACHYCARDIA

Supraventricular arrhythmias begin above the bundle of His; this means that supraventricular arrhythmias include rhythms that begin in the SA node, atrial tissue, or the AV junction. The term *supraventricular tachycardia* (SVT) includes supraventricular rhythms with a ventricular rate

TABLE 4.3	Characteristics of Multifocal Atrial Tachycardia
Rhythm	Irregular as the pacemaker site shifts from the SA node to ectopic atrial locations or AV junction
Rate	Faster than 100 beats/min
P waves	One P wave before each QRS but the size, shape, and direction of the P wave may change from beat to beat; may be upright, inverted, biphasic, rounded, flat, pointed, notched, or buried in the QRS complex; at least three different P-wave configurations (seen in same lead) are required for a diagnosis of multifocal atrial tachycardia
PR interval	Varies as the pacemaker site shifts from the SA node to ectopic atrial locations or the AV junction
QRS duration	0.11 sec or less unless abnormally conducted

AV, Atrioventricular; *SA,* sinoatrial.

faster than 100 beats/min at rest (Page et al, 2015). Three examples of SVTs are shown in Fig. 4.8.

 Did You Know?

Some SVTs need the AV node to sustain the rhythm and some do not. For example, AVNRT and AVRT require the AV node as part of the reentry circuit to continue the tachycardia. Other SVTs use the AV node only to conduct the rhythm to the ventricles. For example, atrial tachycardia, atrial flutter, and AFib arise from a site (or sites) within the atria; they do not need the AV node to sustain the rhythm.

The onset of SVT symptoms often begins in adulthood and can affect the quality of life depending on the frequency and duration of episodes and whether symptoms occur not only with exercise but also at rest (Page et al, 2015). Complaints of

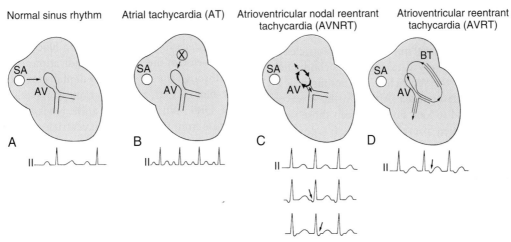

Normal sinus rhythm   Atrial tachycardia (AT)   Atrioventricular nodal reentrant tachycardia (AVNRT)   Atrioventricular reentrant tachycardia (AVRT)

Fig. 4.8 Types of supraventricular tachycardias. A, Normal sinus rhythm is shown here as a reference. B, With atrial tachycardia (AT), a focus (X) outside the sinoatrial (SA) node fires off automatically at a rapid rate. C, With atrioventricular (AV) nodal reentrant tachycardia (AVNRT), the cardiac stimulus originates as a wave of excitation that spins around the AV junctional area. As a result, P waves may be buried in the QRS or appear immediately before or just after the QRS complex *(arrows)* because of nearly simultaneous activation of the atria and ventricles. D, A similar type of reentrant (circus movement) mechanism in Wolff-Parkinson-White syndrome. This mechanism is referred to as *atrioventricular reentrant tachycardia (AVRT)*. Note the P wave in lead II somewhat after the QRS complex. *BT*, Bypass tract. (From Goldberger AL: *Clinical electrocardiography: a simplified approach*, ed 7, St. Louis, 2006, Mosby.)

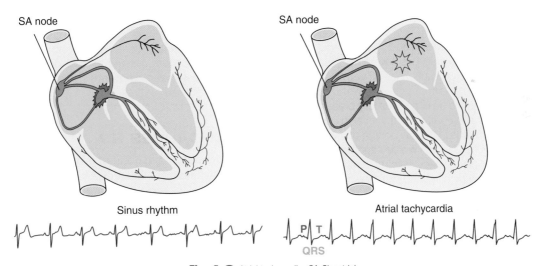

Fig. 4.9 Atrial tachycardia. *SA*, Sinoatrial.

lightheadedness are common. A drop in blood pressure typically occurs during SVT and is greatest in the first 10 to 30 seconds, normalizing within 30 to 60 seconds despite minimal changes in heart rate (Page et al, 2015).

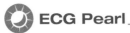 **ECG Pearl**

It is important to look closely for P waves in all dysrhythmias, but it is very important when trying to figure out the origin of a tachycardia. If P waves are not visible in one lead, try looking in another before finalizing your rhythm diagnosis.

Atrial Tachycardias

Atrial tachycardia (AT) is a regular rhythm that arises from an ectopic focus in the atria at a rate faster than 100 beats/min and does not require the participation of the AV node to maintain the dysrhythmia (Ellenbogen & Stambler, 2014) (Fig. 4.9). This rapid atrial rate overrides the SA node and becomes the pacemaker. AT is often precipitated by a PAC. When three or more PACs occur in a row at a rate of more than 100 beats/min, AT is present.

HOW DO I RECOGNIZE IT?

[Objectives 8, 9]

With AT, conduction of the atrial impulse to the ventricles is often 1:1. This means that every atrial impulse is conducted through the AV node to the ventricles. This results in a P wave preceding each QRS complex. Although the P waves appear upright, they tend to look different from those seen when the impulse is initiated from the SA node. It is possible for an AT to have negative P waves in the inferior leads if it arises from the lower part of the atrium. Because conducted impulses travel through the ventricles in the usual manner, the QRS complexes appear normal. The ECG characteristics of AT are shown in Table 4.4.

The term *paroxysmal* describes a rhythm that starts or ends suddenly. AT that starts or ends suddenly is called **paroxysmal supraventricular tachycardia (PSVT)**, once known as **paroxysmal atrial tachycardia** (Fig. 4.10). PSVT may last for minutes, hours, or days. If the onset or end of PSVT is not observed on the ECG, the dysrhythmia is simply called *SVT*.

With very rapid atrial rates, the AV node begins to filter some of the impulses coming to it. By doing so, it protects the ventricles from excessively rapid rates. When the AV node selectively filters conduction of some of these impulses, the rhythm is called *paroxysmal supraventricular (or atrial) tachycardia with block*. PSVT with block is often associated with disease of the AV node, medications that slow conduction through the AV node, or digitalis toxicity. When PSVT with block exists, more than one P wave is present before each QRS. When the AV node blocks every other atrial impulse from traveling to the ventricles the rhythm is called *PSVT with 2:1 block* (Fig. 4.11).

There is more than one type of AT. ATs may be caused by an automatic, triggered, or reentrant mechanism (Zimetbaum, 2016). MAT has already been discussed. AT that begins in a small area (focus) within the atria is called *focal AT*. **Focal atrial tachycardia** often presents with PSVT. *Automatic AT*, also called *ectopic AT*, is a type of focal AT in which a small cluster of cells with abnormal automaticity fire. The impulse is spread from the cluster of cells to the surrounding atrium and then to the ventricles via the AV node. P waves look different from sinus P waves, but they are still related to the QRS complex. Vagal maneuvers do not usually stop the tachycardia, but they may slow the ventricular rate.

TABLE 4.4	Characteristics of Atrial Tachycardia
Rhythm	Regular
Rate	101 to 250 beats/min
P waves	One P wave precedes each QRS complex in lead II; these P waves differ in shape from sinus P waves; an isoelectric baseline is usually present between P waves; if the atrial rhythm originates in the low portion of the atrium, P waves will be negative in the inferior leads; with rapid rates, it may be difficult to distinguish P waves from T waves
PR interval	May be shorter or longer than normal; may be difficult to measure because P waves may be hidden in the T waves of preceding beats
QRS duration	0.11 sec or less unless abnormally conducted

> ### CLINICAL CORRELATION
>
> Although correct use of the term *paroxysmal* requires observing the onset or cessation of the dysrhythmia and identification of the underlying rhythm that preceded it, some practitioners use the term to describe the sudden onset or cessation of a patient's *symptoms* associated with the dysrhythmia.

WHAT CAUSES IT?

Atrial tachycardia can occur in people with normal hearts or in those with organic heart disease. AT may be related to an acute event such as the following:

- Acute illness with excessive catecholamine release
- Digitalis toxicity
- Electrolyte imbalance
- Heart disease including coronary artery disease (CAD), valvular disease, cardiomyopathies, and congenital heart disease

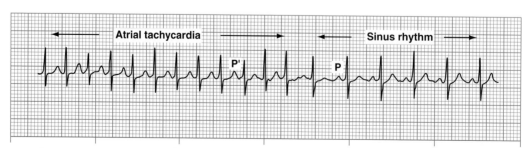

Fig. 4.10 Paroxysmal supraventricular tachycardia that ends spontaneously with the abrupt resumption of sinus rhythm. The P waves of the tachycardia (rate: about 150 beats/min) are superimposed on the preceding T waves. (From Goldberger AL: *Clinical electrocardiography: a simplified approach*, ed 7, St. Louis, 2006, Mosby.)

- Infection
- Pulmonary embolism
- Stimulant use (e.g., caffeine, albuterol, theophylline, cocaine)

The autonomic nervous system is associated with initiating or triggering some ATs (Ellenbogen & Stambler, 2014). Reports of AT triggered by belching, changes in posture, and swallowing, and the termination of AT with a Valsalva maneuver or with the administration of beta-blockers support the probable association between autonomic nervous system activity and AT in some patients (Ellenbogen & Stambler, 2014).

 CLINICAL CORRELATION

The signs and symptoms experienced by a patient with a tachycardia depend on the ventricular rate, how long the tachycardia lasts, the patient's general health, and the presence of underlying heart disease. The faster the heart rate, the more likely the patient is to have signs and symptoms resulting from the rapid rate.

WHAT DO I DO ABOUT IT?

[Objective 8]

Assessment findings and symptoms associated with AT vary widely and may include the following:

- Acute changes in mental status
- Asymptomatic
- Dizziness or lightheadedness
- Dyspnea
- Fatigue
- Fluttering sensation in the chest
- Hypotension
- Ischemic chest discomfort
- Palpitations
- Signs of shock
- Syncope or near syncope

When taking the patient's history, try to find out how often the episodes occur, how long they last, and possible triggers. If the patient complains of palpitations, find out if they are regular or irregular. Palpitations that occur regularly with a sudden onset and end usually are the result of AVNRT or AVRT. Irregular palpitations may be the result of premature complexes, AFib, or MAT. Tachycardias may cause syncope because the rapid ventricular rate decreases cardiac output and blood flow to the brain. Syncope is most likely to occur just after the onset of a rapid AT or when the rhythm stops abruptly. Predisposed people may experience angina or heart failure.

A rhythm that lasts from 3 beats up to 30 seconds is a *nonsustained rhythm*. A *sustained rhythm* is one that lasts more than 30 seconds. If episodes of AT are short, the patient may be asymptomatic. If AT is sustained and the patient is symptomatic because of the rapid rate, treatment should include applying a pulse oximeter and administering oxygen (if indicated), obtaining the patient's vital signs, and establishing intravenous (IV) access. A 12-lead ECG should be obtained. If the patient is not hypotensive, vagal maneuvers may be tried. Vagal maneuvers are discussed later. Although vagal maneuvers are rarely successful, they may be attempted in an effort to terminate the rhythm or slow conduction through the AV node. If vagal maneuvers fail, antiarrhythmic medications should be tried if the patient is hemodynamically stable. Adenosine can be useful to either restore sinus rhythm or diagnose the tachycardia mechanism in patients with suspected focal AT (Page et al, 2015).

Beta-blockers and calcium channel blockers (e.g., diltiazem, verapamil) may be ordered to slow the ventricular rate (Page et al, 2015). If AT is sustained and causing persistent signs of hemodynamic compromise, IV adenosine may be ordered and, if it is ineffective or if administration is not feasible, synchronized cardioversion should be performed (Page et al, 2015). Synchronized cardioversion is discussed later in this chapter.

PSVT with AV block often occurs because of excess digitalis. In these cases, the patient's ventricular rate is not excessively fast. The drug should be withheld and serum digoxin levels obtained. Long-term medication therapy may include the use of calcium channel blockers or beta-blockers.

When AT is difficult to control and causes serious signs and symptoms, radiofrequency catheter ablation may be necessary. When catheter ablation is performed, electrophysiologic studies are done to locate the abnormal pathways and reentry circuits in the heart. Once localized, a special ablation catheter is placed at the site of the abnormal pathway. Low-energy, high-frequency current is

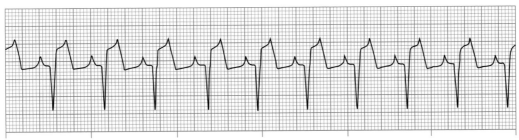

Fig. 4.11 Atrial tachycardia with 2:1 block. P waves are clearly seen before the QRS complexes. Others are hidden in the T waves. The atrial rate is 180 beats/min, and the ventricular rate is 90 beats/min. (From Andreoli TE, Benjamin I, Griggs R, et al: *Andreoli and Carpenter's Cecil essentials of medicine*, Philadelphia, 2011, Saunders.)

delivered through this catheter. With each burst of energy from the catheter, an area of tissue is destroyed (ablated). The energy is applied in various areas until the unwanted pathway is no longer functional and the circuit is broken. ATs occasionally can recur at a different site after a successful ablation.

 Drug Pearl _____

Adenosine

- Adenosine slows the rate of the sinoatrial node, slows conduction time through the AV node, can interrupt reentry pathways that involve the AV node, and can restore sinus rhythm in SVT. Reentry circuits are the underlying mechanism for many episodes of SVT. Adenosine acts at specific receptors to cause a temporary block of conduction through the AV node, interrupting these reentry circuits. A 12-lead electrocardiogram recording is desirable when adenosine is used.

- Adenosine has an onset of action of 10 to 40 seconds and a duration of 1 to 2 minutes. Because of its short half-life (i.e., 10 seconds), the medication is administered intravenously as rapidly as possible (i.e., over a period of seconds) and *immediately* followed with a saline flush.

VAGAL MANEUVERS

[Objective 10]

Vagal maneuvers are methods used to stimulate baroreceptors in the internal carotid arteries and the aortic arch. The stimulation of these receptors results in reflex stimulation of the vagus nerve and the release of acetylcholine. Acetylcholine prolongs the effective refractory period of the AV node, thereby slowing conduction through the AV node and interrupting the reentrant circuit.

Carotid sinus massage, also called **carotid sinus pressure**, is a vagal maneuver that is performed with the patient's neck extended. Steady pressure is applied to the right or left carotid sinus just underneath the angle of the jaw for 5 to 10 seconds (Page et al, 2015) (Fig. 4.12). The pressure applied directly stretches the wall of the carotid sinus, thereby stimulating the baroreceptors (Lederer, 2012). Carotid sinus pressure should be avoided in older adults and in patients who have a history of stroke, known carotid artery stenosis, or a carotid **bruit** on auscultation (Olgin, 2008). Simultaneous, bilateral carotid pressure is not recommended. Because many organizations stipulate that carotid massage only be performed by a physician, it is prudent to check your agency's policy with regard to this procedure.

Application of a cold stimulus to the face (e.g., a washcloth soaked in iced water, a cold pack, or crushed ice mixed with water in a plastic bag or glove) is another type of vagal maneuver that is based on the classic diving reflex. This is done for up to 10 seconds. When using this method, do not obstruct the patient's mouth or nose or apply pressure to the eyes. The use of a cold stimulus to the face is often effective in children but seldom in adults.

The Valsalva maneuver is a type of vagal maneuver during which the patient is instructed to make a forced expiratory effort against a closed glottis. This increases intrathoracic pressure and stretches the aorta, stimulates the aortic baroreceptors, and triggers vagus nerve activation (Lederer, 2012). The patient may be asked to blow through an occluded straw or take a deep breath and bear down as if having a bowel movement.

 CLINICAL CORRELATION

Research has shown improved success rates when performing a Valsalva maneuver with the patient supine while forcefully exhaling for at least 15 seconds (Walker & Cutting, 2010). More recently, a modified Valsalva maneuver has shown improved success with conversion to sinus rhythm. With this procedure, the patient is placed in a semi-recumbent position and asked to blow into a 10-mL syringe until the plunger moves (Appelboam et al, 2015). The patient is then immediately moved to a supine position with passive leg elevation by a staff member at 45-degrees for 15 seconds and then returned to a semi-recumbent position for 45 seconds before reassessment of the patient's cardiac rhythm. Conversion to sinus rhythm was significantly more common in the modified-maneuver group (43%) than in the control group (17%) (Appelboam et al, 2015).

SYNCHRONIZED CARDIOVERSION

[Objective 11]

Synchronized cardioversion is the delivery of a shock to the heart by means of a defibrillator to terminate a rapid dysrhythmia. A *synchronized* shock means the shock is

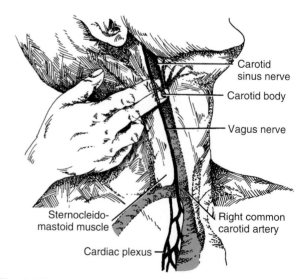

Fig. 4.12 Carotid sinus massage. The carotid sinus (carotid body) is located at the bifurcation of the carotid artery at the angle of the jaw. (From Conover MB: *Understanding electrocardiography,* ed 7, St. Louis, 1995.)

timed to avoid the relative refractory period of the cardiac cycle. When the sync control is pressed, the machine searches for the QRS complex. When a QRS complex is detected, the monitor places a flag or sync marker on that complex. It may appear as an oval, square, line, or highlighted triangle on the ECG display, depending on the machine used. To deliver a shock, press and hold the shock button on the defibrillator until a message appears on the screen indicating that the shock has been delivered. If using standard paddles, press and hold the shock control on each paddle until the message is seen.

Indications

Because the machine must be able to detect a QRS complex in order to sync, synchronized cardioversion is used to treat rhythms that have a clearly identifiable QRS complex and a rapid ventricular rate in patients who show signs of hemodynamic compromise. Examples of rhythms treated with cardioversion include narrow-QRS tachycardias, AFib, atrial flutter, and monomorphic ventricular tachycardia. Elective cardioversion should not be performed in patients with evidence of digoxin toxicity, severe hypokalemia, or other electrolyte imbalances until these factors are corrected (January et al, 2014).

Atrioventricular Nodal Reentrant Tachycardia

[Objective 12]

Atrioventricular nodal reentrant tachycardia (AVNRT) is the most common type of SVT (Mani & Pavri, 2014). Patients with AVNRT have two pathways within the AV node that

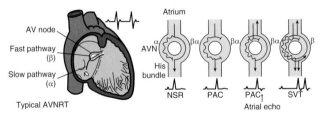

Fig. 4.13 Schematic for supraventricular tachycardia (SVT) resulting from atrioventricular (AV) nodal reentry (AVNRT). *AV,* AV node; *NSR,* normal sinus rhythm; *PAC,* premature atrial complex. (From Braunwald E, Goldman L, Menz C: *Primary cardiology,* ed 2, Philadelphia, 2003, Saunders.)

conduct impulses at different speeds and recover at different rates (Zimetbaum, 2016). Under the right conditions, these fast and slow pathways can form an electrical circuit or loop (Fig. 4.13). As one side of the loop is recovering, the other is firing.

Typical AVNRT, also termed *slow–fast tachycardia*, is usually caused by single or multiple PACs. It is estimated that 80% of AVNRTs are of the slow–fast type (Mani & Pavri, 2014). This means that a PAC, having found the fast pathway refractory, conducts the impulse to the ventricles by means of the slow pathway. This is reflected by a prolonged PR interval on the ECG. If the fast pathway has recovered, the impulse can conduct rapidly up the fast pathway and depolarize the atria, resulting in an echo beat (Mani & Pavri, 2014). The impulse can then reenter the slow pathway to conduct again. If this pattern continues, AVNRT is initiated, resulting in a very rapid and regular ventricular rhythm ranging from 150 to 250 beats/min.

A less common type of AVNRT is called *atypical AVNRT*, also known as *fast–slow tachycardia*. Atypical AVNRT is often initiated by a premature complex that conducts down the fast pathway and returns by means of the slow pathway.

HOW DO I RECOGNIZE IT?

Look at the example of AVNRT in Fig. 4.14. You can see narrow-QRS complexes that occur at a regular rate of 168 beats/min. P waves are not clearly seen. Because AVNRT begins in the area of the AV node, the impulse spreads to the atria and ventricles at almost the same time. This results in P waves that are usually hidden in the QRS complex. If the ventricles are stimulated first and then the atria, a negative (inverted) P wave will appear after the QRS in leads II, III, and aVF. When the atria are depolarized after the ventricles, the P wave typically distorts the end of the QRS complex. The PR interval is not measurable because P waves are not seen before the QRS complex.

In our example of AVNRT, you can see ST-segment depression. ST-segment changes (usually depression) are common in patients with SVTs. In most patients, these ST-segment changes are thought to be the result of repolarization changes. However, in older adults and those with a high likelihood of ischemic heart disease, ST-segment changes may represent ECG changes consistent with an acute coronary syndrome. The patient should be watched closely.

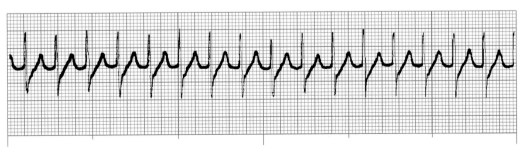

Fig. 4.14 Atrioventricular nodal reentrant tachycardia.

TABLE **4.5**	Characteristics of Atrioventricular Nodal Reentrant Tachycardia
Rhythm	Ventricular rhythm is usually very regular
Rate	150 to 250 beats/min; typically 180 to 200 beats/min in adults
P waves	Often hidden in the QRS complex; if the ventricles are stimulated first and then the atria, a negative (inverted) P wave will appear after the QRS in leads II, III, and aVF; when the atria are depolarized after the ventricles, the P wave typically distorts the end of the QRS complex
PR interval	P waves are not seen before the QRS complex; therefore, the PR interval is not measurable
QRS duration	0.11 sec or less unless abnormally conducted

Appropriate laboratory tests and a 12-lead ECG should be obtained to rule out infarction as needed. The ECG characteristics of AVNRT are summarized in Table 4.5.

WHAT CAUSES IT?

Although AVNRT can occur at any age, it often presents in young adulthood, occurring more often in women than in men (Zimetbaum, 2016). Whether a person is born with a tendency to have AVNRT or whether it develops later in life for an unknown reason has not been clearly determined. AVNRT is most often seen in young adults who have no structural heart disease or ischemic heart disease. It also occurs in patients with COPD, CAD, valvular heart disease, heart failure, and digitalis toxicity. AVNRT can be triggered by hypoxia, stress, anxiety, caffeine, smoking, sleep deprivation, and many medications. AVNRT can cause angina or myocardial infarction (MI) in patients with CAD.

WHAT DO I DO ABOUT IT?

Because AVNRT may be short-lived or sustained, treatment depends on the duration of the tachycardia and severity of the patient's signs and symptoms. Assessment findings and symptoms that may be associated with rapid ventricular rates may include the following:

- Chest pain or pressure
- Dizziness
- Dyspnea
- Heart failure
- Lightheadedness
- Nausea
- Neck pulsations
- Nervousness, anxiety
- Palpitations (common)
- Signs of shock
- Syncope
- Weakness

If the patient is stable but symptomatic and the symptoms are the result of the rapid heart rate, apply a pulse oximeter and administer supplemental oxygen, if indicated. Obtain the patient's vital signs, establish IV access, and obtain a 12-lead ECG. While continuously monitoring the patient's ECG, attempt a vagal maneuver if there are no contraindications. AVNRT is usually responsive to vagal maneuvers. If vagal maneuvers do not slow the rate or cause conversion of the tachycardia to a sinus rhythm, the first antiarrhythmic given is adenosine. The administration of calcium channel blockers or beta-blockers is indicated when AVNRT fails to convert to sinus rhythm or if it recurs. It has been estimated that 80% to 98% of stable patients with SVT respond to pharmacologic therapy with adenosine, diltiazem, or verapamil (Page et al, 2015).

An unstable patient is one who has signs and symptoms of hemodynamic compromise. Examples of these signs and symptoms include acute changes in mental status, chest pain or discomfort, hypotension, shortness of breath, pulmonary congestion, heart failure, acute MI, and signs of shock. If the patient is unstable, treatment should include application of a pulse oximeter and administration of supplemental oxygen (if indicated), IV access, and sedation (if the patient is awake and time permits) followed by synchronized cardioversion.

Recurrent AVNRT may require treatment with a long-acting calcium channel blocker or beta-blocker. Antiarrhythmics such as amiodarone may also be used. Recurrent episodes vary in frequency, duration, and severity from several times a day to every 2 to 3 years. Patients who are resistant to drug therapy or who do not wish to remain on lifelong medications for the dysrhythmia are candidates for radiofrequency catheter ablation. Catheter ablation has become the treatment of choice in the management of patients with symptomatic recurrent episodes of AVNRT. It is successful in permanently interrupting the circuit and curing the dysrhythmia in most cases.

Atrioventricular Reentrant Tachycardia

[Objective 13]

Atrioventricular reentrant tachycardia (AVRT) is the next most common type of SVT. The term **preexcitation** refers to a rhythm that originates above the ventricles and transmits an impulse along a pathway outside the AV node and the AV bundle. As a result, this supraventricular impulse excites the ventricles earlier than would be expected if the impulse had traveled through the normal conduction system.

During fetal development, strands of myocardial tissue form connections between the atria and the ventricles, outside of the normal conduction system. These strands normally become nonfunctional shortly after birth; however, in patients with preexcitation syndrome, these connections persist. Because these connections bypass part or all of the normal conduction system, they are called **accessory pathways** or *bypass tracts* (Fig. 4.15). Some people have more than one accessory pathway. Anatomically, accessory pathways are most commonly found in the left side of the heart (Leitch & Barlow, 2010).

With AVRT, the reentrant circuit involves four components—the atrium, the normal AV node, the ventricle, and an accessory pathway (Saksena et al, 2012). Several types of accessory pathways have been described. The location of the accessory pathway and the conductive properties of the

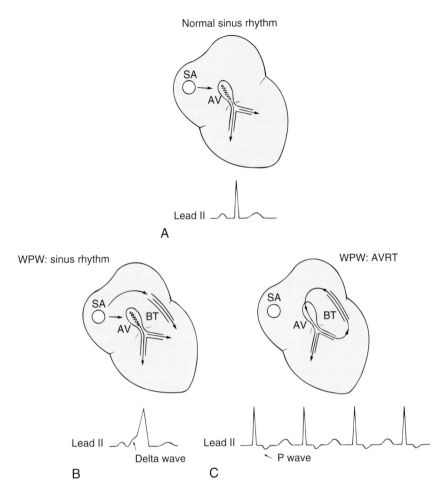

Fig. 4.15 Normal and abnormal conduction pathways. A, Conduction during sinus rhythm in the normal heart spreads from the sinoatrial (SA) node to the atrioventricular (AV) node and then down the bundle branches. The *jagged line* indicates physiologic slowing of conduction in the AV node. B, With Wolff-Parkinson-White (WPW) pattern, an abnormal accessory conduction pathway called a bypass tract (BT) connects the atria and ventricles. With WPW, during sinus rhythm, the electrical impulse is conducted quickly down the bypass tract, preexciting the ventricles before the impulse arrives via the AV node. Consequently, the PR interval is short, and the QRS complex is wide, with slurring at its onset (delta wave). C, WPW predisposes patients to develop an atrioventricular reentrant tachycardia (AVRT), in which a premature atrial beat may spread down the normal pathway to the ventricles, travel back up the bypass tract, and recirculate down the AV node again. This reentrant loop can repeat itself over and over, resulting in a tachycardia. Notice the normal QRS complex and often negative P wave in lead II during this type of bypass-tract tachycardia. (From Goldberger AL: *Clinical electrocardiography: a simplified approach,* ed 7, St. Louis, 2006, Mosby.)

pathway and AV node determine the extent of preexcitation (Hamdan, 2010). Unlike the AV node, an accessory pathway does not have the ability to slow or reduce the number of atrial impulses transmitted to the ventricles; therefore, patients with preexcitation syndromes are prone to tachydysrhythmias, including PSVT, AVRT, and AFib. The number of atrial impulses reaching the ventricles may approach 300 to 350 beats/min, which significantly increases the risk of development of ventricular fibrillation.

The most common form of preexcitation is the **Wolff-Parkinson-White (WPW) pattern**. The WPW pattern includes a triad of findings that consist of the following: (1) A short PR interval, (2) a delta wave, and (3) a wide QRS complex (Fig. 4.16). A patient is said to have WPW syndrome when a WPW preexcitation pattern is present on the ECG and a tachydysrhythmia occurs that is related to the accessory pathway (Olgin & Zipes, 2012).

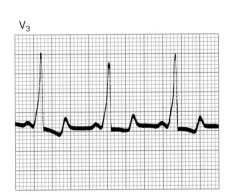

Fig. 4.16 Typical Wolff-Parkinson-White (WPW) pattern showing a short PR interval, delta wave, wide QRS complex, and secondary ST and T-wave changes. (From Chou T, Ramaiah LS: *Electrocardiography in clinical practice: adult and pediatric,* ed 4, Philadelphia, 1996, Saunders.)

HOW DO I RECOGNIZE IT?

The ECG characteristics of WPW described here are usually seen when the patient is *not* having a tachycardia. WPW syndrome usually goes undetected until it manifests in a patient as a tachycardia.

When WPW is associated with a sinus rhythm, the P wave looks normal. The PR interval is short (less than 0.12 second) because the impulse travels very quickly across the accessory pathway, bypassing the normal delay in the AV node. As the impulse crosses the insertion point of the accessory pathway in the ventricular muscle, that part of the ventricle is stimulated earlier (preexcited) than if the impulse had followed the normal conduction pathway through the bundle of His and Purkinje fibers. On the ECG, preexcitation of the ventricles can be seen as a **delta wave** in some leads. A delta wave is an initial slurred deflection at the beginning of the QRS complex that may be positive or negative. It reflects the relatively slow ventricular depolarization over the accessory pathway (Fig. 4.17) (Mark et al, 2009).

 ECG Pearl _____

Recognizing the Wolff-Parkinson-White Pattern

- Delta wave
- Short PR interval
- Widening of the QRS complex

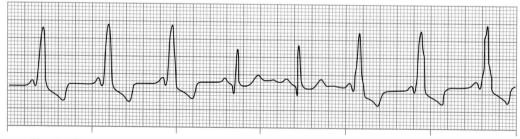

	Normal conduction	WPW
A		Delta / or
B		Delta / or

Fig. 4.17 Characteristic findings with the Wolff-Parkinson-White (WPW) pattern (short PR interval, QRS widening, and delta wave) compared with normal conduction. A, The usual appearance of WPW in leads in which the QRS complex is mainly upright. B, The usual appearance of WPW when the QRS is predominantly negative. Negative delta waves may simulate pathologic Q waves, mimicking myocardial infarction. (From Grauer K: *A practical guide to ECG interpretation*, ed 2, St. Louis, 1998, Mosby.)

Normally, conduction through the Purkinje fibers is very fast. In WPW, the spread of the impulse is slow because it must spread from working cell to working cell in the ventricular muscle. This is because the accessory pathway bypasses the specialized cells of the heart's conduction system. Because the impulse spreads slowly through the working cells, the delay in conduction results in a QRS that is usually more than 0.12 second in duration. The QRS complex seen in WPW is actually a combination of the impulse that preexcites the ventricles through the accessory pathway and the impulse that follows the normal conduction pathway through the AV node (Hamdan, 2010). As a result, the end (i.e., terminal) portion of the QRS usually looks normal. However, because the ventricles are activated abnormally, they repolarize abnormally. This is seen on the ECG as changes in the ST segment and T wave. The direction of the ST segment and T wave is usually opposite the direction of the delta wave and QRS complex, which can mimic ECG signs of myocardial ischemia or injury. An example of WPW is shown in Fig. 4.18. The ECG characteristics of WPW are summarized in Table 4.6.

WHAT CAUSES IT?

WPW syndrome is more common among men than among women, and most people with WPW syndrome have no associated heart disease. WPW syndrome is one of the most common causes of tachydysrhythmias in infants and children. Although the accessory pathway in WPW syndrome is believed to be congenital in origin, symptoms associated with preexcitation often do not appear until the patient is a teenager or during young adulthood.

WHAT DO I DO ABOUT IT?

Although some people with AVRT never have symptoms, common signs and symptoms associated with AVRT and a rapid ventricular rate include the following:

- Anxiety
- Chest discomfort
- Dizziness
- Lightheadedness
- Palpitations (common)
- Shortness of breath during exercise
- Signs of shock
- Weakness

Fig. 4.18 Rhythm strip showing an example of intermittent preexcitation. The first three beats show preexcitation. This is followed by abrupt normalization of the QRS complex in the next two beats. The preexcitation pattern returns for the final three beats. (From Zipes DP, Jalife J: *Cardiac electrophysiology: from cell to bedside*, ed 3, Philadelphia, 2000, Saunders.)

If a delta wave is noted on the ECG but the patient is asymptomatic, no specific treatment is required (Hamdan, 2010). If the patient is symptomatic because of the rapid ventricular rate, treatment will depend on how unstable the patient is, the width of the QRS complex (i.e., wide or narrow), and the regularity of the ventricular rhythm. Consultation with a cardiologist is recommended when caring for a patient with AVRT.

Vagal maneuvers are recommended if the patient is stable and there are no contraindications (Page et al, 2015). Medications such as adenosine, digoxin, diltiazem, and verapamil should be avoided. These medications are contraindicated because they slow or block conduction across the AV node, but they may speed up conduction through the accessory pathway, thereby resulting in a further *increase* in the ventricular rate (Link et al, 2015). Although the potential for beta-blockers to enhance conduction across an accessory pathway is controversial, caution should be exercised in the use of these drugs in patients with AFib associated with preexcitation (Fuster et al, 2011). If the patient is unstable, preparations should be made for synchronized cardioversion.

ATRIAL FLUTTER

[Objective 14]
Atrial flutter is a reentrant rhythm in which an irritable site within the atria fires regularly at a very rapid rate.

How Do I Recognize It?

Typical atrial flutter, also known as *common atrial flutter* or *counterclockwise atrial flutter*, is caused by reentry in which an impulse circles around a large area of tissue, such as the entire right atrium, in a counterclockwise direction (January et al, 2014) (Fig. 4.19). Atrial waveforms are produced that resemble the teeth of a saw or a picket fence; these are called *flutter waves* or **F waves**. F waves are predominantly negative in leads II, III, and aVF and positive in V_1 (Fuster et al, 2011). The atrial rate typically ranges from 240 to 300 beats/min (January et al, 2014). Because P waves are not observed in atrial flutter, the PR interval is not measurable. The QRS complex is usually 0.11 second or less because atrial flutter is a supraventricular rhythm, and the impulse is conducted normally through the AV junction and Purkinje fibers. However, if flutter waves are buried in the QRS complex or if an intraventricular conduction delay exists, the QRS will appear wide (i.e., greater than 0.11 second).

With atypical atrial flutter, the impulse circulates in a clockwise direction, resulting in F waves that are

TABLE **4.6**	Characteristics of Wolff-Parkinson-White Pattern
Rhythm	Regular, unless associated with AFib
Rate	Usually 60 to 100 beats/min if the underlying rhythm is sinus in origin
P waves	Normal and positive in lead II unless WPW is associated with AFib
PR interval	If P waves are observed, 0.12 sec or less, because the impulse travels very quickly across the accessory pathway, bypassing the normal delay in the AV node
QRS duration	Usually more than 0.12 sec; slurred upstroke of the QRS complex (delta wave) may be seen in one or more leads

AFib, Atrial fibrillation; *AV,* atrioventricular; *WPW,* Wolff-Parkinson-White.

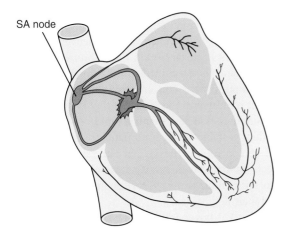

Sinus rhythm

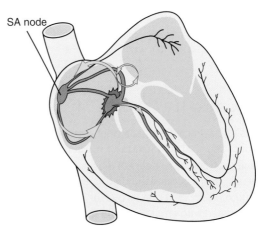

Atrial flutter

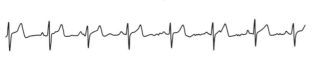

Fig. 4.19 Atrial flutter. *F,* Flutter wave; *SA,* sinoatrial.

predominantly positive in leads II, III, and aVF and negative in V_1. The mechanism of atypical atrial flutter may be related to incisional scars from previous cardiac surgeries involving atrial tissue, previous atrial ablation, idiopathic fibrosis in areas of the atrium, or other anatomic or functional barriers to conduction in the atria (Goel et al, 2013; Olgin & Zipes, 2012). It is important to recognize that the F-wave descriptions provided for typical and atypical atrial flutter are not always reliable with regard to the location of the reentry circuit or the type of atrial flutter (January et al, 2014).

With atrial flutter, an irritable focus within the atrium typically depolarizes at a rate of 300 beats/min. If each impulse were transmitted to the ventricles, the ventricular rate would equal 300 beats/min. The healthy AV node protects the ventricles from these extremely fast atrial rates. Normally, the AV node cannot conduct faster than about 180 impulses/min. Thus, at an atrial rate of 300 beats/min, every other impulse arrives at the AV node while it is still refractory. The resulting ventricular response of 150 beats/min is called *2:1 conduction*. (The ratio of the atrial rate [300 beats/min] to the ventricular rate [150 beats/min] is 2 to 1.) Atrial flutter with an atrial rate of 300 beats/min and a ventricular rate of 100 beats/min results in 3:1 conduction, 75 beats/min results in 4:1 conduction, 50 beats/min results in 6:1 conduction, and so on. Although conduction ratios in atrial flutter are often even (i.e., 2:1, 4:1, 6:1), variable conduction can also occur, which produces an irregular ventricular rhythm. In individuals with an accessory pathway, atrial flutter may be associated with 1:1 conduction because the AV node is bypassed, producing extremely rapid ventricular rates. When atrial flutter is present with 2:1 conduction, it may be difficult to tell the difference between atrial flutter and sinus tachycardia, AT, AVNRT, AVRT, or SVT. The ECG characteristics of atrial flutter are shown in Table 4.7.

 ECG Pearl

Atrial flutter or AFib that has a rapid ventricular rate is described as *uncontrolled*. Atrial flutter or AFib with a rapid ventricular response is commonly called *Aflutter with RVR* or *AFib with RVR*.

What Causes It?

Atrial flutter is often precipitated by a brief episode of AT or by AFib (January et al, 2014). It may last for seconds to hours and occasionally persists for 24 hours or longer. Chronic atrial flutter is unusual. This is because the rhythm usually converts to sinus rhythm or AFib, either on its own or with treatment. Conditions associated with atrial flutter are shown in Box 4.1.

What Do I Do About It?

Patients with atrial flutter commonly present with complaints of palpitations, difficulty breathing, fatigue, or chest discomfort. The severity of signs and symptoms associated

TABLE **4.7**	Characteristics of Atrial Flutter
Rhythm	Atrial regular; ventricular regular or irregular depending on AV conduction and blockade
Rate	The atrial rate typically ranges from 240 to 300 beats/min; the ventricular rate varies and is determined by AV blockade; the ventricular rate will usually not exceed 180 beats/min as a result of the intrinsic conduction rate of the AV junction
P waves	No identifiable P waves; saw-toothed "flutter" waves are present
PR interval	Not measurable
QRS duration	0.11 sec or less but may be widened if flutter waves are buried in the QRS complex or if abnormally conducted

AV, Atrioventricular.

Box **4.1**	Conditions Associated with Atrial Flutter

- Cardiac surgery
- Cardiomyopathy
- Chronic lung disease
- Complication of myocardial infarction
- Digitalis or quinidine toxicity
- Hyperthyroidism
- Ischemic heart disease
- Mitral or tricuspid valve stenosis or regurgitation
- Pericarditis or myocarditis
- Pulmonary embolism

with atrial flutter vary, depending on the ventricular rate, how long the rhythm has been present, and the patient's cardiovascular status. It is best to consult a cardiologist when considering treatment options.

Vagal maneuvers may help to identify the rhythm by temporarily slowing AV conduction and revealing the underlying flutter waves (Fig. 4.20). When vagal maneuvers are used in the management of atrial flutter, the response is usually sudden slowing and then a return to the former rate. Vagal maneuvers will not usually convert atrial flutter because the reentry circuit is located in the atria, not the AV node.

If atrial flutter is associated with a rapid ventricular rate and the patient is stable but symptomatic, treatment is usually aimed at controlling the ventricular rate with medications such as beta-blockers (e.g., esmolol, metoprolol, propranolol) or nondihydropyridine calcium channel blockers (e.g., verapamil, diltiazem).

Synchronized cardioversion should be considered for any patient with atrial flutter who has serious signs and symptoms because of the rapid ventricular rate (e.g., hypotension, signs of shock, or heart failure) (Link et al, 2015). If synchronized cardioversion is performed, atrial flutter can be successfully converted to a sinus rhythm with the use of low energy levels.

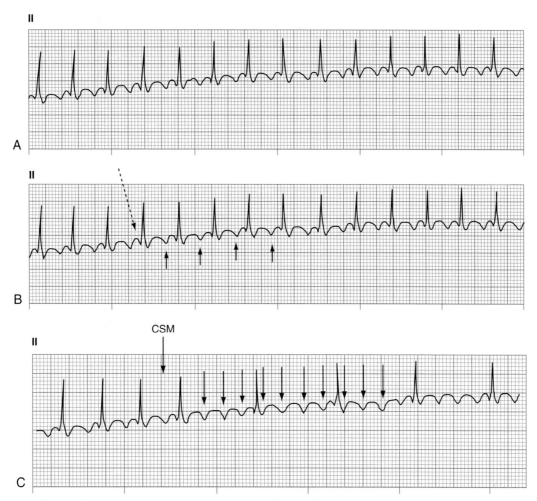

Fig. 4.20 Atrial flutter. A, Rhythm strip showing a narrow-QRS tachycardia with a ventricular rate just under 150 beats/min. B, The same rhythm shown in *A* with *arrows* added indicating possible atrial activity. C, When carotid sinus massage (CSM) is performed, the rate of conduction through the atrioventricular (AV) node slows, revealing atrial flutter. (From Grauer K: *A practical guide to ECG interpretation,* ed 2, St. Louis, 1998, Mosby.)

ATRIAL FIBRILLATION

[Objective 15]

AFib is the most common dysrhythmia treated in clinical practice and the most common dysrhythmia for which patients are hospitalized (Morady & Zipes, 2015). AFib occurs because of abnormal automaticity in one or several rapidly firing sites in the atria or reentry involving one or more circuits in the atria (Fig. 4.21). Irritable sites in the atria fire at a rate of 300 to 600 times per minute. These rapid impulses cause the muscles of the atria to quiver (i.e., fibrillate), thereby resulting in ineffectual atrial contraction, decreased stroke volume, a subsequent decrease in cardiac output, and a loss of atrial kick. The ventricular response to AFib depends on the electrophysiologic properties of the AV node and other conducting tissues, the level of sympathetic and parasympathetic tone, the presence or absence of accessory pathways, and the action of drugs (Fuster et al, 2011). AFib may occur alone or in association with other atrial dysrhythmias (January et al, 2014).

How Do I Recognize It?

With AFib, the AV node attempts to protect the ventricles from the hundreds of impulses bombarding it per minute. It does this by blocking many of the impulses generated by the irritable sites in the atria. The ventricular rate and rhythm are determined by the degree of blocking by the AV node of these rapid impulses.

Look at the example of AFib in Fig. 4.22. One of the first things you notice is that the ventricular rhythm is irregular. With AFib, atrial depolarization occurs very irregularly, which results in an irregular ventricular rhythm. The ventricular rhythm associated with AFib is described as irregularly irregular because there is no pattern to the irregularity. Because the ventricular rhythm is irregular, we will use the 6-second method of rate calculation to determine the ventricular rate, which is about 80 beats/min.

Because of the quivering of the atrial muscle and because there is no uniform wave of atrial depolarization in AFib, there is no P wave. Instead, you see a baseline that looks erratic (i.e., wavy). This corresponds with the rapid atrial rate. These wavy deflections are called *fibrillatory waves or* **f waves**. Some clinicians refer to fibrillatory waves of large amplitude as *coarse* fibrillatory waves and those of small amplitude as *fine* fibrillatory waves. This distinction has no clinical relevance.

We cannot measure a PR interval because there is no P wave. The QRS complex is narrow (i.e., measuring 0.08 to 0.10 second) because the impulse started above the bifurcation of the bundle of His and was conducted normally through the AV node and bundle and Purkinje fibers. We cannot measure a QT interval because T waves are not clearly seen.

AFib may be confused with MAT because both rhythms are irregular; however, P waves, although varying in size, shape, and direction, are clearly visible in MAT and a distinct isoelectric period is seen between P waves (Page et al, 2015). Suspect toxicity caused by digitalis, beta-blockers, or calcium channel blockers if AFib occurs with a slow, regular ventricular rate. This can occur when a patient who has AFib is prescribed medications to slow the ventricular rate. Excess medication can cause third-degree AV block (Fig. 4.23). When AFib is present with a third-degree AV

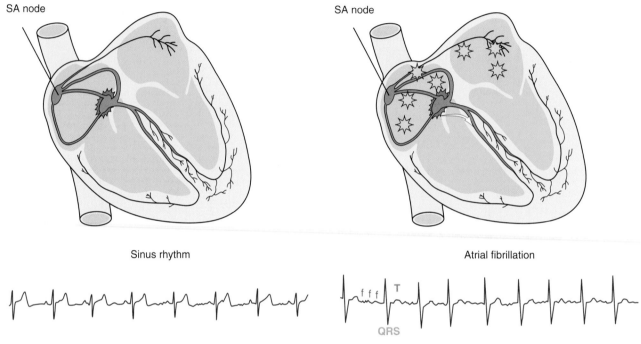

Sinus rhythm

Atrial fibrillation

Fig. 4.21 Atrial fibrillation. *f,* Fibrillatory wave; *SA,* sinoatrial.

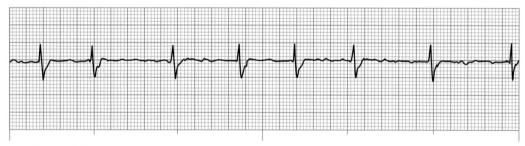

Fig. 4.22 Atrial fibrillation with a ventricular response of 80 beats/min. (From Aehlert B: *ECG study cards,* St. Louis, 2004, Mosby.)

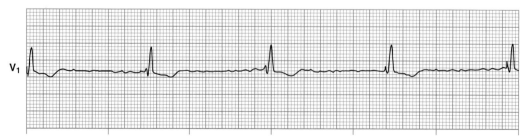

Fig. 4.23 Atrial fibrillation with third-degree atrioventricular block. The ventricular rate is slow and regular because of the block. (From Goldberger AL: *Clinical electrocardiography: a simplified approach,* ed 7, St. Louis, 2006, Mosby.)

block, the diagnosis of AFib is made on the basis of the presence of f waves (Morady & Zipes, 2015). The ECG characteristics of AFib are shown in Table 4.8.

What Causes It?

Although most patients with AFib have some form of cardiovascular disease, AFib can occur in patients without detectable heart disease or related symptoms. Examples of conditions that predispose patients to AFib appear in Table 4.9.

Patients who experience AFib are at increased risk of atrial thrombus formation, leading to stroke, peripheral thromboembolism, or both (January et al, 2014). Because the atria do not contract effectively and expel all of the blood within them, blood may pool within these chambers and form clots. A clot may dislodge on its own or because of conversion of AFib to a sinus rhythm.

What Do I Do About It?

AFib may occur as a self-limiting episode, it may come and go, or it may exist as a sustained rhythm. About 25% of patients who experience AFib are asymptomatic (Morady & Zipes, 2015). When symptoms are present, the severity of the signs and symptoms associated with AFib vary with the ventricular rate (either too fast or too slow), the loss of effective atrial contraction, sympathetic activation, and the beat-to-beat variability in ventricular

filling (January et al, 2014). Examples of common symptoms include fatigue (the most common symptom), chest discomfort or pain, dizziness, effort intolerance, lightheadedness, palpitations, shortness of breath, and heart failure.

Obtaining a thorough medical history and patient assessment are important. When obtaining the patient's history, asking about the number of episodes of AFib, their frequency, the nature of the patient's symptoms, and possible triggers may help to determine the pattern of the dysrhythmia.

Treatment decisions are based on the ventricular rate, the duration of the rhythm, the patient's general health, and how he or she is tolerating the rhythm. It is best to consult a cardiologist when considering specific therapies.

Rate control and rhythm control are the two primary treatment strategies used to control symptoms of AFib. With rate control, the patient remains in AFib, but the ventricular rate is controlled to decrease acute symptoms, reduce signs of ischemia, and reduce or prevent signs of heart failure from developing. With rhythm control, sinus rhythm is reestablished.

If AFib is associated with a rapid ventricular rate and the patient is stable but symptomatic, treatment is usually aimed at controlling the ventricular rate with medications such as beta-blockers (e.g., esmolol, metoprolol, propranolol) or nondihydropyridine calcium channel blockers (e.g., verapamil, diltiazem). Synchronized cardioversion should be considered if the patient with AFib has serious signs and symptoms because of the rapid ventricular rate. Because pharmacologic or electric cardioversion carries a risk of thromboembolism, anticoagulation is recommended before attempting conversion of AFib to a sinus rhythm when the duration of the AFib exceeds 48 hours (January et al, 2014). Catheter ablation is recommended for selected patients with AFib, such as those who have AFib with WPW syndrome and a history of syncope caused by the rapid heart rate. A summary of atrial rhythm characteristics can be found in Tables 4.10 and 4.11.

TABLE 4.8	Characteristics of Atrial Fibrillation
Rhythm	Ventricular rhythm usually irregularly irregular
Rate	Atrial rate usually 300 to 600 beats/min; ventricular rate variable
P waves	No identifiable P waves, fibrillatory waves present; erratic, wavy baseline
PR interval	Not measurable
QRS duration	0.11 sec or less unless abnormally conducted

TABLE 4.9	Conditions That Predispose Patients to Atrial Fibrillation		
Cardiovascular Conditions	**Noncardiovascular Conditions**	**Iatrogenic Causes**
• Coronary artery disease • Congenital heart disease (especially atrial septal defect in adults) • Dilated cardiomyopathy • Heart failure • Hypertension • Hypertrophic cardiomyopathy • Pericardial disease • Rheumatic heart disease • Valvular disease (especially mitral valve disease)	• Acute and chronic alcohol abuse • Autonomic stimulation • Diabetes mellitus • Electrocution • Hyperthyroidism • Obesity • Pulmonary diseases (i.e., chronic obstructive pulmonary disease, pneumonia) • Pulmonary embolism • Sleep apnea	• Antihistamines • Bronchodilating beta agonists • Cardiac and noncardiac surgery • Local anesthetics • Noncardiac diagnostic procedure • Nonprescription cold remedies

TABLE **4.10**	Atrial Rhythms: Summary of Characteristics			
Characteristic	PACs	Wandering Atrial Pacemaker	Atrial Tachycardia	AVNRT
Rhythm	Irregular because of the early beat(s)	May be irregular as pacemaker site shifts from SA node to ectopic atrial locations and AV junction	Regular	Ventricular rhythm is usually very regular
Rate (beats/min)	Usually within normal range, but depends on underlying rhythm	Usually 60 to 100; if rate greater than 100 beats/min, rhythm is called *multifocal atrial tachycardia*	101 to 250	150 to 250
P waves (lead II)	Premature, positive, one precedes each QRS, differ from sinus P waves, may be lost in preceding T wave	Size, shape, and direction may change from beat to beat	Atrial P waves differ from sinus P waves; isoelectric baseline usually present between P waves	P waves often hidden in QRS complex
PR interval	May be normal or prolonged	Varies	May be shorter or longer than normal	If P waves are seen, the PRI will usually measure 0.12 to 0.20 sec
QRS duration	0.11 sec or less unless abnormally conducted	0.11 sec or less unless abnormally conducted	0.11 sec or less unless abnormally conducted	0.11 sec or less unless abnormally conducted

AV, Atrioventricular; *AVNRT,* atrioventricular nodal reentrant tachycardia; *PAC,* premature atrial complex; *PRI,* PR interval; *SA,* sinoatrial.

TABLE **4.11**	Atrial Rhythms: Summary of Characteristics		
Characteristic	Atrial Flutter	Atrial Fibrillation (AFib)	Wolff-Parkinson-White (WPW) Pattern
Rhythm	Atrial regular, ventricular regular or irregular	Ventricular rhythm usually irregularly irregular	Regular, unless associated with AFib
Rate (beats/min)	Atrial rate typically 240 to 300; ventricular rate variable—determined by AV blockade	Atrial rate 300 to 600; ventricular rate variable	60 to 100 if the underlying rhythm is sinus in origin
P waves (lead II)	No identifiable P waves; saw-toothed "flutter" waves present	No identifiable P waves; fibrillatory waves present; erratic, wavy baseline	Normal and positive unless WPW is associated with AFib
PR interval	Not measurable	Not measurable	If P waves are seen, less than 0.12 sec
QRS duration	0.11 sec or less unless abnormally conducted	0.11 sec or less unless abnormally conducted	Usually greater than 0.12 sec; delta wave may be seen in one or more leads

AV, Atrioventricular.

STOP & REVIEW

True/False

Indicate whether the statement is true or false.

_____ **1.** MAT is another name for AFib.

_____ **2.** Synchronized cardioversion is recommended in the treatment of frequent PACs.

_____ **3.** Proper identification of wandering atrial pacemaker requires at least three different P waves, seen in the same lead.

Multiple Choice

Identify the choice that best completes the statement or answers the question.

_____ **4.** All supraventricular dysrhythmias
  a. involve accessory pathways.
  b. begin above the bifurcation of the bundle of His.
  c. begin below the bifurcation of the bundle of His.
  d. require the AV node's participation to sustain the dysrhythmia.

_____ **5.** On the ECG, an impulse that begins in the atria and occurs earlier than the next expected sinus beat will appear as a
  a. P wave that appears after the QRS complex.
  b. QRS measuring more than 0.11 second in duration.
  c. P wave with a PR interval measuring more than 0.20 second.
  d. P wave that may appear in the T wave of the preceding beat.

_____ **6.** A compensatory pause is a
  a. series of waveforms.
  b. delay that occurs following a premature beat that resets the SA node.
  c. period during the cardiac cycle during which cardiac cells can be stimulated to conduct an electrical impulse if exposed to a stronger than normal stimulus.
  d. period during the cardiac cycle during which cardiac cells cannot be stimulated to conduct an electrical impulse, no matter how strong the stimulus.

_____ **7.** The most common type of SVT is
  a. atrial flutter.
  b. AT.
  c. AVRT.
  d. AVNRT.

_____ **8.** Signs and symptoms experienced during a tachydysrhythmia are usually primarily related to
  a. atrial irritability.
  b. vasoconstriction.
  c. slowed conduction through the AV node.
  d. decreased ventricular filling time and stroke volume.

_____ **9.** The WPW pattern is associated with a
  a. short PR interval, delta wave, and wide QRS complex.
  b. long PR interval, delta wave, and normal QRS complex.
  c. long PR interval, flutter waves, and narrow QRS complex.
  d. short PR interval, fibrillatory waves, and narrow QRS complex.

_____ **10.** Which of the following ECG characteristics distinguishes atrial flutter from other atrial dysrhythmias?
  a. The presence of fibrillatory waves
  b. P waves of varying size and amplitude
  c. The presence of delta waves before the QRS
  d. The "saw-tooth" or "picket-fence" appearance of waveforms before the QRS

_____ **11.** In AFib, the PR interval is usually
  a. not measurable.
  b. within normal limits.
  c. less than 0.20 second in duration.
  d. more than 0.20 second in duration.

_____ **12.** Which of the following dysrhythmias is most likely to be associated with a reduction in cardiac output and loss of atrial kick?
  a. AFib
  b. Sinus tachycardia
  c. PACs
  d. Wandering atrial pacemaker

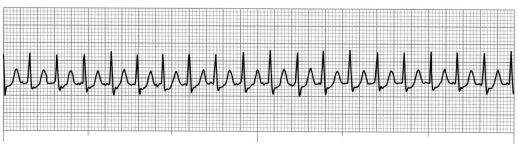

Fig. 4.24 (From Aehlert B: *ECG study cards,* St. Louis, 2004, Mosby.)

Questions 13 through 17 pertain to the following scenario.

A 35-year-old woman is complaining of palpitations.

_____ **13.** The patient is alert and oriented to person, place, time, and event. Her blood pressure is 144/82 mm Hg, and her ventilations are 18 breaths/min and unlabored. She appears anxious and states her "heart is racing." Which of the following statements is correct with regard to assessment of this patient?

    a. Despite the patient's age, palpitations generally indicate the presence of cardiac disease.

    b. A complaint of palpitations is a cause for concern only if they are of sudden onset and their rhythm is irregular.

    c. A complaint of palpitations is always associated with evidence of a rhythm disturbance on the cardiac monitor.

    d. Information relayed by the patient can provide important clues about her cardiovascular status.

_____ **14.** A pulse oximeter has been applied. The patient's oxygen saturation on room air is 97%. The cardiac monitor reveals the rhythm above (Figure 4.24). This rhythm, recorded in lead II, is

    a. sinus tachycardia.

    b. AVNRT.

    c. AVRT.

    d. AFib.

_____ **15.** The PR interval in Fig. 4.24

    a. is 0.06 second.

    b. is 0.12 second.

    c. is 0.20 second.

    d. cannot be measured.

_____ **16.** The QT interval in Fig. 4.24

    a. is 0.16 second.

    b. is 0.24 second.

    c. is 0.38 second.

    d. cannot be measured.

_____ **17.** Intravenous access has been established. A repeat set of vital signs reveals the following: blood pressure, 140/82 mm Hg; pulse, 188 beats/min; and ventilations, 20 breaths/min. The patient's anxiety has increased. She denies chest discomfort and shortness of breath. Her skin is pink and warm but moist. On the basis of the information provided, you should anticipate orders for which of the following?

    a. Immediate sedation

    b. Attempt vagal maneuvers

    c. Synchronized cardioversion

    d. Administer intravenous atropine

Matching

Match the terms below with their descriptions by placing the letter of each correct answer in the space provided.

a. Atrial kick

b. Premature

c. Beta-blockers

d. Accessory pathway

e. Trigeminy

f. Bruit

g. Adenosine

h. Delta wave

i. Uncontrolled

j. Nonconducted PAC

k. Atrial flutter

l. Aberrantly conducted PAC

m. Anticoagulant

n. Erratic

o. AFib

p. Vagal maneuvers

q. Palpitations

r. Stroke

s. Preexcitation

t. Multiform atrial rhythm

u. Bigeminy

_____ **18.** A dysrhythmia that requires at least three different P waves, seen in the same lead, for proper diagnosis

_____ **19.** Common complaint in a patient with a rapid heart rate

_____ **20.** Term used to describe a rhythm that originates above the ventricles and sends an impulse along a pathway outside the AV node and bundle of His.

_____ **21.** Baseline appearance in AFib
_____ **22.** ECG finding associated with WPW pattern
_____ **23.** Patients who experience AFib are at increased risk of having this.
_____ **24.** Blood pushed into the ventricles because of atrial contraction
_____ **25.** An extra bundle of working myocardial tissue that forms a connection between the atria and ventricles outside the normal conduction system
_____ **26.** Methods used to stimulate the vagus nerve in an attempt to slow conduction through the AV node, resulting in slowing of the heart rate
_____ **27.** This dysrhythmia has an irregularly irregular ventricular rhythm with no identifiable P waves.
_____ **28.** Atrial flutter or fibrillation with a rapid ventricular rate
_____ **29.** Every other beat comes from somewhere other than the SA node.
_____ **30.** An early P wave with no QRS following it
_____ **31.** Earlier than expected
_____ **32.** These should be avoided in the presence of severe underlying pulmonary disease.
_____ **33.** Blowing or swishing sound within a vessel
_____ **34.** The name given a PAC associated with a wide QRS complex
_____ **35.** Drug of choice for AVNRT
_____ **36.** This dysrhythmia has saw-tooth waveforms instead of P waves.
_____ **37.** Every third beat comes from somewhere other than the SA node.
_____ **38.** Before elective cardioversion, prophylactic treatment with a(n) ___ is recommended for the patient in atrial flutter or fibrillation.

Short Answer

39. PAT is visible on a patient's cardiac monitor. What does "paroxysmal" mean?

_____
_____
_____

40. Explain why patients who experience AFib are at increased risk of having a stroke.

_____
_____
_____

Atrial Rhythms—Practice Rhythm Strips

Use the five steps of rhythm interpretation to interpret each of the following rhythm strips. All rhythms were recorded in lead II unless otherwise noted.

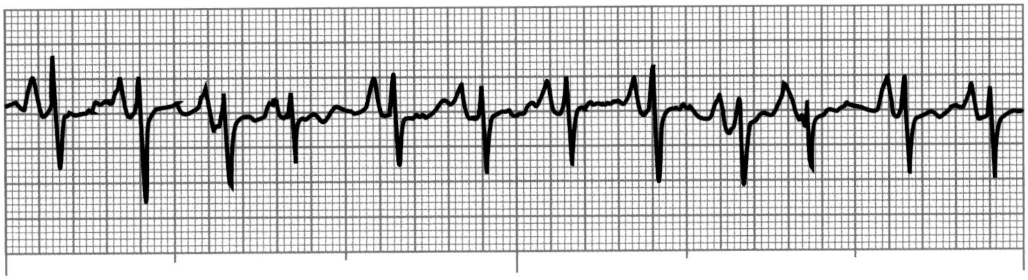

Fig. 4.25

41. Fig. 4.25
Rhythm: _____ Rate: _____ P waves: _____

PR interval: _____ QRS duration: _____ QT interval: _____

Interpretation: _____

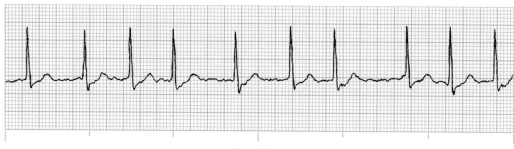

Fig. 4.26

42. **Fig. 4.26.** This rhythm strip is from an 85-year-old man complaining of chest pain and shortness of breath.

Rhythm: _____ Rate: _____ P waves: _____

PR interval: _____ QRS duration: _____ QT interval: _____

Interpretation: _____

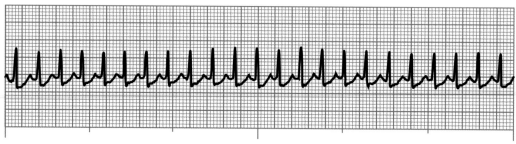

Fig. 4.27 (From Aehlert B: *ECG study cards*, St. Louis, 2004, Mosby.)

43. **Fig. 4.27.** This rhythm strip is from a 53-year-old woman with an altered level of responsiveness.

Rhythm: _____ Rate: _____ P waves: _____

PR interval: _____ QRS duration: _____ QT interval: _____

Interpretation: _____

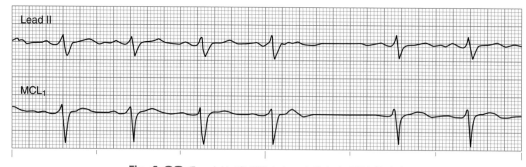

Fig. 4.28 (From Aehlert B: *ECG study cards*, St. Louis, 2004, Mosby.)

44. **Fig. 4.28.** These rhythm strips are from an 82-year-old man complaining of back pain.

Rhythm: _____ Rate: _____ P waves: _____

PR interval: _____ QRS duration: _____ QT interval: _____

Interpretation: _____

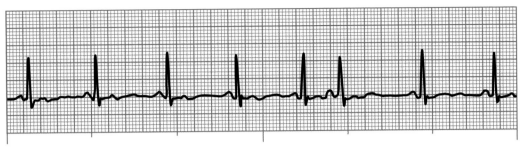

Fig. 4.29 (From Aehlert B: *ECG study cards,* St. Louis, 2004, Mosby.)

45. Fig. 4.29

Rhythm: _____ Rate: _____ P waves: _____

PR interval: _____ QRS duration: _____ QT interval: _____

Interpretation: _____

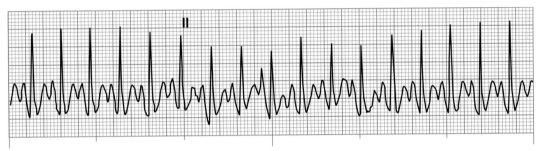

Fig. 4.30 (From Aehlert B: *ECG study cards,* St. Louis, 2004, Mosby.)

46. Fig. 4.30

Rhythm: _____ Rate: _____ P waves: _____

PR interval: _____ QRS duration: _____ QT interval: _____

Interpretation: _____

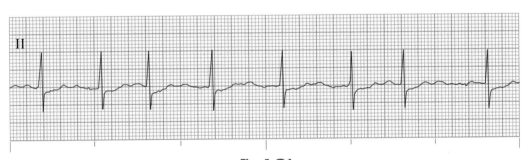

Fig. 4.31

47. Fig. 4.31

Rhythm: _____ Rate: _____ P waves: _____

PR interval: _____ QRS duration: _____ QT interval: _____

Interpretation: _____

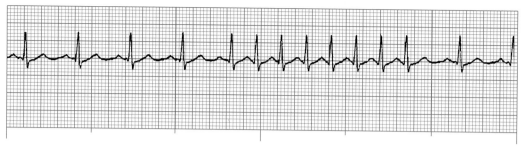

Fig. 4.32

48. **Fig. 4.32**

Rhythm: _____ Rate: _____ P waves: _____

PR interval: _____ QRS duration: _____ QT interval: _____

Interpretation: _____

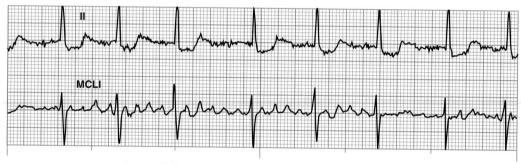

Fig. 4.33 (From Aehlert B: *ECG study cards*, St. Louis, 2004, Mosby.)

49. **Fig. 4.33**. These rhythm strips are from a 74-year-old woman with difficulty breathing.

Rhythm: _____ Rate: _____ P waves: _____

PR interval: _____ QRS duration: _____ QT interval: _____

Interpretation: _____

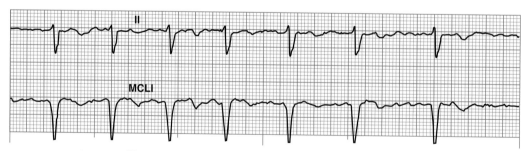

Fig. 4.34 (From Aehlert B: *ECG study cards*, St. Louis, 2004, Mosby.)

50. **Fig. 4.34**. These rhythm strips are from a 78-year-old man complaining of shortness of breath.

Rhythm: _____ Rate: _____ P waves: _____

PR interval: _____ QRS duration: _____ QT interval: _____

Interpretation: _____

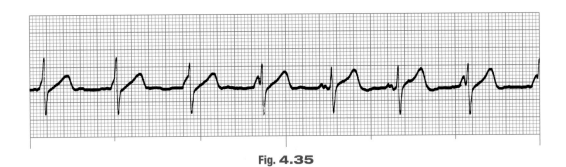

Fig. 4.35

51. **Fig. 4.35**

   Rhythm: _____ Rate: _____ P waves: _____

   PR interval: _____ QRS duration: _____ QT interval: _____

   Interpretation: _____

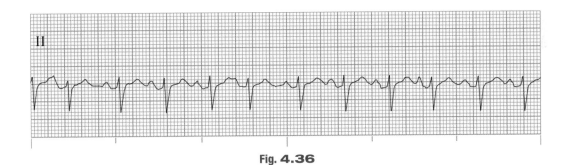

Fig. 4.36

52. **Fig. 4.36**

   Rhythm: _____ Rate: _____ P waves: _____

   PR interval: _____ QRS duration: _____ QT interval: _____

   Interpretation: _____

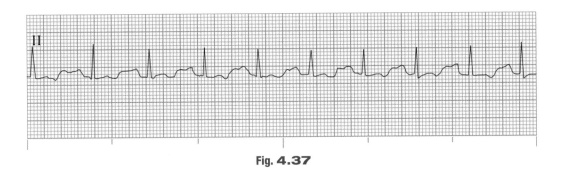

Fig. 4.37

53. **Fig. 4.37**. This rhythm strip is from a 45-year-old man who is complaining of chest pain.

   Rhythm: _____ Rate: _____ P waves: _____

   PR interval: _____ QRS duration: _____ QT interval: _____

   Interpretation: _____

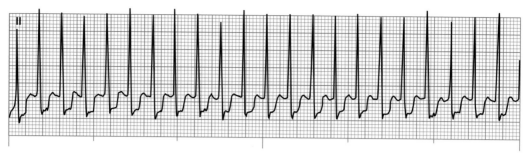

Fig. 4.38 (From Aehlert B: *ECG study cards,* St. Louis, 2004, Mosby.)

54. Fig. 4.38. This rhythm strip is from a 14-year-old adolescent complaining of chest pain.

Rhythm: _____ Rate: _____ P waves: _____

PR interval: _____ QRS duration: _____ QT interval: _____

Interpretation: _____

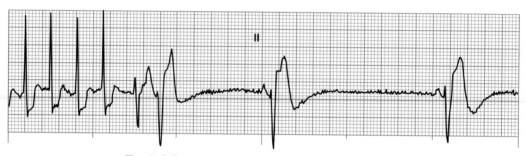

Fig. 4.39 (From Aehlert B: *ECG study cards,* St. Louis, 2004, Mosby.)

55. Fig. 4.39. This rhythm strip is from the same 14-year-old patient as in Fig. 4.38. This rhythm was observed after 6 mg of intravenous adenosine.

Rhythm: _____ Rate: _____ P waves: _____

PR interval: _____ QRS duration: _____ QT interval: _____

Interpretation: _____

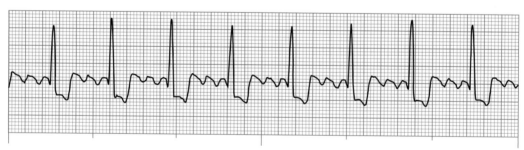

Fig. 4.40 (From Aehlert B: *ECG study cards,* St. Louis, 2004, Mosby.)

56. Fig. 4.40

Rhythm: _____ Rate: _____ P waves: _____

PR interval: _____ QRS duration: _____ QT interval: _____

Interpretation: _____

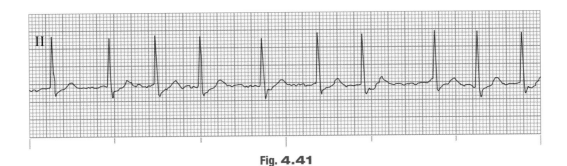

Fig. 4.41

57. **Fig. 4.41**

Rhythm: _____ Rate: _____ P waves: _____

PR interval: _____ QRS duration: _____ QT interval: _____

Interpretation: _____

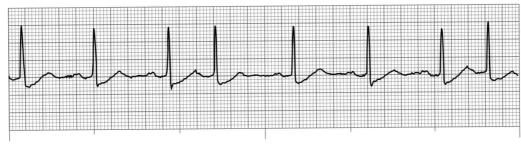

Fig. 4.42 (From Aehlert B: *ECG study cards,* St. Louis, 2004, Mosby.)

58. **Fig. 4.42**. This rhythm strip is from a 72-year-old man complaining of nausea and lightheadedness.

Rhythm: _____ Rate: _____ P waves: _____

PR interval: _____ QRS duration: _____ QT interval: _____

Interpretation: _____

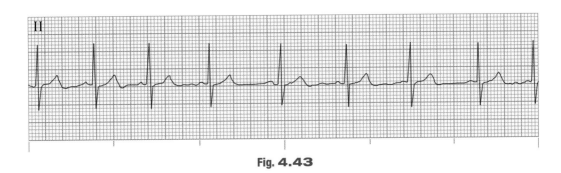

Fig. 4.43

59. **Fig. 4.43**. This rhythm strip is from a 6-year-old boy immediately after a seizure.

Rhythm: _____ Rate: _____ P waves: _____

PR interval: _____ QRS duration: _____ QT interval: _____

Interpretation: _____

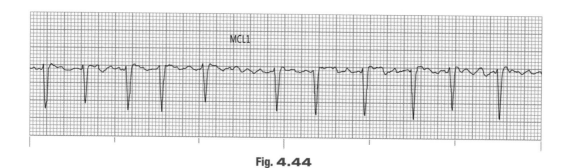

Fig. 4.44

60. **Fig. 4.44**

Rhythm: _____ Rate: _____ P waves: _____

PR interval: _____ QRS duration: _____ QT interval: _____

Interpretation: _____

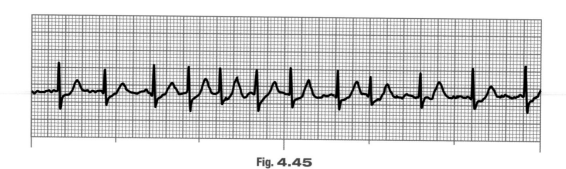

Fig. 4.45

61. **Fig. 4.45**

Rhythm: _____ Rate: _____ P waves: _____

PR interval: _____ QRS duration: _____ QT interval: _____

Interpretation: _____

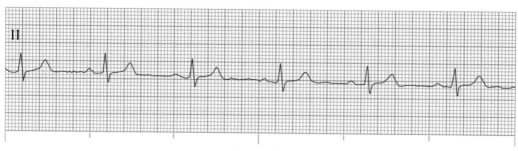

Fig. 4.46

62. **Fig. 4.46**. This rhythm strip is from a 54-year-old man who had a syncopal episode.

Rhythm: _____ Rate: _____ P waves: _____

PR interval: _____ QRS duration: _____ QT interval: _____

Interpretation: _____

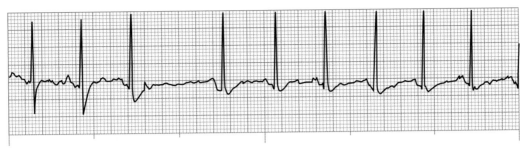

Fig. 4.47 (From Aehlert B: *ECG study cards,* St. Louis, 2004, Mosby.)

63. **Fig. 4.47**. This rhythm strip is from a 57-year-old man with no cardiac history.

Rhythm: _____ Rate: _____ P waves: _____

PR interval: _____ QRS duration: _____ QT interval: _____

Interpretation: _____

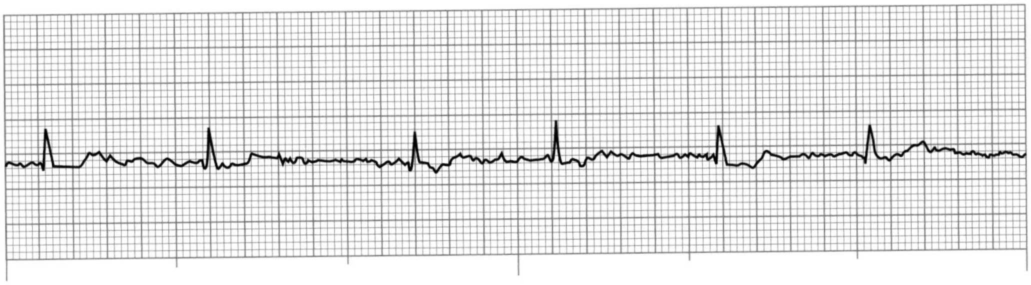

Fig. 4.48 (From Aehlert B: *ECG study cards,* St. Louis, 2004, Mosby.)

64. **Fig. 4.48**

Rhythm: _____ Rate: _____ P waves: _____

PR interval: _____ QRS duration: _____ QT interval: _____

Interpretation: _____

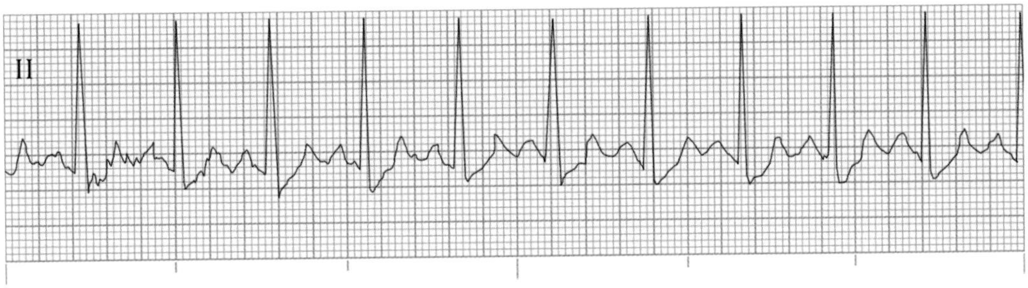

Fig. 4.49

65. **Fig. 4.49**. This rhythm strip is from a 67-year-old woman found unresponsive on the side of the road. Outdoor temperature was 112°F. Her blood pressure was 238/110 mm Hg, and her ventilatory rate was 60 breaths/min.

Rhythm: _____ Rate: _____ P waves: _____

PR interval: _____ QRS duration: _____ QT interval: _____

Interpretation: _____

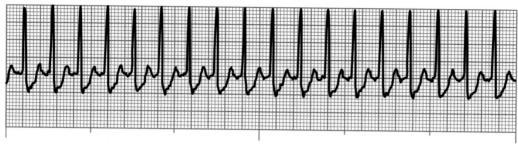

Fig. 4.50 (From Aehlert B: *ECG study cards,* St. Louis, 2004, Mosby.)

66. **Fig. 4.50.** This rhythm strip is from a 67-year-old woman complaining of dizziness and a "funny feeling" in her chest.

Rhythm: _____ Rate: _____ P waves: _____

PR interval: _____ QRS duration: _____ QT interval: _____

Interpretation: _____

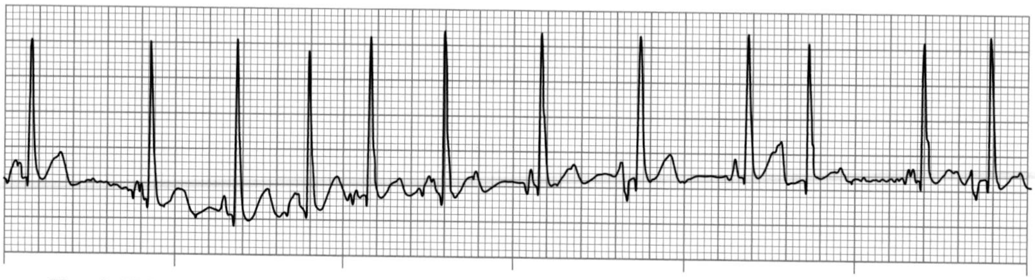

Fig. 4.51 (From Braunwald E, Libby P, Zipes DP, et al: *Heart disease: a textbook of cardiovascular medicine,* ed 6, St. Louis, 2001, Mosby.)

67. **Fig. 4.51**

Rhythm: _____ Rate: _____ P waves: _____

PR interval: _____ QRS duration: _____ QT interval: _____

Interpretation: _____

III

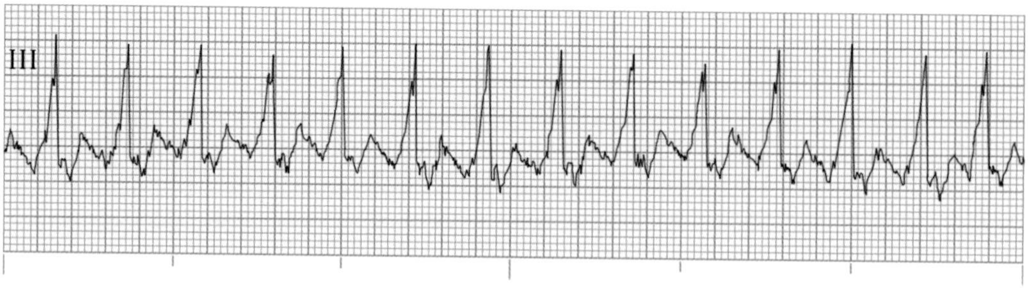

Fig. 4.52

68. **Fig. 4.52.** This rhythm strip is from an 81-year-old woman who experienced a massive myocardial infarction.

Rhythm: _____ Rate: _____ P waves: _____

PR interval: _____ QRS duration: _____ QT interval: _____

Interpretation: _____

Lead II (continuous)

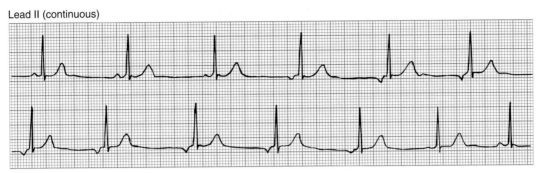

Fig. 4.53 (From Goldberger AL: *Clinical electrocardiography: a simplified approach,* ed 7, St. Louis, 2006, Mosby.)

69. Fig. 4.53

Rhythm: _____ Rate: _____ P waves: _____

PR interval: _____ QRS duration: _____ QT interval: _____

Interpretation: _____

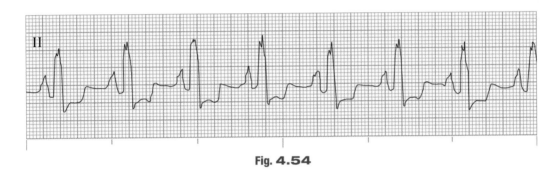

Fig. 4.54

70. Fig. 4.54. This rhythm strip is from a 62-year-old woman complaining of chest pain. She reported a history of three previous heart attacks and had undergone a three-vessel coronary artery bypass graft 10 years ago.

Rhythm: _____ Rate: _____ P waves: _____

PR interval: _____ QRS duration: _____ QT interval: _____

Interpretation: _____

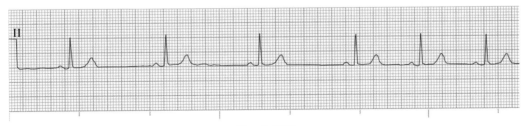

Fig. 4.55

71. Fig. 4.55

Rhythm: _____ Rate: _____ P waves: _____

PR interval: _____ QRS duration: _____ QT interval: _____

Interpretation: _____

STOP & REVIEW / ANSWERS

1. F. AFib may be confused with MAT because both rhythms are irregular; however, P waves, although varying in size, shape, and direction, are clearly visible in MAT. With AFib, there is no uniform wave of atrial depolarization; thus, there is no P wave. Instead, wavy deflections called *fibrillatory waves* or *f waves* are present.
OBJ: Describe the ECG characteristics, possible causes, signs and symptoms, and initial emergency care for MAT.

2. F. Electrical therapy, such as synchronized cardioversion, is not indicated in the treatment of PACs. Examples of rhythms treated with cardioversion include narrow-QRS tachycardias, AFib, atrial flutter, and monomorphic ventricular tachycardia. Frequent PACs are treated by correcting the underlying cause.
OBJ: Discuss the indications for synchronized cardioversion.

3. T. Wandering atrial pacemaker requires at least three different P waves, seen in the same lead, for proper diagnosis.
OBJ: Describe the ECG characteristics, possible causes, signs and symptoms, and initial emergency care for wandering atrial pacemaker (multiform atrial rhythm).

4. B. A supraventricular rhythm is one that originates from a site above the bifurcation of the bundle of His, such as the SA node, atria, or AV junction.
OBJ: N/A

5. D. When compared with the P-P intervals of the underlying rhythm, a PAC is premature—occurring before the next expected sinus P wave. PACs are identified by early (premature) P waves, positive (upright) P waves (in lead II) that differ in shape from sinus P waves (atrial P waves may be flattened, notched, pointed, biphasic, or lost in the preceding T wave), and early P waves that may or may not be followed by a QRS complex.
OBJ: Describe the ECG characteristics, possible causes, signs and symptoms, and initial emergency care for PACs.

6. B. A compensatory pause is a delay that occurs after a premature beat that resets the SA node. A series of waveforms is called a complex. The period during the cardiac cycle during which cardiac cells can be stimulated to conduct an electrical impulse if exposed to a stronger than normal stimulus describes the relative refractory period. The period during the cardiac cycle during which cardiac cells cannot be stimulated to conduct an electrical impulse, no matter how strong the stimulus describes the absolute refractory period.
OBJ: Explain the difference between a compensatory and noncompensatory pause.

7. D. AVNRT, which is caused by reentry in the area of the AV node, is the most common type of SVT.
OBJ: Describe the ECG characteristics, possible causes, signs and symptoms, and initial emergency care for AVNRT.

8. D. Signs and symptoms experienced during a tachydysrhythmia are usually primarily related to a decrease in the length of time spent in diastole. Remember that as the heart rate increases, there is less time for the ventricles to fill and less blood for the ventricles to pump out with each contraction. Thus, an excessively fast heart rate can lead to decreased cardiac output.

9. A. The WPW pattern includes a triad (meaning three) of ECG findings that consist of the following: (1) A short PR interval, (2) a delta wave, and (3) a wide QRS complex. In addition, secondary ST-segment and T-wave changes are often present.
OBJ: Describe the ECG characteristics, possible causes, signs and symptoms, and initial emergency care for AVRT.

10. D. With atrial flutter, atrial waveforms are produced that resemble the teeth of a saw, or a picket fence; these are called *flutter waves* or *F waves*.
OBJ: Describe the ECG characteristics, possible causes, signs and symptoms, and initial emergency care for atrial flutter.

11. A. Because there are no P waves associated with AFib, a PR interval cannot be measured.
OBJ: Describe the ECG characteristics, possible causes, signs and symptoms, and initial emergency care for AFib.

12. A. With AFib, rapid impulses cause the muscles of the atria to quiver (fibrillate). This results in ineffectual atrial contraction, decreased stroke volume, a subsequent decrease in cardiac output, and loss of atrial kick.
OBJ: Describe the ECG characteristics, possible causes, signs and symptoms, and initial emergency care for AFib.

13. D. Information relayed by the patient as part of the history can provide important clues to her cardiovascular (and pulmonary) status. Ask questions to find out the patient's description of her symptoms, when and how often they occur, how long they last, possible triggers, and what measures she has taken to relieve them. A complaint of palpitations warrants timely assessment and intervention, whether or not their rhythm is regular. It is important to determine if chest pain or discomfort, difficulty breathing, or shortness of breath accompanies her palpitations. Some practitioners recommend having the patient "tap out" the rhythm of the palpitations to help determine rhythmicity. Palpitations that occur regularly with a sudden onset and end usually are caused by AVNRT or AVRT. Irregular palpitations may be the result of premature complexes, AFib, or MAT. Patients may report palpitations even when there is no evidence of a rhythm disturbance on the cardiac monitor. This occurs most often in patients with anxiety disorders. Although symptoms such as

chest pain or discomfort, dyspnea, palpitations, edema, and syncope are classic symptoms of cardiac disease, they may also occur because of other organ system diseases (e.g., musculoskeletal, pulmonary, renal, and gastrointestinal).
OBJ: Describe the ECG characteristics, possible causes, signs and symptoms, and initial emergency care for AVNRT.

14. B. The rhythm shown is AVNRT at 188 beats/min.
OBJ: Describe the ECG characteristics, possible causes, signs and symptoms, and initial emergency care for AVNRT.

15. D. Because there are no P waves visible in Fig. 4.24, the PR interval cannot be measured.
OBJ: Define and describe the significance of each of the following as they relate to cardiac electrical activity: P wave, QRS complex, T wave, U wave, PR segment, TP segment, ST segment, PR interval, QRS duration, and QT interval.

16. B. The QT interval in Fig. 4.24 measures 0.24 second.
OBJ: Define and describe the significance of each of the following as they relate to cardiac electrical activity: P wave, QRS complex, T wave, U wave, PR segment, TP segment, ST segment, PR interval, QRS duration, and QT interval.

17. B. The patient is symptomatic but *stable*. Vagal maneuvers may be attempted. If vagal maneuvers were unsuccessful, anticipate orders for IV administration of adenosine. Sedation and cardioversion would be appropriate if the patient was *unstable* (showing signs of hemodynamic compromise). Because atropine is administered to increase heart rate and this patient is already tachycardic, it is contraindicated in this patient situation.
OBJ: Describe the ECG characteristics, possible causes, signs and symptoms, and initial emergency care for AVNRT.

18. T
19. Q
20. S
21. N
22. H
23. R
24. A
25. D
26. P
27. O
28. I
29. U
30. J
31. B
32. C
33. F
34. L
35. G
36. K
37. E
38. M

39. The term *paroxysmal* is used to describe a rhythm that starts or ends suddenly. Some practitioners use this term to describe the sudden onset or end of a patient's symptoms.
OBJ: Explain the terms paroxysmal atrial tachycardia and paroxysmal supraventricular tachycardia.

40. Because the atria do not contract effectively and expel all of the blood within them, blood may pool within them and form clots. A clot may dislodge on its own or because of conversion to a sinus rhythm. A stroke can result if a clot moves from the atria and lodges in an artery in the brain.
OBJ: Describe the ECG characteristics, possible causes, signs and symptoms, and initial emergency care for AFib.

Practice Rhythm Strip Answers

Note: Because of the distortion of ECGs that can occur during printing, a range of acceptable measurements is provided in the rhythm strip answers throughout this textbook.

41. Fig. 4.25
Rhythm: Irregular
Rate: 120 beats/min
P waves: Sinus P waves look alike; P waves of beats 4 and 10 are early
PR interval: 0.16 second
QRS duration: 0.08 to 0.10 second
QT interval: 0.28 second
Interpretation: Sinus tachycardia at 120 beats/min with PACs (beats 4 and 10)

42. Fig. 4.26
Rhythm: Irregular
Rate: 110 beats/min
P waves: Fibrillatory waves present
PR interval: None
QRS duration: 0.08 to 0.10 second
QT interval: 0.28 to 0.32 second
Interpretation: AFib at 110 beats/min

43. Fig. 4.27
Rhythm: Regular
Rate: 231 beats/min
P waves: None visible; hidden in T waves
PR interval: None
QRS duration: 0.06 to 0.08 second
QT interval: 0.24 second
Interpretation: AVNRT at 231 beats/min with ST-segment depression

44. Fig. 4.28
Rhythm: Irregular
Rate: 71 beats/min (sinus beats)
P waves: Upright before each QRS; one early P wave distorts the T wave of beat 4 (most clearly seen in lead MCL1)
PR interval: 0.20 second (lead II)
QRS duration: 0.12 second (lead II)
QT interval: 0.40 to 0.44 second (lead II)
Interpretation: Sinus rhythm at 71 beats/min with a wide QRS and a nonconducted PAC

45. **Fig. 4.29**

Rhythm: Irregular

Rate: 80 beats/min (sinus beats)

P waves: Upright before each QRS; an early P wave appears with beat 6

PR interval: 0.12 second (sinus beats)

QRS duration: 0.06 to 0.08 second (sinus beats)

QT interval: 0.24 second (sinus beats)

Interpretation: Sinus rhythm at 80 beats/min with a PAC (beat 6)

46. **Fig. 4.30**

Rhythm: Regular

Rate: 177 beats/min

P waves: Upright before each QRS

PR interval: 0.12 second

QRS duration: 0.06 to 0.08 second

QT interval: 0.20 to 0.24 second

Interpretation: Sinus tachycardia at 177 beats/min

47. **Fig. 4.31**

Rhythm: Irregular

Rate: 80 beats/min

P waves: Fibrillatory waves present

PR interval: None

QRS duration: 0.08 second

QT interval: Unable to determine; T waves are not consistently visible

Interpretation: AFib at 80 beats/min

48. **Fig. 4.32**

Rhythm: Irregular

Rate: 97 beats/min (sinus beats), 200 beats/min (PSVT)

P waves: Upright before each QRS (sinus beats); hidden in T waves (PSVT)

PR interval: 0.16 second (sinus beats)

QRS duration: 0.08 second

QT interval: 0.24 to 0.32 second

Interpretation: Sinus rhythm at 97 beats/min with a PAC precipitating a run of PSVT at 200 beats/min, back to a sinus rhythm at 97 beats/min

49. **Fig. 4.33**

Rhythm: Irregular

Rate: 80 beats/min

P waves: Flutter waves of varying ratios present

PR interval: None

QRS duration: 0.08 to 0.10 second

QT interval: Unable to determine

Interpretation: Atrial flutter at 80 beats/min

50. **Fig. 4.34**

Rhythm: Irregular

Rate: 70 beats/min

P waves: Fibrillatory waves present

PR interval: None

QRS duration: 0.10 to 0.12 second

QT interval: 0.32 second

Interpretation: AFib at 70 beats/min

51. **Fig. 4.35**

Rhythm: Regular

Rate: 70 beats/min

P waves: Upright before each QRS but vary in shape

PR interval: Varies

QRS duration: Varies

QT interval: 0.44 second

Interpretation: Underlying rhythm is sinus, but pacemaker site varies; ventricular rate about 70 beats/min; patient with known WPW syndrome; note the delta waves

52. **Fig. 4.36**

Rhythm: Irregular

Rate: 120 beats/min

P waves: Sinus P waves look alike; early P waves of beats 2 and 6 distort the T waves of the preceding beats

PR interval: 0.16 to 0.18 second (sinus beats)

QRS duration 0.08 to 0.10 second

QT interval 0.26 to 0.28 second

Interpretation Sinus tachycardia at 120 beats/min with two PACs (beats 2 and 6)

53. **Fig. 4.37**

Rhythm: Irregular (all beats but the first are regular)

Rate: 94 beats/min

P waves: Uniform and upright before each QRS

PR interval: 0.20 to 0.22 second

QRS duration: 0.06 second

QT interval: 0.32 second

Interpretation: Sinus rhythm at 94 beats/min with inverted T waves (because the rhythm is technically irregular, the rhythm could be interpreted as sinus arrhythmia)

54. **Fig. 4.38**

Rhythm: Regular

Rate: 214 beats/min

P waves: None visible; hidden in T waves

PR interval: None

QRS duration: 0.06 second

QT interval: 0.20 to 0.24 second

Interpretation: AVNRT at 214 beats/min with ST-segment depression

55. **Fig. 4.39**

Rhythm: Regular to irregular as rhythm conversion occurs

Rate: 214 beats/min (AVNRT) to about 30 beats/min (sinus beats)

P waves: None visible with AVNRT; upright before QRS with sinus beats

PR interval: 0.12 to 0.16 second (sinus beats)

QRS duration: 0.06 second (AVNRT, last sinus beat)

QT interval: 0.28 second (sinus beats)

Interpretation: AVNRT at 214 beats/min with ST-segment depression; rhythm conversion evidenced by a sinus beat, a possible PAC, and then sinus bradycardia at about 30 beats/min

56. **Fig. 4.40**
Rhythm: Regular
Rate: 85 beats/min
P waves: Flutter waves present
PR interval: None
QRS duration: 0.06 second
QT interval: Unable to determine
Interpretation: Atrial flutter at 85 beats/min with ST-segment depression

57. **Fig. 4.41**
Rhythm: Irregular
Rate: 100 beats/min
P waves: Fibrillatory waves present
PR interval: None
QRS duration: 0.06 to 0.10 second
QT interval: 0.32 second
Interpretation: AFib at 100 beats/min

58. **Fig. 4.42**
Rhythm: Irregular
Rate: 80 beats/min
P waves: Sinus P waves look alike; early P waves of beats 4 and 8 distort the T waves of the preceding beats
PR interval: 0.20 second (sinus beats)
QRS duration: 0.06 to 0.08 second
QT interval: 0.40 second
Interpretation: Sinus rhythm at 80 beats/min with two PACs (beats 4 and 8) and ST-segment depression

59. **Fig. 4.43**
Rhythm: Irregular
Rate: 90 beats/min (within normal limits for age)
P waves: Upright before each QRS; P wave amplitude varies among beats
PR interval: 0.08 to 0.16 second
QRS duration: 0.08 second
QT interval: 0.32 second
Interpretation: Sinus arrhythmia at 90 beats/min

60. **Fig. 4.44**
Rhythm: Irregular
Rate: 110 beats/min
P waves: Flutter waves present
PR interval: None
QRS duration: 0.08 to 0.10 second
QT interval: Unable to determine
Interpretation: Atrial flutter at 110 beats/min

61. **Fig. 4.45**
Rhythm: Irregular
Rate: 120 beats/min
P waves: Fibrillatory waves present
PR interval: None
QRS duration: 0.08 second
QT interval: 0.28 to 0.32 second
Interpretation: AFib at 120 beats/min

62. **Fig. 4.46**
Rhythm: Regular
Rate: 60 beats/min
P waves: Uniform and upright before each QRS
PR interval: 0.20 second
QRS duration: 0.08 second
QT interval: 036 second
Interpretation: Sinus rhythm at 60 beats/min

63. **Fig. 4.47**
Rhythm: Irregular
Rate: 90 beats/min
P waves: Upright before each QRS but some vary in shape and amplitude; an early P wave appears after beat 3
PR interval: 0.12 to 0.18 second
QRS duration: 0.08 second
QT interval: 0.28 to 0.30 sec; unable to clearly determine because of artifact
Interpretation: Sinus rhythm at 90 beats/min with a nonconducted PAC

64. **Fig. 4.48**
Rhythm: Irregular
Rate: 60 beats/min
P waves: Fibrillatory waves present
PR interval: None
QRS duration: 0.06 to 0.08 second
QT interval: Unable to determine
Interpretation: AFib at 60 beats/min

65. **Fig. 4.49**
Rhythm: Regular
Rate: 107 beats/min
P waves: Upright before each QRS; artifact present
PR interval: 0.16 to 0.18 second
QRS duration: 0.08 to 0.10 second
QT interval: 0.28 to 0.32 second; artifact present
Interpretation: Sinus tachycardia at 107 beats/min with ST-segment depression

66. **Fig. 4.50**
Rhythm: Regular
Rate: 177 beats/min
P waves: None visible; hidden in T waves
PR interval: None
QRS duration: 0.06 to 0.10 second
QT interval: 0.24 second
Interpretation: AVNRT at 177 beats/min with ST-segment depression

67. **Fig. 4.51**
Rhythm: Irregular
Rate: 120 beats/min
P waves: Vary in size, shape, and direction
PR interval: Varies
QRS duration: 0.08 to 0.10 second
QT interval: 0.24 to 0.28 second
Interpretation: MAT at 120 beats/min

68. Fig. 4.52

Rhythm: Irregular
Rate: 140 beats/min
P waves: Flutter waves visible despite artifact
PR interval: None
QRS duration: 0.12 to 0.16 second
QT interval: Unable to determine
Interpretation: Atrial flutter with a ventricular response of 140 beats/min

69. Fig. 4.53

Rhythm: Irregular
Rate: 50 beats/min (top strip)
P waves: Vary in size, shape, and direction
PR interval: Varies
QRS duration: 0.06 to 0.08 second
QT interval: 0.40 to 0.44 second
Interpretation: Wandering atrial pacemaker at 50 beats/min

70. Fig. 4.54

Rhythm: Regular
Rate: 75 beats/min
P waves: Upright before each QRS but vary in size and shape
PR interval: 0.16 to 0.18 second
QRS duration: 0.12 to 0.14 second
QT interval: 0.36 second
Interpretation: Sinus rhythm at 75 beats/min with wide, notched QRS complexes, ST-segment depression, and inverted T waves

71. Fig. 4.55

Rhythm: Irregular
Rate: 60 beats/min
P waves: Upright before each QRS but some vary in amplitude
PR interval: 0.14 to 0.16 second
QRS duration: 0.06 to 0.08 second
QT interval: 0.38 to 0.42 second
Interpretation: Sinus arrhythmia at 60 beats/min

REFERENCES

Appelboam, A., Reuben, A., Mann, C., Gagg, J., Ewings, P., Barton, A., & REVERT trial collaborators. (2015). Postural modification to the standard Valsalva manoeuvre for emergency treatment of supraventricular tachycardias (REVERT): a randomised controlled trial. *Lancet, 386*(10005), 1747–1753.

Ellenbogen, K. A., & Stambler, B. S. (2014). Atrial tachycardia. In D. P. Zipe & J. Jalife (Eds.), *Cardiac electrophysiology: From cell to bedside* (6th ed.) (pp. 699–722). Philadelphia: Saunders.

Fuster, V., Rydén, L. E., Cannom, D. S., Crijns, H. J., Curtis, A. B., Ellenbogen, K. A., & Wann, L. S. (2011). 2011 ACCF/AHA/HRS focused updates incorporated into the ACC/AHA/ESC 2006 guidelines for the management of patients with atrial fibrillation. *J Am Coll Cardiol, 57*(11), 1330–1337.

Goel, R., Srivathsan, K., & Mookadam, M. (2013). Supraventricular and ventricular arrhythmias. *Primary care, 40*(1), 43–71.

Hamdan, M. H. (2010). Cardiac arrhythmias. In T. E. Andreoli, I. J. Benjamin, R. C. Griggs, & E. J. Wing (Eds.), *Andreoli and Carpenter's Cecil essentials of medicine* (8th ed.) (pp. 118–144). Philadelphia: Saunders.

January, C. T., Wann, L. S., Alpert, J. S., Calkins, H., Cigarroa, J. E., Cleveland, J. C., & Yancy, C. W. (2014). 2014 AHA/ACC/HRS guideline for the management of patients with atrial fibrillation: a report of the American College of Cardiology/American Heart Association Task Force on Practice Guidelines and the Heart Rhythm Society. *J Am Coll Cardiol, 64*(21), e1–e76.

Lederer, W. J. (2012). Cardiac electrophysiology and the electrocardiogram. In W. F. Boron & E. L. Boulpaep (Eds.), *Medical physiology: A cellular and molecular approach* (2nd ed.) (pp. 504–528). Philadelphia: Saunders.

Leitch, J. W., & Barlow, M. (2010). Pre-excitation syndromes. In M. H. Crawford, J. P. DiMarco, & W. J. Paulus (Eds.), *Cardiology* (3rd ed.) (pp. 821–834). Philadelphia: Elsevier.

Link, M. S., Berkow, L. C., Kudenchuk, P. J., Halperin, H. R., Hess, E. P., Moitra, V. K., & Donnino, M. W. (2015, Oct). *2015 American Heart Association Guidelines for CPR & ECC*. Retrieved Oct 30, 2015, from American Heart Association. Web-based Integrated Guidelines for Cardiopulmonary Resuscitation and Emergency Cardiovascular Care – Part 7: Adult Advanced Cardiovascular Life Support Eccguidelines.heart.org.

Mani, B. C., & Pavri, B. B. (2014). Dual atrioventricular nodal pathways physiology: a review of relevant anatomy, electrophysiology, and electrocardiographic manifestations. *Indian Pacing Electrophysiol J, 14*(1), 12–25.

Mark, D. G., Brady, W. J., & Pines, J. M. (2009). Preexcitation syndromes: diagnostic consideration in the ED. *Am J Emerg Med, 27*(7), 878–888.

Morady, F., & Zipes, D. P. (2015). Atrial fibrillation: Clinical features, mechanisms, and management. In D. L. Mann, D. P. Zipes, P. Libby, R. O. Bonow, & E. Braunwald (Eds.), *Braunwald's heart disease: A textbook of cardiovascular medicine* (10th ed.) (pp. 798–820). Philadelphia: Saunders.

Olgin, J. E. (2008). Approach to the patient with suspected arrhythmia. In L. Goldman & D. Ausiello (Eds.), *Cecil medicine* (23rd ed.) (pp. 394–400). Philadelphia: Saunders.

Olgin, J., & Zipes, D. P. (2012). Specific arrhythmias: Diagnosis and treatment. In R. O. Bonow, D. L. Mann D. P. Zipes, & P. Libby (Eds.), *Braunwald's heart disease: A textbook of cardiovascular medicine* (9th ed.) (pp. 771–824). Philadelphia: Saunders.

Page, R. L., Joglar, J. A., Caldwell, M. A., Calkins, H., Conti, J. B., Deal, B. J., & Al-Khatib, S. M. (2015). 2015 ACC/AHA/HRS guideline for the management of adult patients with supraventricular tachycardia. *Circulation, 132*(14), 1–131.

Saksena, S., Bharati, S., Lindsay, B. D., & Levy, S. (2012). Paroxysmal supraventricular tachycardia and pre-excitation syndromes. In S. Saksena & A. J. Camm (Eds.), *Electrophysiological disorders of the heart* (2nd ed.) (pp. 531–558). Philadelphia: Saunders.

Walker, S., & Cutting, P. (2010). Impact of a modified Valsalva manoeuvre in the termination of paroxysmal supraventricular tachycardia. *Emerg Med J, 27*(4), 287–291.

Zimetbaum, P. (2016). Cardiac arrhythmias with supraventricular origin. In L. Goldman & A. I. Schafer (Eds.), *Goldman's Cecil medicine* (25th ed.) (pp. 356–366). Philadelphia: Saunders.

Junctional Rhythms

5

LEARNING OBJECTIVES

After reading this chapter, you should be able to:

1. Describe the electrocardiogram (ECG) characteristics, possible causes, signs and symptoms, and initial emergency care for premature junctional complexes (PJCs).
2. Describe the ECG characteristics and possible causes for junctional escape beats.
3. Explain the difference between PJCs and junctional escape beats.
4. Describe the ECG characteristics, possible causes, signs and symptoms, and initial emergency care for a junctional escape rhythm.
5. Describe the ECG characteristics, possible causes, signs and symptoms, and initial emergency care for an accelerated junctional rhythm.
6. Describe the ECG characteristics, possible causes, signs and symptoms, and initial emergency care for junctional tachycardia.

KEY TERMS

accelerated junctional rhythm: Dysrhythmia originating in the atrioventricular (AV) bundle with a rate between 61 and 100 beats/min

atrioventricular bundle: The bundle of His

atrioventricular node: A group of cells that conduct an electrical impulse through the heart; located in the floor of the right atrium immediately behind the tricuspid valve and near the opening of the coronary sinus

bundle of His: Fibers located in the upper portion of the interventricular septum that conduct an electrical impulse through the heart

junctional bradycardia: A rhythm that begins in the AV bundle with a rate of less than 40 beats/min

junctional escape rhythm: A rhythm that begins in the AV bundle; characterized by a very regular ventricular rate of 40 to 60 beats/min

junctional tachycardia: A rhythm that begins in the AV bundle with a ventricular rate of more than 100 beats/min

retrograde: Moving backward; moving in the opposite direction to that which is considered normal

INTRODUCTION

The **atrioventricular node** (AV node) is a group of specialized cells located in the lower part of the right atrium above the base of the tricuspid valve (Fig. 5.1). The AV node's main job is to delay an electrical impulse. This allows the atria to contract and complete filling of the ventricles with blood before the next ventricular contraction.

After passing through the AV node, the electrical impulse enters the **bundle of His**. The bundle of His, also called the *common bundle* or the **AV bundle**, is located in the upper part of the interventricular septum. It connects the AV node with the right and left bundle branches. The bundle of His has pacemaker cells that are capable of discharging at a rhythmic rate of 40 to 60 beats/min. The AV node and the nonbranching portion of the bundle of His are called the *AV junction* (Fig. 5.2). The bundle of His conducts the electrical impulse to the bundle branches.

Remember that the sinoatrial (SA) node is normally the heart's pacemaker. The AV junction may assume responsibility for pacing the heart if:

- The SA node fails to discharge (e.g., sinus arrest).
- An impulse from the SA node is generated but blocked as it exits the SA node (e.g., SA block).
- The rate of discharge of the SA node is slower than that of the AV junction (e.g., a sinus bradycardia or the slower phase of a sinus arrhythmia).
- An impulse from the SA node is generated and is conducted through the atria but is not conducted to the ventricles (e.g., an AV block).

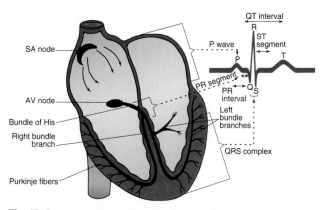

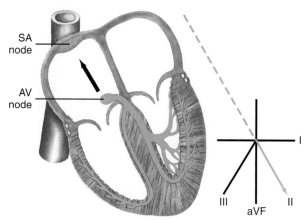

Fig. 5.1 The atrioventricular (AV) node is located in the lower portion of the right atrium. The bundle of His is located in the upper part of the interventricular septum. *SA*, Sinoatrial. (From Ignatavicius DD, Workman LM: *Medical-surgical nursing: patient-centered collaborative care*, ed 8, Philadelphia, 2016, Saunders.)

Fig. 5.3 If the atrioventricular (AV) junction paces the heart, the electrical impulse must travel in a backward (retrograde) direction to activate the atria. If a P wave is seen, it will be inverted in leads II, III, and aVF because the impulse is traveling away from the positive electrode. *SA*, Sinoatrial. (From Grauer K: *A practical guide to ECG interpretation*, ed 2, St. Louis, 1998, Mosby.)

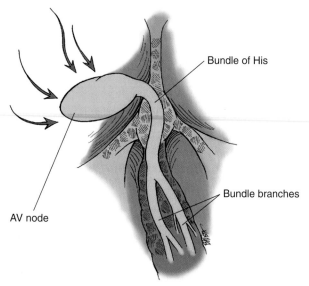

Fig. 5.2 The atrioventricular (AV) junction.

Rhythms that begin in the AV junction used to be called *nodal rhythms* until electrophysiologic studies proved the AV node does not contain pacemaker cells. The cells nearest the bundle of His are actually responsible for secondary pacing function. Rhythms originating from the AV junction are now called *junctional dysrhythmias*.

If the AV junction paces the heart, the electrical impulse must travel in a backward (**retrograde**) direction to activate the atria. If a P wave is seen, it will be inverted in leads II, III, and aVF because the impulse is traveling away from the positive electrode (Fig. 5.3). If the atria depolarize before the ventricles, an inverted P wave will be seen *before* the QRS complex, and the PR interval will usually measure 0.12 second or less (Fig. 5.4). The PR interval is shorter than usual because an impulse that begins in the AV junction does not have to travel as far to stimulate the ventricles. If the atria and ventricles depolarize at the same time, a P wave will not be visible because it will be hidden in the QRS complex. When the atria are depolarized after the ventricles, the P wave typically distorts the end of the QRS complex, and an inverted P wave will appear *after* the QRS. The QRS duration associated with a rhythm that begins in the AV junction measures 0.11 second or less if conduction through the bundle branches, Purkinje fibers, and ventricles is normal.

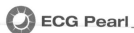 **ECG Pearl** _____

P waves are usually positive (i.e., upright) in lead I. Inverted P waves may be seen in some, all, or none of the chest leads.

PREMATURE JUNCTIONAL COMPLEXES

How Do I Recognize Them?

[Objective 1]

A PJC occurs when an irritable site (i.e., focus) within the AV junction fires before the next SA node impulse is ready to fire. This interrupts the sinus rhythm. Because the impulse is conducted through the ventricles in the usual manner, the QRS complex will usually measure 0.11 second or less. PJCs are sometimes called *premature junctional extrasystoles*. A noncompensatory (incomplete) pause often follows a PJC. This pause represents the delay during which the SA node resets its rhythm for the next beat. PJCs may occur in patterns—couplets, bigeminy, trigeminy, and quadrigeminy.

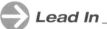 **Lead In** _____

Distinguishing PACs from PJCs

You can usually tell the difference between a PAC and a PJC by the P wave. A PAC typically has an upright P wave before the QRS complex in leads II, III, and aVF. A P wave may or may not be present with a PJC. If a P wave is present, it is inverted (retrograde) and may precede or follow the QRS. PJCs can be misdiagnosed when the P wave of a PAC is buried in the preceding T wave.

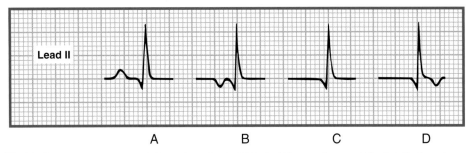

Fig. 5.4 A, With a sinus rhythm, the P wave is positive (upright) in lead II because the wave of depolarization is moving toward the positive electrode. The P wave associated with a junctional beat (in lead II) may be inverted (retrograde) and appear before the QRS B, be hidden by the QRS C, or appear after the QRS D. (From Grauer K: *A practical guide to ECG interpretation*, ed 2, St. Louis, 1998, Mosby.)

Junctional complexes may come early (before the next expected sinus beat) or late (after the next expected sinus beat). If the complex is *early*, it is called a *premature junctional complex*. If the complex is *late*, it is called a *junctional escape beat*. To determine if a complex is early or late, we need to see at least two sinus beats in a row to establish the regularity of the underlying rhythm.

Let's look at Fig. 5.5. Looking at the overall rhythm, it appears to be irregular. Because the rhythm is irregular, we estimate the rate using the 6-second method of rate calculation at 140 beats/min. All QRS complexes appear to be narrow, so we assume that all impulses started from above the ventricles. Using a pen or pencil, mark an "S" for SA node above each normal-looking P wave. Mark a "J" for junctional above those P waves that are inverted or absent. When you are finished, you should have a "J" marked over the P waves in beats 2, 5, 8, and 11. The rest of the P waves should be marked with an "S." Now take your calipers or a piece of paper and mark the third and fourth complexes in Fig. 5.5. We already determined that these complexes came from the SA node. These beats reflect the underlying rhythm. We now know that the underlying rhythm is a sinus tachycardia at about 140 beats/min. Now move your calipers or paper to the right. If beat 5 occurred on time (i.e., when the next sinus beat was expected), it will line up with your calipers or paper. The fifth complex is early; it occurred *before* the next expected sinus beat; therefore, this complex is a PJC. The other beats that have an inverted P wave before the QRS are also PJCs.

A PJC is not an entire rhythm; rather, it is a single beat. When identifying a rhythm, be sure to specify the underlying rhythm and the origin of the ectopic beat(s). In this rhythm strip, we found that the underlying rhythm was a sinus tachycardia at about 140 beats/min. All of the ectopic beats were early and came from the AV junction; therefore, we interpret this rhythm strip as sinus tachycardia at 140 beats/min with frequent PJCs. The ECG characteristics of PJCs are shown in Table 5.1.

What Causes Them?

Premature junctional complexes are less common than either PACs or PVCs. Causes of PJCs are shown in Box 5.1.

What Do I Do About Them?

PJCs do not normally require treatment because most individuals who have PJCs are asymptomatic. However, PJCs may lead to symptoms of palpitations or the feeling of skipped beats. Lightheadedness, dizziness, and other signs of decreased cardiac output can occur if PJCs are frequent. If PJCs occur because of ingestion of stimulants or digitalis toxicity, these substances should be withheld.

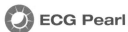 **ECG Pearl** _____

Keep in mind that inverted P waves are normal in lead V_1. To determine if a beat or rhythm came from the AV junction using this lead, look for a short PR interval. Use lead II, III, or aVF to confirm your findings.

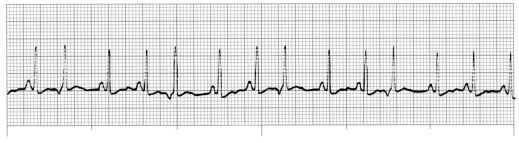

Fig. 5.5 Sinus tachycardia at 140 beats/min with frequent premature junctional complexes.

TABLE 5.1	Characteristics of Premature Junctional Complexes
Rhythm	Irregular because of the premature beats
Rate	Usually within normal range but depends on underlying rhythm
P waves	May occur before, during, or after the QRS; if visible, the P wave is inverted in leads II, III, and aVF
PR interval	If a P wave occurs before the QRS, the PR interval will usually be 0.12 sec or less; if no P wave occurs before the QRS, there will be no PR interval
QRS duration	0.11 sec or less unless abnormally conducted

Box 5.1	Causes of Premature Junctional Complexes

- Acute coronary syndromes
- Digitalis toxicity
- Electrolyte imbalance
- Heart failure
- Mental and physical fatigue
- Rheumatic heart disease
- Stimulants (e.g., caffeine, tobacco, cocaine)
- Valvular heart disease

JUNCTIONAL ESCAPE BEATS OR RHYTHM

How Do I Recognize It?

[Objectives 2, 3, 4]

A junctional escape beat begins in the AV junction and appears *late* (i.e., after the next expected sinus beat). Junctional escape beats frequently occur during episodes of sinus arrest or follow pauses of nonconducted PACs. Look at Fig. 5.6. Looking at the rhythm strip, you can see that the rhythm is irregular. There are three normal-looking beats on the left and two more on the far right. In the center of the strip is an odd-looking beat that appears in the middle of a long pause between beats 3 and 5. Looking more closely at beats 1, 2, 3, 5, and 6, you can see

an upright P wave before each QRS complex. These beats came from the SA node. On the basis of this information, we know that the underlying rhythm is sinus in origin. Using your calipers or a piece of paper, mark the first and second complexes. When you move the calipers or paper to the right, you can see that beat 4 came *late*—that is, after the next expected sinus beat.

Now let's try to figure out where beat 4 came from and why. If you put your finger over beat 4, can you explain what happened? The long pause between beats 3 and 5 is an episode of sinus arrest. Remember that if the SA node fails to initiate an impulse, an escape pacemaker site (i.e., the AV junction or ventricles) should assume responsibility for pacing the heart. Look closely at beat 4. The QRS complex is narrow, and there is no P wave before the QRS complex. The narrow QRS complex and absence of a positive P wave before the QRS complex tells us the beat came from the AV junction. Because the beat is *late*, it is a junctional escape beat. If beat 4 had been *early*, we would call it a PJC. What happened here? The SA node fired in beats 1, 2, and 3. When the sinus did not fire again when it should have, the AV junction kicked in and fired. Thus, a junctional escape beat is *protective*—preventing cardiac standstill. This beat is followed by two sinus beats. Complete identification of the events that occurred in this rhythm strip would be as follows: Sinus rhythm at 60 beats/min with an episode of sinus arrest and a junctional escape beat. The ECG characteristics of junctional escape beats are shown in Table 5.2.

 ECG Pearl

Junctional escape beats and rhythms occur when the SA node fails to pace the heart or AV conduction fails.

A junctional *rhythm* is several sequential junctional escape *beats*. The terms *junctional rhythm* and **junctional escape rhythm** are used interchangeably. Remember that the intrinsic rate of the AV junction is 40 to 60 beats/min. Because a junctional rhythm starts from above the ventricles, the QRS complex is usually narrow, and its rhythm is very regular.

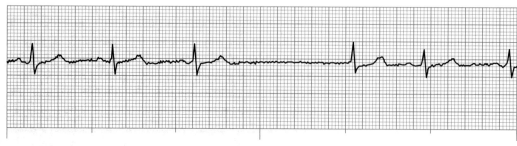

Fig. 5.6 Sinus rhythm at 60 beats/min with an episode of sinus arrest and a junctional escape beat. (From Aehlert B: *ECG study cards,* St. Louis, 2004, Mosby.)

If the AV junction paces the heart at a rate slower than 40 beats/min, the resulting rhythm is called a **junctional bradycardia**. This may seem confusing because the AV junction's normal pacing rate of 40 to 60 beats/min *is* bradycardic. However, the term *junctional bradycardia* refers to a rate slower than normal for the AV junction. Fig. 5.7 is a continuous rhythm strip. In *A*, you can see inverted (i.e., retrograde) P waves before the QRS complexes. In *B*, note the change in the location of the P waves. In the first beat, the retrograde P wave is seen before the QRS. In the second beat, no P wave is seen. In the remaining beats, the P wave is seen after the QRS complexes. The ECG characteristics of a junctional rhythm are shown in Table 5.3.

What Causes It?

Junctional escape beats frequently occur during episodes of sinus arrest or after pauses of nonconducted PACs.

Junctional escape beats may also be observed in healthy individuals during sinus bradycardia. Causes of a junctional rhythm include the following:

- Acute coronary syndromes (particularly inferior wall myocardial infarction [MI])
- Effects of medications (e.g., beta-blockers, digitalis, diltiazem, quinidine, verapamil)
- Hypoxia
- Immediately after cardiac surgery
- Increased parasympathetic tone
- Rheumatic heart disease
- SA node disease
- Valvular disease

TABLE 5.2	Characteristics of Junctional Escape Beats
Rhythm	Irregular because of *late* beats
Rate	Usually within normal range but depends on underlying rhythm
P waves	May occur before, during, or after the QRS; if visible, the P wave is inverted in leads II, III, and aVF
PR interval	If a P wave occurs before the QRS, the PR interval will usually be 0.12 sec or less; if no P wave occurs before the QRS, there will be no PR interval
QRS duration	0.11 sec or less unless abnormally conducted

TABLE 5.3	Characteristics of Junctional Escape Rhythm
Rhythm	Very regular
Rate	40 to 60 beats/min
P waves	May occur before, during, or after the QRS; if visible, the P wave is inverted in leads II, III, and aVF
PR interval	If a P wave occurs before the QRS, the PR interval will usually be 0.12 sec or less; if no P wave occurs before the QRS, there will be no PR interval
QRS duration	0.11 sec or less unless abnormally conducted

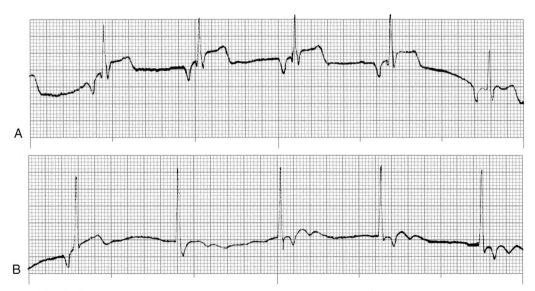

Fig. 5.7 Junctional escape rhythm. Continuous strips. A, Note the inverted (retrograde) P waves before the QRS complexes. B, Note the change in the location of the P waves. In the first beat, the retrograde P wave is seen before the QRS. In the second beat, no P wave is seen. In the remaining beats, the P wave is seen after the QRS complexes. (From Aehlert B: *ECG study cards,* St. Louis, 2004, Mosby.)

What Do I Do About It?

The patient may be asymptomatic with a junctional escape rhythm, or he or she may experience signs and symptoms that may be associated with the slow heart rate and decreased cardiac output. Treatment depends on the cause of the dysrhythmia and the patient's presenting signs and symptoms. Signs and symptoms may include weakness, chest pain or pressure, syncope, an altered level of consciousness, and hypotension. If the dysrhythmia is caused by digitalis toxicity, this medication should be withheld. If the patient's signs and symptoms are related to the slow heart rate, treatment should include application of a pulse oximeter and administration of supplemental oxygen, if indicated. Establish intravenous (IV) access and obtain a 12-lead ECG. Atropine, given IV, is typically the first medication given for symptomatic bradycardia. Reassess the patient's response and continue monitoring the patient.

ACCELERATED JUNCTIONAL RHYTHM

How Do I Recognize It?

[Objective 5]

If the AV junction speeds up and fires at a rate of 61 to 100 beats/min, the resulting rhythm is called an **accelerated junctional rhythm**. This rhythm is caused by abnormal automaticity of the bundle of His. The only ECG difference between a junctional rhythm and an accelerated junctional rhythm is the increase in the ventricular rate. An example of an accelerated junctional rhythm is shown in Fig. 5.8. The ECG characteristics of this rhythm are shown in Table 5.4, and Box 5.2 offers a snapshot of junctional rhythms.

What Causes It?

Causes of this dysrhythmia include acute MI, cardiac surgery, chronic obstructive pulmonary disease, digitalis toxicity, hypokalemia, and rheumatic fever.

What Do I Do About It?

The patient is usually asymptomatic because the ventricular rate is 61 to 100 beats/min; however, the patient should be

TABLE 5.4	Characteristics of Accelerated Junctional Rhythm
Rhythm	Very regular
Rate	61 to 100 beats/min
P waves	May occur before, during, or after the QRS; if visible, the P wave is inverted in leads II, III, and aVF
PR interval	If a P wave occurs before the QRS, the PR interval will usually be 0.12 sec or less; if no P wave occurs before the QRS, there will be no PR interval
QRS duration	0.11 sec or less unless abnormally conducted

Box 5.2	Junctional Dysrhythmias at a Glance
• Junctional rhythm: 40 to 60 beats/min • Accelerated junctional rhythm: 61 to 100 beats/min • Junctional tachycardia: 101 to 180 beats/min	

monitored closely. If the rhythm is caused by digitalis toxicity, this medication should be withheld.

JUNCTIONAL TACHYCARDIA

How Do I Recognize It?

[Objective 6]

Junctional tachycardia is an ectopic rhythm that begins in the pacemaker cells found in the bundle of His. When three or more sequential PJCs occur at a rate of more than 100 beats/min, a junctional tachycardia exists. Junctional tachycardias can be regular or irregular with variable conduction to the atria (Page et al, 2015). *Nonparoxysmal* (i.e., gradual onset) *junctional tachycardia* is a benign dysrhythmia that is usually associated with a gradual increase in rate (i.e., a warm-up pattern) to more than 100 beats/min. It rarely exceeds 120 beats/min (Zimetbaum, 2016). *Paroxysmal junctional tachycardia*, which is also known as *focal* or *automatic junctional tachycardia*, is an uncommon dysrhythmia that starts and ends suddenly and that is often precipitated by a PJC. The ventricular rate for paroxysmal junctional tachycardia is generally faster, at a rate of 140 beats/min or more. When the ventricular rate is greater than 150 beats/min, it is difficult to distinguish junctional tachycardia from

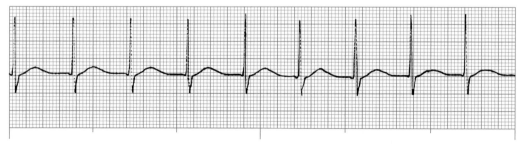

Fig. 5.8 Accelerated junctional rhythm at 93 beats/min.

other supraventricular tachycardias. An example of junctional tachycardia is shown in Fig. 5.9. The ECG characteristics of this rhythm are shown in Table 5.5.

What Causes It?

Junctional tachycardia is uncommon in adults and more common in children (Kumar et al, 2006). When it occurs, it is generally caused by abnormal automaticity or triggered activity (Kumar et al, 2006). Junctional tachycardia may occur because of an acute coronary syndrome, digitalis toxicity, heart failure, or theophylline administration.

What Do I Do About It?

Patients experiencing a junctional tachycardia may be asymptomatic. With sustained ventricular rates of 150 beats/min or more, the patient may complain of fatigue, palpitations, or chest discomfort or may experience syncope. Symptoms are most common at the onset of the dysrhythmia (Zimetbaum, 2016). Because of the fast ventricular rate, the ventricles may be unable to fill completely, which results in decreased cardiac output. The more rapid the rate, the greater the incidence of symptoms because of increased myocardial oxygen demand. Junctional tachycardia associated with an acute coronary syndrome may do the following:

- Cause heart failure, hypotension, or cardiogenic shock
- Extend the size of an MI
- Increase myocardial ischemia
- Increase the frequency and severity of chest pain
- Predispose the patient to ventricular dysrhythmias

Treatment depends on the severity of the patient's signs and symptoms, and expert consultation is advised. If the patient tolerates the rhythm, observation is often all that is needed. If the patient is symptomatic because of the rapid rate, initial treatment should include application of a pulse oximeter and administration of supplemental oxygen, if indicated. Establish IV access and obtain a 12-lead ECG. Because it is often difficult to distinguish junctional tachycardia from other narrow-QRS tachycardias, vagal maneuvers and, if necessary, IV adenosine may be ordered to help determine the origin of the rhythm. If the rhythm is the result of digitalis toxicity, the medication should be withheld. If the rhythm is the result of theophylline administration, the infusion should be slowed or stopped. A beta-blocker or calcium channel blocker may be ordered (if no contraindications exist) to slow conduction through the AV node and thereby slow the ventricular rate. A summary of junctional rhythm characteristics appears in Table 5.6.

 Drug Pearl _____

Patients who do not tolerate treatment with antiarrhythmic medications or who have recurring episodes of junctional tachycardia may be referred for radiofrequency ablation.

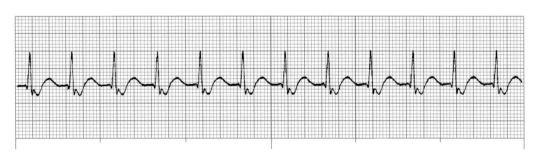

Fig. 5.9 Junctional tachycardia at 115 beats/min.

TABLE 5.5	Characteristics of Junctional Tachycardia
Rhythm	Ventricular rhythm may be regular or irregular
Rate	101 to 180 beats/min
P waves	May occur before, during, or after the QRS; if visible, the P wave is inverted in leads II, III, and aVF
PR interval	If a P wave occurs before the QRS, the PR interval will usually be 0.12 sec or less; if no P wave occurs before the QRS, there will be no PR interval
QRS duration	0.11 sec or less unless abnormally conducted

TABLE 5.6	Junctional Rhythms: Summary of Characteristics				
Characteristic	PJCs	Junctional Escape Beat	Junctional Escape Rhythm	Accelerated Junctional Rhythm	Junctional Tachycardia
Rhythm	Irregular because of *premature* beats	Irregular because of *late* beats	Regular	Regular	Regular or irregular
Rate (beats/min)	Usually within normal range but depends on underlying rhythm	Usually within normal range but depends on underlying rhythm	40 to 60	61 to 100	101 to 180
P waves (leads II, III, aVF)	May occur before, during, or after the QRS; if visible, the P wave is inverted	May occur before, during, or after the QRS; if visible, the P wave is inverted	May occur before, during, or after the QRS; if visible, the P wave is inverted	May occur before, during, or after the QRS; if visible, the P wave is inverted	May occur before, during, or after the QRS; if visible, the P wave is inverted
PR interval	If a P wave occurs before the QRS, the PR interval will usually be 0.12 sec or less; if no P wave occurs before the QRS, there will be no PR interval	If a P wave occurs before the QRS, the PR interval will usually be 0.12 sec or less; if no P wave occurs before the QRS, there will be no PR interval	If a P wave occurs before the QRS, the PR interval will usually be 0.12 sec or less; if no P wave occurs before the QRS, there will be no PR interval	If a P wave occurs before the QRS, the PR interval will usually be 0.12 sec or less; if no P wave occurs before the QRS, there will be no PR interval	If a P wave occurs before the QRS, the PR interval will usually be 0.12 sec or less; if no P wave occurs before the QRS, there will be no PR interval
QRS duration	0.11 sec or less unless abnormally conducted	0.11 sec or less unless abnormally conducted	0.11 sec or less unless abnormally conducted	0.11 sec or less unless abnormally conducted	0.11 sec or less unless abnormally conducted

PJC, Premature junctional complex.

STOP & REVIEW

True/False

Indicate whether the statement is true or false.

_____ **1.** Premature junctional complexes are more common than PACs or PVCs.

_____ **2.** A PJC produces a positive (upright) P wave in leads II, III, and aVF that comes before, during, or after the QRS complex.

_____ **3.** The intrinsic rate of the AV junction is 20 to 40 beats/min.

Multiple Choice

Identify the choice that best completes the statement or answers the question.

_____ **4.** The term *junctional bradycardia* is used to describe a rhythm that is junctional in origin with
  a. an atrial rate of 40 to 60 beats/min.
  b. an atrial rate slower than 60 beats/min.
  c. a ventricular rate of 40 to 60 beats/min.
  d. a ventricular rate slower than 40 beats/min.

_____ **5.** A _____ pause often follows a PJC and represents the delay during which the SA node resets its rhythm for the next beat.
  a. noncompensatory (incomplete)
  b. compensatory (complete)

_____ **6.** In rhythms originating from the AV junction, the QRS duration is typically _____ or less unless an intraventricular conduction delay exists.
  a. 0.04 second
  b. 0.11 second
  c. 0.14 second
  d. 0.20 second

_____ **7.** An accelerated junctional rhythm is identified by a regular ventricular response occurring at a rate of
  a. 20 to 40 beats/min.
  b. 40 to 60 beats/min.
  c. 61 to 100 beats/min.
  d. 101 to 180 beats/min.

_____ **8.** Select the *incorrect* statement regarding junctional dysrhythmias.
  a. A junctional rhythm may be seen in acute coronary syndromes.
  b. An accelerated junctional rhythm is a potentially life-threatening dysrhythmia.
  c. The ventricular rhythm associated with a junctional rhythm is typically very regular.
  d. The QRS complex of a PJC is typically markedly different from the QRS complex of a beat conducted by the SA node.

_____ **9.** The primary waveform used to differentiate PJCs from PACs is the
  a. P wave.
  b. Q wave.
  c. R wave.
  d. T wave.

_____ **10.** In a junctional rhythm viewed in lead II, where is the location of the P wave on the ECG if ventricular depolarization precedes atrial depolarization?
  a. Before the QRS complex
  b. During the QRS complex
  c. After the QRS complex

Questions 11 to 14 pertain to the following scenario.

A 63-year-old man is complaining of dizziness that began about 45 minutes ago while he was cleaning his garage. Because the patient's oxygen saturation level on room air was 88%, supplemental oxygen is being administered. The cardiac monitor has been applied, revealing the rhythm below. A coworker is attempting to establish intravenous access.

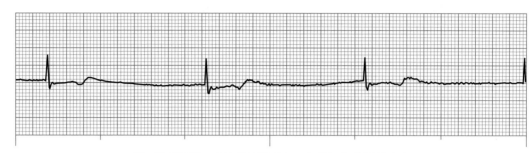

Fig. 5.10 (From Aehlert B: *ECG study cards,* St. Louis, 2004, Mosby.)

_____ **11.** Which of the following statements is true with regard to this patient's cardiac rhythm?
  a. The atrial rhythm is irregular.
  b. There are more P waves than QRS complexes.
  c. The ventricular rhythm is regular and the QRS is wide.
  d. The ventricular rhythm is regular and the QRS is narrow.

_____ **12.** The patient's ventricular rate is
  a. 32 beats/min.
  b. 45 beats/min.
  c. 60 beats/min.
  d. 75 beats/min.

_____ **13.** The rhythm shown on the cardiac monitor is
  a. sinus bradycardia.
  b. junctional bradycardia.
  c. junctional escape rhythm.
  d. accelerated junctional rhythm.

_____ **14.** The patient's blood pressure is 82/50 mm Hg and ventilations are 16 breaths/min. He states that his normal blood pressure is about 130/80 mm Hg. The patient denies chest discomfort and states that he takes no prescription medications. His skin is cool, pink, and moist, and his breath sounds are clear. Intravenous access has been successfully established. On the basis of the information provided, which of the following statements is true regarding this patient situation?
  a. Because the patient is symptomatic with this rhythm, a vagal maneuver should be attempted.
  b. The patient is symptomatic with this rhythm. Obtain a 12-lead ECG and then administer atropine IV.
  c. Therapeutic interventions are not indicated because there is no evidence of ST-segment elevation (STE) on the cardiac monitor.
  d. Although the patient is complaining of dizziness, this symptom does not warrant any further intervention other than cardiac monitoring at this time.

Matching

Match the terms below with their descriptions by placing the letter of each correct answer in the space provided.

a. Retrograde
b. Accelerated junctional rhythm
c. Nodal rhythms
d. Inverted P wave appears before the QRS complex in leads II, III, and aVF
e. Location of the AV node
f. Junctional tachycardia
g. Digitalis
h. Hidden within the QRS complex (not visible)
i. Location of the bundle of His
j. Premature junctional complex

_____ **15.** Lower part of the right atrium above the base of the tricuspid valve
_____ **16.** Name given to a dysrhythmia that originates in the AV junction with a ventricular rate between 101 to 180 beats/min
_____ **17.** Upper part of the interventricular septum
_____ **18.** Location of the P wave on the ECG if atrial and ventricular depolarization occurs simultaneously
_____ **19.** Term formerly used for dysrhythmias that originate in the AV junction

_____ **20.** A beat originating within the AV junction that appears earlier than the next expected sinus beat
_____ **21.** Name given to a dysrhythmia that originates in the AV junction with a ventricular rate between 61 to 100 beats/min
_____ **22.** Occurring in a backward direction
_____ **23.** Location of the P wave on the ECG if atrial depolarization precedes ventricular depolarization
_____ **24.** Excess of this medication is a common cause of junctional dysrhythmias

Short Answer

25. Fill in the blank areas in the table below to help you recall the primary differences among junctional rhythm, accelerated junctional rhythm, and junctional tachycardia.

ECG Finding	Junctional Rhythm	Accelerated Junctional Rhythm	Junctional Tachycardia
Rhythm	Regular	Regular	Regular or irregular
Rate (beats/min)	_____	_____	_____
P waves (lead II)	_____	_____	_____
PR interval	_____	_____	_____
QRS duration	0.11 sec or less unless abnormally conducted	0.11 sec or less unless abnormally conducted	0.11 sec or less unless abnormally conducted

Junctional Rhythms—Practice Rhythm Strips

Use the five steps of rhythm interpretation to interpret each of the following rhythm strips. All rhythms were recorded in lead II unless otherwise noted.

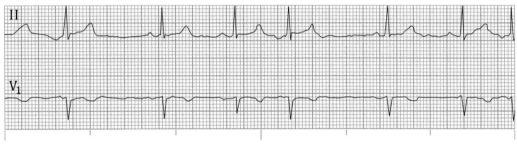

Fig. **5.11**

26. Fig. 5.11

Rhythm: _____ Rate: _____ P waves: _____

PR interval: _____ QRS duration: _____ QT interval: _____

Interpretation: _____

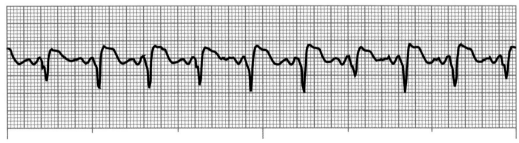

Fig. **5.12**

27. Fig. 5.12. Identify the rhythm (lead III).

Rhythm: _____ Rate: _____ P waves: _____

PR interval: _____ QRS duration: _____ QT interval: _____

Interpretation: _____

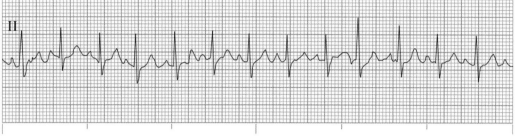

Fig. 5.13

28. **Fig. 5.13**. This rhythm strip is from a 74-year-old woman with chest pain. She rated her pain 9/10.

Rhythm: _____ Rate: _____ P waves: _____

PR interval: _____ QRS duration: _____ QT interval: _____

Interpretation: _____

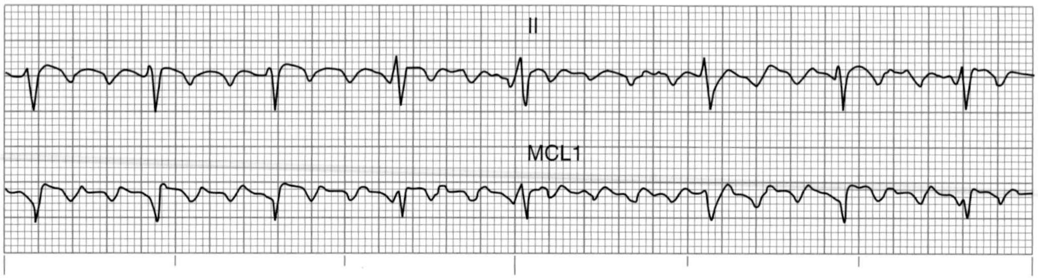

Fig. 5.14 (From Aehlert B: *ECG study cards,* St. Louis, 2004, Mosby.)

29. **Fig. 5.14**

Rhythm: _____ Rate: _____ P waves: _____

PR interval: _____ QRS duration: _____ QT interval: _____

Interpretation: _____

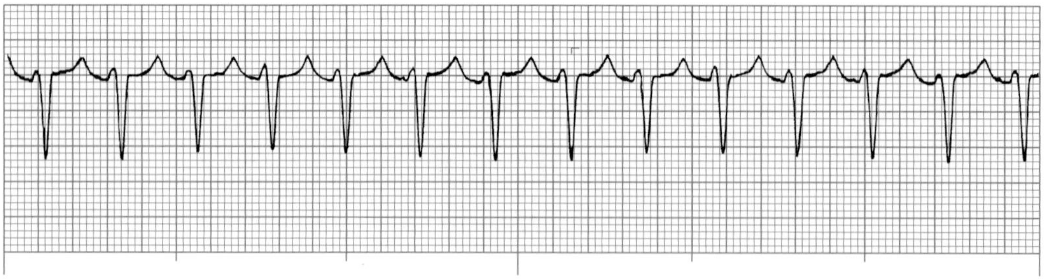

Fig. 5.15

30. **Fig. 5.15**

Rhythm: _____ Rate: _____ P waves: _____

PR interval: _____ QRS duration: _____ QT interval: _____

Interpretation: _____

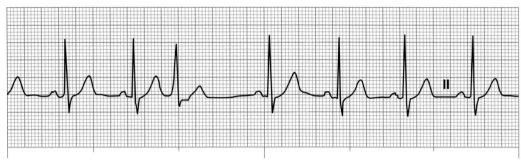

Fig. 5.16 (From Aehlert B: *ECG study cards*, St. Louis, 2004, Mosby.)

31. Fig. 5.16

Rhythm: _____ Rate: _____ P waves: _____

PR interval: _____ QRS duration: _____ QT interval: _____

Interpretation: _____

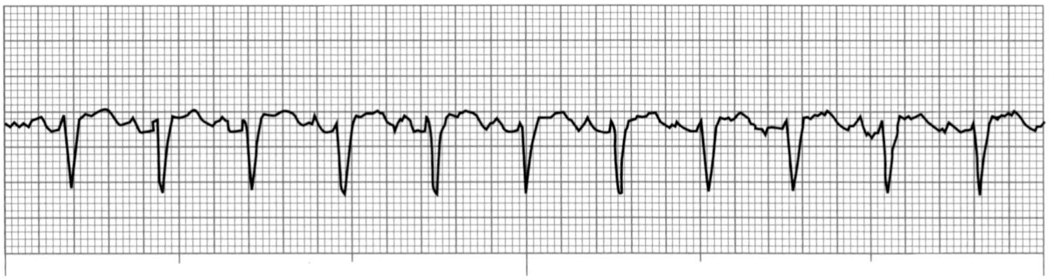

Fig. 5.17 (From Aehlert B: *ECG study cards*, St. Louis, 2004, Mosby.)

32. Fig. 5.17. This rhythm strip is from an 80-year-old woman who states, "The room is spinning."

Rhythm: _____ Rate: _____ P waves: _____

PR interval: _____ QRS duration: _____ QT interval: _____

Interpretation: _____

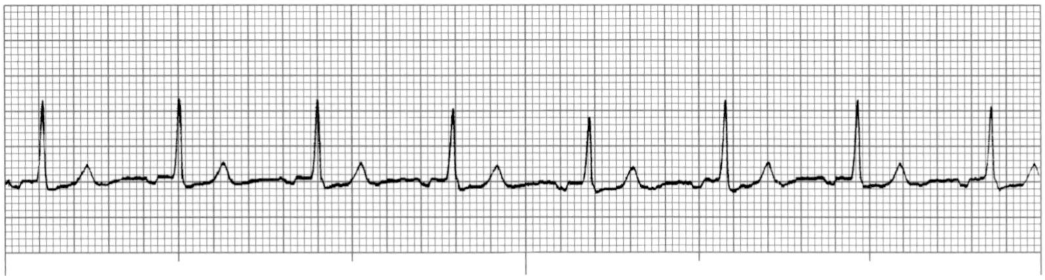

Fig. 5.18

33. Fig. 5.18. This rhythm strip is from an 88-year-old woman who experienced a syncopal episode. Her medical history includes a myocardial infarction 9 years ago, a stroke 5 years ago, hypertension, and diabetes.

Rhythm: _____ Rate: _____ P waves: _____

PR interval: _____ QRS duration: _____ QT interval: _____

Interpretation: _____

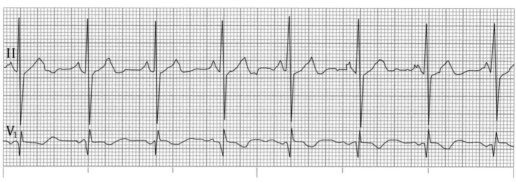

Fig. 5.19

34. **Fig. 5.19**. This rhythm strip is from a 72-year-old man presenting with left-sided weakness. He has a history of a brain tumor.

Rhythm: _____ Rate: _____ P waves: _____

PR interval: _____ QRS duration: _____ QT interval: _____

Interpretation: _____

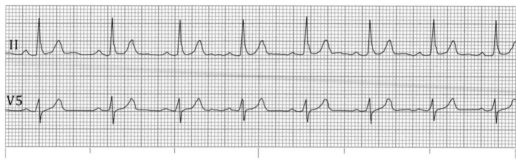

Fig. 5.20

35. **Fig. 5.20**

Rhythm: _____ Rate: _____ P waves: _____

PR interval: _____ QRS duration: _____ QT interval: _____

Interpretation: _____

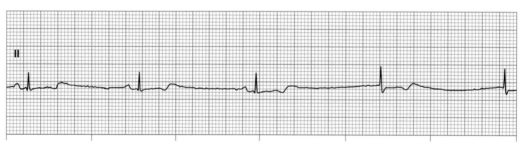

Fig. 5.21 (From Aehlert B: *ECG study cards,* St. Louis, 2004, Mosby.)

36. **Fig. 5.21**

Rhythm: _____ Rate: _____ P waves: _____

PR interval: _____ QRS duration: _____ QT interval: _____

Interpretation: _____

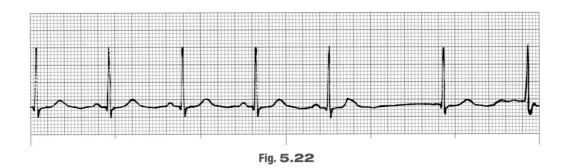

Fig. 5.22

37. **Fig. 5.22**

Rhythm: _____ Rate: _____ P waves: _____

PR interval: _____ QRS duration: _____ QT interval: _____

Interpretation: _____

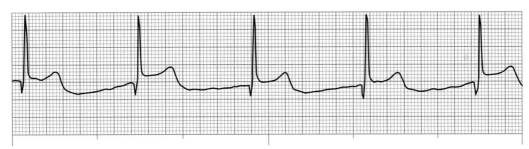

Fig. 5.23 (From Aehlert B: *ECG study cards,* St. Louis, 2004, Mosby.)

38. **Fig. 5.23**

Rhythm: _____ Rate: _____ P waves: _____

PR interval: _____ QRS duration: _____ QT interval: _____

Interpretation: _____

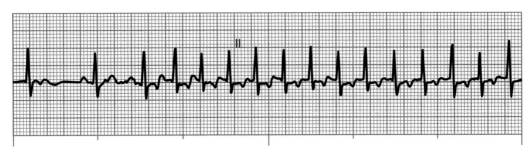

Fig. 5.24 (From Aehlert B: *ECG study cards,* St. Louis, 2004, Mosby.)

39. **Fig. 5.24**. This rhythm strip is from a 43-year-old woman who was complaining of palpitations. The patient had a history of supraventricular tachycardia and stated that she could not tolerate adenosine.

Rhythm: _____ Rate: _____ P waves: _____

PR interval: _____ QRS duration: _____ QT interval: _____

Interpretation: _____

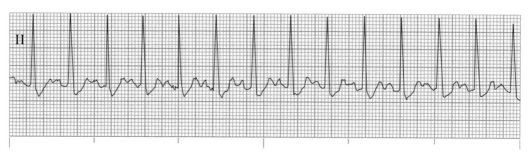

Fig. 5.25

40. **Fig. 5.25**. This rhythm strip is from a 43-year-old man after a seizure.

Rhythm: _____ Rate: _____ P waves: _____

PR interval: _____ QRS duration: _____ QT interval: _____

Interpretation: _____

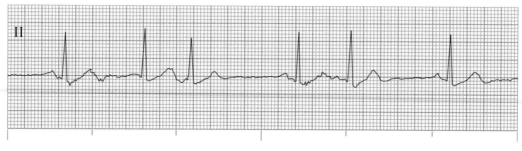

Fig. 5.26

41. **Fig. 5.26**

Rhythm: _____ Rate: _____ P waves: _____

PR interval: _____ QRS duration: _____ QT interval: _____

Interpretation: _____

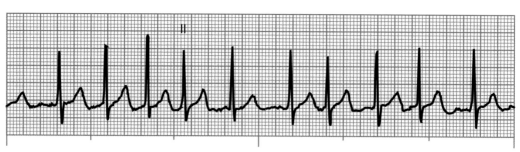

Fig. 5.27 (From Aehlert B: *ECG study cards*, St. Louis, 2004, Mosby.)

42. **Fig. 5.27**. This rhythm strip is from a 96-year-old man complaining of chest pain and palpitations.

Rhythm: _____ Rate: _____ P waves: _____

PR interval: _____ QRS duration: _____ QT interval: _____

Interpretation: _____

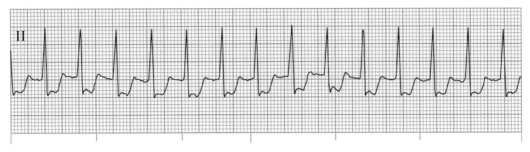

Fig. 5.28

43. **Fig. 5.28**. This rhythm strip is from a 79-year-old man complaining of palpitations. His initial blood pressure was 112/84 mm Hg. His second blood pressure, 8 minutes after the first, was 78/P mm Hg.

   Rhythm: _____ Rate: _____ P waves: _____

   PR interval: _____ QRS duration: _____ QT interval: _____

   Interpretation: _____

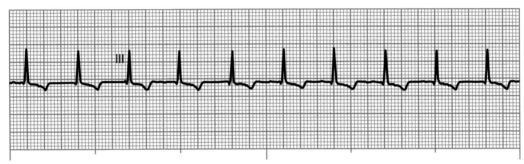

Fig. 5.29 (From Aehlert B: *ECG study cards,* St. Louis, 2004, Mosby.)

44. **Fig. 5.29**

   Rhythm: _____ Rate: _____ P waves: _____

   PR interval: _____ QRS duration: _____ QT interval: _____

   Interpretation: _____

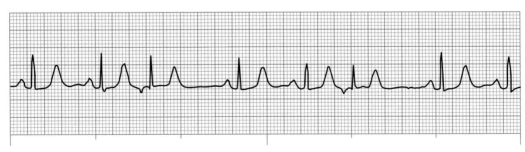

Fig. 5.30 (From Aehlert B: *ECG study cards,* St. Louis, 2004, Mosby.)

45. **Fig. 5.30**

   Rhythm: _____ Rate: _____ P waves: _____

   PR interval: _____ QRS duration: _____ QT interval: _____

   Interpretation: _____

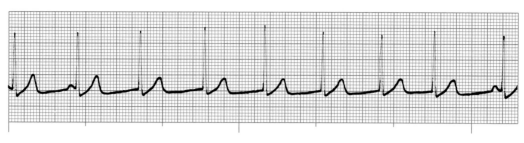

Fig. 5.31

46. **Fig. 5.31**

Rhythm: _____ Rate: _____ P waves: _____

PR interval: _____ QRS duration: _____ QT interval: _____

Interpretation: _____

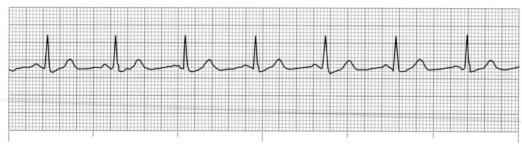

Fig. 5.32 (From Aehlert B: *ECG study cards,* St. Louis, 2004, Mosby.)

47. **Fig. 5.32**. This rhythm strip (lead I) is from a 51-year-old man found unresponsive. He had a history of esophageal varices and gastrointestinal bleeding.

Rhythm: _____ Rate: _____ P waves: _____

PR interval: _____ QRS duration: _____ QT interval: _____

Interpretation: _____

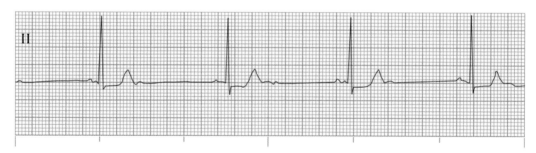

Fig. 5.33

48. **Fig. 5.33**

Rhythm: _____ Rate: _____ P waves: _____

PR interval: _____ QRS duration: _____ QT interval: _____

Interpretation: _____

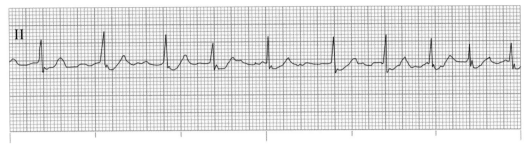

Fig. 5.34

49. **Fig. 5.34**. This rhythm strip is from a 75-year-old man complaining of chest pain that had been present for 20 minutes. He rated his pain 8/10.

Rhythm: _____ Rate: _____ P waves: _____

PR interval: _____ QRS duration: _____ QT interval: _____

Interpretation: _____

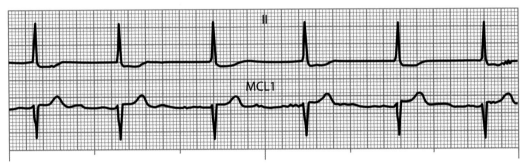

Fig. 5.35 (From Aehlert B: *ECG study cards,* St. Louis, 2004, Mosby.)

50. **Fig. 5.35**. This rhythm strip is from a 76-year-old woman complaining of weakness.

Rhythm: _____ Rate: _____ P waves: _____

PR interval: _____ QRS duration: _____ QT interval: _____

Interpretation: _____

STOP & REVIEW / ANSWERS

1. F. Premature junctional complexes are less common than either PACs or PVCs.
OBJ: Describe the ECG characteristics, possible causes, signs and symptoms, and initial emergency care for PJCs.

2. F. A P wave may or may not be present with a PJC. If a P wave is present, it is inverted (retrograde) and may precede or follow the QRS. PJCs can be misdiagnosed when the P wave of a PAC is buried in the preceding T wave.
OBJ: Describe the ECG characteristics, possible causes, signs and symptoms, and initial emergency care for PJCs.

3. F. The AV node and the nonbranching portion of the bundle of His are called the AV *junction*. The bundle of His has pacemaker cells that are capable of discharging at a rhythmic rate of 40 to 60 beats/min.
OBJ: Describe the location, the function, and (where appropriate) the intrinsic rate of the following structures: SA node, AV bundle, and Purkinje fibers.

4. D. If the AV junction paces the heart at a rate slower than 40 beats/min, the resulting rhythm is called a *junctional bradycardia*. This may seem confusing because the AV junction's normal pacing rate (40 to 60 beats/min) is bradycardic. However, the term *junctional bradycardia* refers to a rate slower than normal for the AV junction.
OBJ: Describe the ECG characteristics, possible causes, signs and symptoms, and initial emergency care for a junctional escape rhythm.

5. A. A noncompensatory (incomplete) pause often follows a PJC. This pause represents the delay during which the SA node resets its rhythm for the next beat.
OBJ: Explain the difference between a compensatory and noncompensatory pause.

6. B. The QRS duration associated with a rhythm that begins in the AV junction measures 0.11 second or less if conduction through the bundle branches, Purkinje fibers, and ventricles is normal.
OBJ: Describe the ECG characteristics, possible causes, signs and symptoms, and initial emergency care for a junctional escape rhythm.

7. C. An accelerated junctional rhythm is a dysrhythmia originating in the AV bundle with a ventricular rate between 61 and 100 beats/min.
OBJ: Describe the ECG characteristics, possible causes, signs and symptoms, and initial emergency care for an accelerated junctional rhythm.

8. B. The patient who has an accelerated junctional rhythm is usually asymptomatic because the ventricular rate is 61 to 100 beats/min, which is the same rate as a sinus rhythm.
OBJ: Describe the ECG characteristics, possible causes, signs and symptoms, and initial emergency care for an accelerated junctional rhythm.

9. A. You can usually tell the difference between a PAC and a PJC by the P wave. A PAC typically has an upright P wave before the QRS complex in leads II, III, and aVF. A P wave may or may not be present with a PJC. If a P wave is present, it is inverted (retrograde) and may precede or follow the QRS.
OBJ: Describe the ECG characteristics, possible causes, signs and symptoms, and initial emergency care for PJCs.

10. C. If the AV junction paces the heart, the electrical impulse must travel in a backward (retrograde) direction to activate the atria. If a P wave is seen, it will be inverted in leads II, III, and aVF because the impulse is traveling away from the positive electrode. If the atria depolarize before the ventricles, an inverted P wave will be seen *before* the QRS complex, and the PR interval will usually measure 0.12 second or less. The PR interval is shorter than usual because an impulse that begins in the AV junction does not have to travel as far to stimulate the ventricles. If the atria and ventricles depolarize at the same time, a P wave will not be visible because it will be hidden in the QRS complex. When the atria are depolarized after the ventricles, the P wave typically distorts the end of the QRS complex, and an inverted P wave will appear *after* the QRS.
OBJ: Describe the ECG characteristics, possible causes, signs and symptoms, and initial emergency care for a junctional escape rhythm.

11. D. In this rhythm strip, the atrial rate and rhythm cannot be determined because P waves are not visible. The ventricular rhythm is regular and the QRS is narrow, measuring 0.08 second.
OBJ: Describe the ECG characteristics, possible causes, signs and symptoms, and initial emergency care for a junctional escape rhythm.

12. A. The patient's ventricular rate is about 32 beats/min (1500 divided by 46.5).
OBJ: Identify how heart rates, durations, and amplitudes may be determined from ECG recordings.

13. B. The cardiac monitor shows a junctional bradycardia at 32 beats/min with ST-segment depression and inverted T waves.
OBJ: Describe the ECG characteristics, possible causes, signs and symptoms, and initial emergency care for a junctional escape rhythm.

14. B. Although there is no evidence of STE on the cardiac monitor, this patient is symptomatic with his slow heart rate as evidenced by his dizziness and hypotension. Treatment of a patient with symptomatic bradycardia should include application of a pulse oximeter and administration of supplemental oxygen (if indicated) and establishing IV access, which have already been

done. Next, obtain a 12-lead ECG and then administer atropine IV. Reassess the patient's response to your
interventions and continue to monitor the patient.
Because vagal maneuvers are used to attempt to slow
the heart rate of some *tachycardias* and this patient is
bradycardic, vagal maneuvers are contraindicated in
this situation.

OBJ: Describe the ECG characteristics, possible causes, signs
and symptoms, and initial emergency care for a junctional
escape rhythm.

15. E
16. F
17. I
18. H
19. C
20. J
21. B
22. A
23. D
24. G

25. ANS:

ECG Finding	Junctional Rhythm	Accelerated Junctional Rhythm	Junctional Tachycardia
Rhythm	Regular	Regular	Regular or irregular
Rate (beats/min)	**40 to 60**	**61 to 100**	**101 to 180**
P waves (lead II)	**May occur before, during, or after the QRS; if visible, the P wave is inverted**	**May occur before, during, or after the QRS; if visible, the P wave is inverted**	**May occur before, during, or after the QRS; if visible, the P wave is inverted**
PR interval	**If a P wave occurs before the QRS, the PR interval will usually be 0.12 sec or less; if no P wave occurs before the QRS, there will be no PR interval**	**If a P wave occurs before the QRS, the PR interval will usually be 0.12 sec or less; if no P wave occurs before the QRS, there will be no PR interval**	**If a P wave occurs before the QRS, the PR interval will usually be 0.12 sec or less; if no P wave occurs before the QRS, there will be no PR interval**
QRS duration	0.11 sec or less unless abnormally conducted	0.11 sec or less unless abnormally conducted	0.11 sec or less unless abnormally conducted

OBJ: Describe the ECG characteristics, possible causes, signs and symptoms, and initial emergency care for junctional
escape rhythm, accelerated junctional rhythm, and junctional tachycardia.

Practice Rhythm Strip Answers

Note: Because of the distortion of ECGs that can occur during printing, a range of acceptable measurements is provided in the
rhythm strip answers throughout this textbook.

26. **Fig. 5.11**
Rhythm: Irregular
Rate: 70 beats/min
P waves: Sinus P waves look alike; P waves of beats 1, 4,
and 7 are early and inverted
PR interval: 0.12 to 0.16 second (sinus beats)
QRS duration: 0.06 second
QT interval: 0.36 second
Interpretation: Sinus rhythm at 70 beats/min with PJCs
(junctional trigeminy)

27. **Fig. 5.12**
Rhythm: Regular
Rate: 100 beats/min
P waves: Inverted before each QRS
PR interval: 0.12 to 0.16 second

QRS duration: 0.08 to 0.10 second
QT interval: 0.28 to 0.32 second
Interpretation: Accelerated junctional rhythm at 100
beats/min with STE

28. **Fig. 5.13**
Rhythm: Irregular
Rate: 130 beats/min
P waves: Upright before each QRS, but the shape and
amplitude of some differ; P wave of beat 10 is early and
hidden in the T wave of the preceding beat
PR interval: 0.14 second
QRS duration: 0.06 to 0.08 second
QT interval: 0.28 second
Interpretation: Sinus tachycardia at 130 beats/min with
a PAC

29. **Fig. 5.14**
    Rhythm: Irregular
    Rate: 80 beats/min
    P waves: Flutter waves present
    PR interval: None
    QRS duration: 0.08 to 0.10 second
    QT interval: Unable to determine
    Interpretation: Atrial flutter at 80 beats/min

30. **Fig. 5.15**
    Rhythm: Regular
    Rate: 136 beats/min
    P waves: None visible; hidden in T waves
    PR interval: Unable to determine
    QRS duration: 0.10 to 0.12 second
    QT interval: 0.32 to 0.36 second
    Interpretation: Narrow-QRS tachycardia, probably junctional tachycardia, at 136 beats/min

31. **Fig. 5.16**
    Rhythm: Irregular
    Rate: 70 beats/min
    P waves: Sinus P waves are upright and some are notched; P wave of beat 3 is early, inverted, and appears after the QRS
    PR interval: 0.16 second
    QRS duration: 0.08 to 0.10 second
    QT interval: 0.36 second
    Interpretation: Sinus rhythm at 70 beats/min with a PJC (beat 3 is the PJC)

32. **Fig. 5.17**
    Rhythm: Regular
    Rate: 115 beats/min
    P waves: Upright before each QRS but some differ in shape
    PR interval: 0.12 to 0.16 second
    QRS duration: 0.12 second
    QT interval: 0.32 second
    Interpretation: Sinus tachycardia at 115 beats/min with a wide QRS and STE

33. **Fig. 5.18**
    Rhythm: Regular
    Rate: 75 beats/min
    P waves: Inverted before each QRS
    PR interval: 0.16 second
    QRS duration: 0.06 to 0.08 second
    QT interval: 0.32 to 0.36 second
    Interpretation: Accelerated junctional rhythm at 75 beats/min

34. **Fig. 5.19**
    Rhythm: Regular
    Rate: 75 beats/min
    P waves: Upright before each QRS
    PR interval: 0.12 second
    QRS duration: 0.08 second
    QT interval: 0.36 second
    Interpretation: Sinus rhythm at 75 beats/min

35. **Fig. 5.20**
    Rhythm: Irregular
    Rate: 80 beats/min
    P waves: Upright before each QRS
    PR interval: 0.16 to 0.20 second
    QRS duration: 0.08 second
    QT interval: 0.32 second
    Interpretation: Sinus arrhythmia at 80 beats/min

36. **Fig. 5.21**
    Rhythm: Irregular
    Rate: 33 beats/min (sinus beats); 32 beats/min (junctional beats)
    P waves: Sinus P waves upright before QRS; none visible for junctional beats
    PR interval: 0.16 to 0.20 second (sinus beats)
    QRS duration: 0.04 to 0.06 second
    QT interval: 0.36 to 0.40 second
    Interpretation: Sinus bradycardia at 33 beats/min to junctional bradycardia at 32 beats/min

37. **Fig. 5.22**
    Rhythm: Irregular
    Rate: 70 beats/min
    P waves: Sinus P waves upright before each QRS; an early P wave appears after beat 5 and distorts the T wave; beat 6 has no P wave
    PR interval: 0.16 second
    QRS duration: 0.08 second
    QT interval: 0.36 second
    Interpretation: Sinus rhythm at 70 beats/min with a nonconducted PAC (note distortion of the T wave of the beat preceding the pause) and a junctional escape beat

38. **Fig. 5.23**
    Rhythm: Regular
    Rate: 45 beats/min
    P waves: None visible
    PR interval: None
    QRS duration: 0.08 to 0.11 second
    QT interval: 0.48 to 0.52 second
    Interpretation: Junctional rhythm at 45 beats/min with STE and a prolonged QT interval

39. **Fig. 5.24**
    Rhythm: Irregular; regular during the tachycardia
    Rate: 160 beats/min; 188 beats/min during the tachycardia
    P waves: Inverted after QRS in beat 1; sinus P wave in beats 2 and 3; cannot differentiate with certainty between inverted P waves and inverted T waves in beats associated with the tachycardia
    PR interval: 0.14 to 0.16 second (sinus beats)
    QRS duration: 0.06 to 0.08 second
    QT interval: 0.24 second if the inverted waveforms during the tachycardia are T waves
    Interpretation: Junctional beat, two sinus beats, changing to a narrow QRS tachycardia that is probably junctional tachycardia at 188 beats/min; ST-segment depression

40. **Fig. 5.25**
Rhythm: Regular
Rate: 136 beats/min
P waves: Upright before each QRS; some are notched, some are pointed, others are smooth and rounded
PR interval: 0.14 to 0.16 second
QRS duration: 0.08 second
QT interval: 0.24 to 0.28 second
Interpretation: Sinus tachycardia at 136 beats/min with ST-segment depression

41. **Fig. 5.26**
Rhythm: Irregular
Rate: 60 beats/min
P waves: Upright before sinus beats, early and inverted before the QRS in beat 3, early and upright in beat 5
PR interval: 0.18 to 0.20 second
QRS duration: 0.06 to 0.08 second
QT interval: 0.40 to 0.44 second
Interpretation: Sinus rhythm at 60 beats/min with a PJC (beat 3), a PAC (beat 5), and ST-segment depression; artifact is present

42. **Fig. 5.27**
Rhythm: Irregular
Rate: 100 beats/min
P waves: Fibrillatory waves present
PR interval: None
QRS duration: 0.06 to 0.08 second
QT interval: 0.32 to 0.36 second
Interpretation: Atrial fibrillation at 100 beats/min

43. **Fig. 5.28**
Rhythm: Regular
Rate: 143 beats/min
P waves: None visible before each QRS; cannot differentiate with certainty between inverted P waves and inverted T waves after each QRS
PR interval: None
QRS duration: 0.06 to 0.08 second
QT interval: 0.24 second if the inverted waveforms after each QRS are T waves
Interpretation: Narrow-QRS tachycardia, probably junctional tachycardia, at 143 beats/min with ST-segment depression

44. **Fig. 5.29**
Rhythm: Regular
Rate: 97 beats/min
P waves: None visible
PR interval: None
QRS duration: 0.06 to 0.08 second
QT interval: 0.28 to 0.32 second
Interpretation: Accelerated junctional rhythm at 97 beats/min; inverted T waves

45. **Fig. 5.30**
Rhythm: Irregular
Rate: 80 beats/min

P waves: Sinus P waves are upright; early inverted P waves appear in beats 3 and 6
PR interval: 0.16 second (sinus beats)
QRS duration: 0.04 to 0.06 second (sinus beats)
QT interval: 0.36 to 0.40 second
Interpretation: Sinus rhythm at 80 beats/min with PJCs (beats 3 and 6)

46. **Fig. 5.31**
Rhythm: Irregular
Rate: 79 beats/min (junctional beats)
P waves: Upright before sinus beats; not visible for junctional beats
PR interval: 0.10 second (sinus beats)
QRS duration: 0.04 to 0.06 second
QT interval: 0.32 second
Interpretation: Sinus rhythm changing to an accelerated junctional rhythm at 79 beats/min, back to a sinus rhythm

47. **Fig. 5.32**
Rhythm: Regular
Rate: 73 beats/min
P waves: Upright before each QRS
PR interval: 0.12 second
QRS duration: 0.06 to 0.08 second
QT interval: 0.36 to 0.40 second
Interpretation: Sinus rhythm at 73 beats/min

48. **Fig. 5.33**
Rhythm: Regular
Rate: 40 beats/min
P waves: Low amplitude but upright before each QRS; some are notched
PR interval: 0.12 to 0.16 second
QRS duration: 0.06 to 0.08 second
QT interval: 0.36 to 0.40 second
Interpretation: Sinus bradyarrhythmia at 40 beats/min with ST-segment depression; U waves are present

49. **Fig. 5.34**
Rhythm: Irregular
Rate: 100 beats/min
P waves: Fibrillatory waves present
PR interval: None
QRS duration: 0.06 to 0.08 second
QT interval: 0.28 to 0.32 second
Interpretation: Atrial fibrillation at 100 beats/min with ST-segment depression

50. **Fig. 5.35**
Rhythm: Irregular
Rate: 60 beats/min
P waves: None visible
PR interval: None
QRS duration: 0.04 to 0.06 second
QT interval: 0.32 to 0.36 second
Interpretation: Junctional rhythm at 60 beats/min; STE in MCL_1

REFERENCES

Kumar, U. N., Rao, R. K., & Scheinman, M. M. (2006). The 12-lead electrocardiogram in supraventricular tachycardia. *Cardiol Clin*, *24*(3), 427–437.

Page, R. L., Joglar, J. A., Caldwell, M. A., Calkins, H., Conti, J. B., Deal, B. J., & Al-Khatib, S. M. (2015). 2015 ACC/AHA/HRS guideline for the management of adult patients with supraventricular tachycardia. *Circulation*, *132*(14), 1–131.

Zimetbaum, P. (2016). Cardiac arrhythmias with supraventricular origin. In L. Goldman & A. I. Schafer (Eds.), *Goldman's Cecil medicine* (25th ed.) (pp. 356–366). Philadelphia: Saunders.

Ventricular Rhythms

6

LEARNING OBJECTIVES

After reading this chapter, you should be able to:

1. Describe the electrocardiogram (ECG) characteristics, possible causes, signs and symptoms, and initial emergency care for premature ventricular complexes (PVCs).
2. Explain the terms *bigeminy*, *trigeminy*, *quadrigeminy*, and *run* as used to describe premature complexes.
3. Explain the difference between PVCs and ventricular escape beats.
4. Describe the ECG characteristics of ventricular escape beats.
5. Describe the ECG characteristics, possible causes, signs and symptoms, and initial emergency care for an idioventricular rhythm (IVR).
6. Explain the term *pulseless electrical activity* (PEA).
7. Describe the ECG characteristics, possible causes, signs and symptoms, and initial emergency care for an accelerated idioventricular rhythm (AIVR).
8. Explain the terms *sustained* and *nonsustained ventricular tachycardia* (VT), *monomorphic VT*, and *polymorphic VT* (PMVT).
9. Describe the ECG characteristics, possible causes, signs and symptoms, and initial emergency care for monomorphic VT.
10. Describe the ECG characteristics, possible causes, signs and symptoms, and initial emergency care for PMVT.
11. Describe the ECG characteristics, possible causes, signs and symptoms, and initial emergency care for ventricular fibrillation (VF).
12. State the purpose and indications for defibrillation.
13. Describe the ECG characteristics, possible causes, signs and symptoms, and initial emergency care for asystole.

KEY TERMS

accelerated idioventricular rhythm (AIVR): Dysrhythmia originating in the ventricles with a rate between 41 and 100 beats/min

agonal rhythm: Dysrhythmia similar in appearance to an IVR but occurring at a rate of less than 20 beats/min; dying heart

asystole: A total absence of ventricular electrical activity

automated external defibrillator (AED): A machine with a sophisticated computer system that analyzes a patient's heart rhythm using an algorithm to distinguish shockable rhythms from nonshockable rhythms and providing visual and auditory instructions to the rescuer to deliver an electrical shock, if a shock is indicated.

atrioventricular (AV) dissociation: Any dysrhythmia in which the atria and ventricles beat independently (e.g., VT, complete AV block)

burst: Three or more sequential ectopic beats; also referred to as a "salvo" or "run"

compensatory pause: Pause for which the normal beat after a premature complex occurs when expected; also called a *complete pause*

defibrillation: Delivery of an electrical current across the heart muscle over a very brief period to terminate an abnormal heart rhythm; also called *unsynchronized countershock* or *asynchronous countershock* because the delivery of current has no relationship to the cardiac cycle.

fusion beat: Beat that occurs because of simultaneous activation of one cardiac chamber by two sites (foci); in pacing, the ECG waveform that results when an intrinsic depolarization and a pacing stimulus occur simultaneously and both contribute to depolarization of that cardiac chamber

interpolated PVC: PVC that occurs between two normally conducted QRS complexes and that does not disturb the next ventricular depolarization or sinoatrial (SA) node activity

monomorphic: Having the same shape

polymorphic: Varying in shape

run: Three or more sequential ectopic beats; also referred to as a "salvo" or "burst"

salvo: Three or more sequential ectopic beats; also referred to as a "run" or "burst"

torsades de pointes (TdP): Type of polymorphic VT associated with a prolonged QT interval; the QRS changes in shape, amplitude, and width and appears to twist around the isoelectric line, resembling a spindle

ventricular tachycardia (VT): Dysrhythmia originating in the ventricles with a ventricular rate greater than 100 beats/min

INTRODUCTION

The ventricles are the heart's least efficient pacemaker (Fig. 6.1). If the ventricles function as the heart's pacemaker, they normally generate impulses at a rate of 20 to 40 beats/min. The ventricles may assume responsibility for pacing the heart if the sinoatrial (SA) node fails to discharge, an impulse from the SA node is generated but blocked as it exits the SA node, the rate of discharge of the SA node is slower than that of the ventricles, or an irritable site in either ventricle produces an early beat or rapid rhythm.

The shape of the QRS complex is influenced by the site of origin of the electrical impulse. Normally, an electrical impulse that begins in the SA node, atria, or AV junction results in depolarization of the right and left ventricles at about the same time. The resulting QRS complex is usually narrow, measuring 0.11 second or less in duration.

If an area of either ventricle becomes ischemic or injured, it can become irritable. This irritability affects the manner in which impulses are conducted. Ventricular beats and rhythms can start in any part of the ventricles and may occur because of reentry, abnormal automaticity, or triggered activity (Berger et al, 2016; Garan, 2016). When an ectopic site within a ventricle assumes responsibility for pacing the heart, the electrical impulse bypasses the normal intraventricular conduction pathway. This results in stimulation of the ventricles at slightly different times. As a result, ventricular beats and rhythms usually have QRS complexes that are abnormally shaped and longer than normal (e.g., greater than 0.11 second). If the atria are depolarized after the ventricles, retrograde P waves may be seen.

Because ventricular depolarization is abnormal, ventricular repolarization is also abnormal and results in changes in ST segments and T waves. The T waves are usually in a direction opposite that of the QRS complex; if the major QRS deflection is negative, the ST segment is usually elevated, and the T wave is positive (i.e., upright). If the major QRS deflection is positive, the ST segment is usually depressed, and the T wave is usually negative (i.e., inverted). P waves are usually not seen with ventricular dysrhythmias, but if they are visible, they have no consistent relationship to the QRS complex (i.e., **atrioventricular [AV] dissociation**).

 Lead In _____

Getting the Big Picture

When a ventricular rhythm is present, the appearance of ST segments and T waves in the opposite direction of the last portion of the QRS complex can complicate matters when looking for ECG signs of myocardial injury and infarction. For example, when the QRS complexes of a ventricular rhythm are negative, the ST segment is usually elevated. The resulting ST-segment elevation may be the result of abnormal repolarization and not a result of any infarction-related causes. Assess the patient's clinical presentation and the results of other diagnostic studies in addition to your ECG findings.

PREMATURE VENTRICULAR COMPLEXES

How Do I Recognize Them?

[Objective 1]

A premature ventricular complex (PVC), also called a *premature ventricular extrasystole*, *ventricular premature beat*, or *premature ventricular depolarization*, arises from an irritable site (i.e., focus) within either ventricle. By definition, a PVC is *premature*, occurring earlier than the next expected sinus beat. The shape of the QRS of a PVC depends on the location of the irritable focus within the ventricles (Fig. 6.2). The width of the QRS of a PVC is typically 0.12 second or greater because the PVC causes the ventricles to fire prematurely and in an abnormal manner (Fig. 6.3). The T wave usually points in a direction opposite that of the QRS complex.

A **compensatory pause** often follows a PVC and occurs because the SA node is usually not affected by the PVC

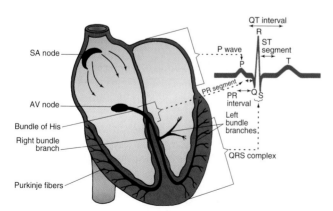

Fig. 6.1 The ventricles are the heart's least efficient pacemaker. *AV,* Atrioventricular; *SA,* sinoatrial. (From Ignatavicius DD, Workman LM: *Medical-surgical nursing: patient-centered collaborative care,* ed 8, Philadelphia, 2016, Saunders.)

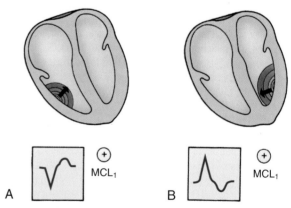

Fig. 6.2 A, Right premature ventricular complex (PVC). The spread of depolarization is from right to left, away from the positive electrode in lead V₁ (MCL₁), resulting in a wide, negative QRS complex. B, Left ventricular PVC. The spread of depolarization is from left to right, toward the positive electrode in lead V₁ (MCL₁). The QRS complex is wide and upright. (From Urden LD, Stacy KM, Lough ME: *Critical care nursing,* ed 8, St. Louis, 2018, Mosby.)

(Fig. 6.4). The SA node discharges at its regular rate and rhythm, including the period during and after the PVC. It is important to note that the presence of a full compensatory pause does not reliably differentiate ventricular ectopy from atrial ectopy; this is because atrial ectopy may produce a similar compensatory pattern if it does not reset the SA node (Crawford & Spence, 1995). In addition, when backward (i.e., retrograde) conduction occurs and a PVC is conducted to the atria, as in slow sinus rates, the PVC can reset the SA node, thereby resulting in a noncompensatory pause (Berger et al, 2016; Crawford & Spence, 1995).

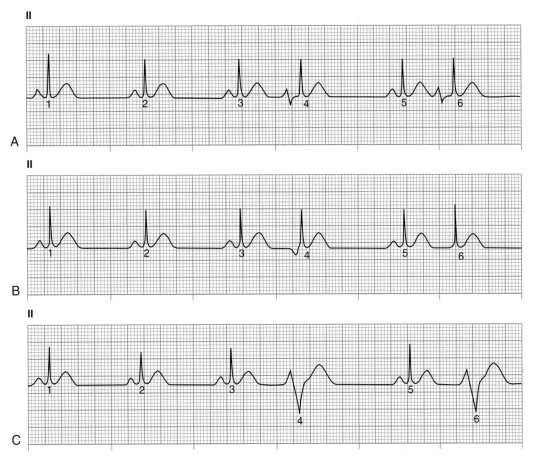

Fig. 6.3 Premature beats. A, Sinus rhythm with premature atrial complexes (PACs). The fourth and sixth beats are preceded by premature P waves that look different from the normally conducted sinus beats. Note that the QRS complex that follows each of these PACs is narrow and identical in appearance to that of the sinus-conducted beats. B, Sinus rhythm with premature junctional complexes (PJCs). The fourth and sixth beats are PJCs. Beat No. 4 is preceded by an inverted P wave with a short PR interval. There is no identifiable atrial activity associated with beat No. 6. C, Sinus rhythm with premature ventricular complexes (PVCs). The fourth and sixth beats are very different in appearance from the normally conducted sinus beats. Beats 4 and 6 are PVCs. They are not preceded by P waves. (From Grauer K: *A practical guide to ECG interpretation,* ed 2, St. Louis, 1998, Mosby.)

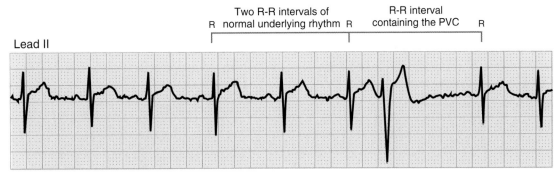

Fig. 6.4 A premature ventricular complex (PVC) is often followed by a full compensatory pause. A compensatory pause is present if the period between the complex before and after a premature beat is the same as two normal R-R intervals. (From Paul S, Hebra JD: *The nurse's guide to cardiac rhythm interpretation: implications for patient care,* Philadelphia, 1998, Saunders.)

A **fusion beat** is a result of an electrical impulse from a supraventricular site (e.g., SA node) discharging at the same time as an ectopic site in the ventricles (Fig. 6.5). Because fusion beats are a result of both supraventricular and ventricular depolarization, these beats do not resemble normally conducted beats, nor do they resemble true ventricular beats.

PATTERNS OF PREMATURE VENTRICULAR COMPLEXES

PVCs may occur alone or in groups (i.e., patterns). PVCs that occur infrequently with no identifiable pattern are called

isolated PVCs. Two consecutive PVCs are called a *pair* or *couplet* (Fig. 6.6). Couplets are also referred to as "two PVCs in a row" or "back-to-back PVCs." The appearance of couplets indicates the ventricular ectopic site is very irritable. Three or more sequential PVCs are termed a **run**, a **salvo**, or a **burst**, and three or more PVCs that occur in a row at a rate of more than 100 beats/min are considered a run of VT.

Ventricular bigeminy describes a rhythm in which every other beat is a PVC (Fig. 6.7); with *ventricular trigeminy*, every third beat is a PVC; and with *ventricular quadrigeminy*, every fourth beat is a PVC.

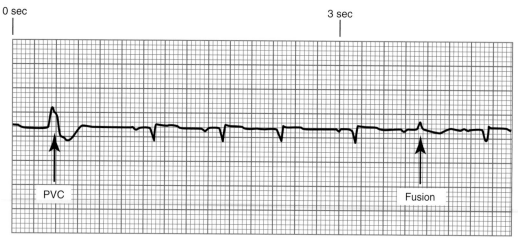

Fig. 6.5 Ventricular fusion beat *(second arrow).* The QRS duration is only 0.08 second, and the shape represents the normal QRS and the previous premature ventricular complex (PVC). (From Urden LD, Stacy KM, Lough ME: *Critical care nursing,* ed 8, St. Louis, 2018, Mosby.)

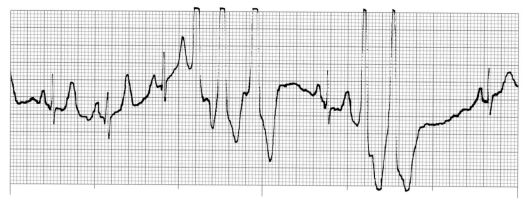

Fig. 6.6 Sinus rhythm with a run of ventricular tachycardia and one episode of ventricular couplets. (From Aehlert B: *ECG study cards,* St. Louis, 2004, Mosby.)

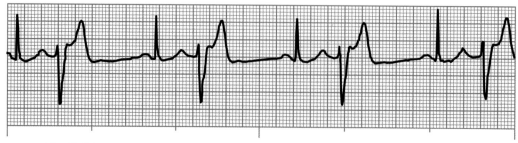

Fig. 6.7 Sinus bradycardia with ventricular bigeminy. (From Aehlert B: *ECG study cards,* St. Louis, 2004, Mosby.)

TYPES OF PREMATURE VENTRICULAR COMPLEXES

Uniform and Multiform Premature Ventricular Complexes

[Objective 2]

PVCs that look alike in the same lead and begin from the same anatomic site (i.e., focus) are called *uniform PVCs* (Fig. 6.8). PVCs that look different from one another in the same lead are called *multiform PVCs* (Fig. 6.9). The terms *unifocal* and *multifocal* are sometimes used to describe PVCs that are similar or different in appearance. Uniform PVCs are unifocal; that is, they arise from the same anatomic site within the ventricles. Multiform PVCs often, but do not always, arise from different anatomic sites; therefore, multiform PVCs are not necessarily multifocal (Goldberger et al, 2013). In general, multiform PVCs are considered more serious than uniform PVCs because they suggest a greater area of irritable myocardial tissue.

A PVC can occur with any supraventricular dysrhythmia. Thus it is important when identifying the rhythm to first describe the patient's underlying rhythm and then describe the ectopic beats present (i.e., "Sinus tachycardia with uniform PVCs at 110 beats/min" or "Sinus tachycardia with multiform PVCs at 120 beats/min").

Interpolated Premature Ventricular Complexes

When a PVC occurs between two normally conducted QRS complexes without interfering with the normal cardiac cycle it is called an **interpolated PVC** (Fig. 6.10). An interpolated PVC does not have a full compensatory pause; rather, it is squeezed between two normally conducted QRS complexes (i.e., the R-R intervals between sinus beats remain the same) and does not disturb the next ventricular depolarization or SA node activity. An interpolated PVC usually occurs when the PVC is very early or when the patient's underlying heart rate is relatively slow.

R-on-T Premature Ventricular Complexes

An R-on-T PVC occurs when the R wave of a PVC falls on the T wave of the preceding beat (Fig. 6.11). Because ventricular repolarization is not yet complete during the last half of the T wave (i.e., the relative refractory period), it is possible

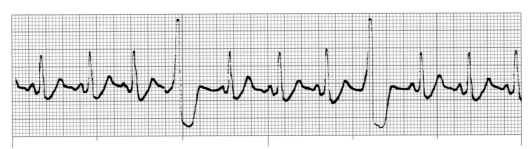

Fig. 6.8 Sinus tachycardia with uniform premature ventricular complexes. (From Aehlert B: *ECG study cards,* St. Louis, 2004, Mosby.)

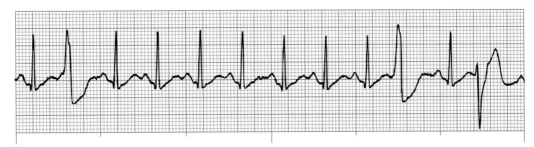

Fig. 6.9 Sinus tachycardia with multiform premature ventricular complexes. (From Aehlert B: *ECG study cards,* St. Louis, 2004, Mosby.)

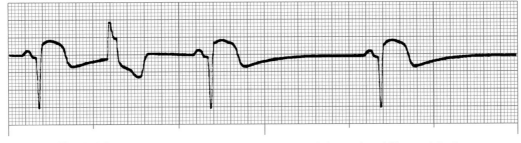

Fig. 6.10 Sinus bradycardia with an interpolated premature ventricular complex and ST-segment elevation.

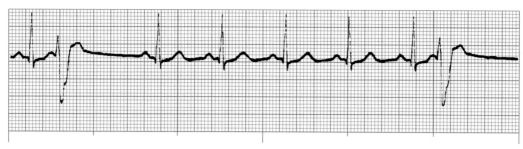

Fig. 6.11 Sinus rhythm with two R-on-T premature ventricular complexes. (From Aehlert B: *ECG study cards,* St. Louis, 2004, Mosby.)

TABLE 6.1	Characteristics of Premature Ventricular Complexes
Rhythm	Irregular because of the premature beats; if the premature ventricular complex (PVC) is an interpolated PVC, the rhythm will be regular
Rate	Usually within normal range, but depends on the underlying rhythm
P waves	Usually absent or, with retrograde conduction to the atria, may appear after the QRS (usually upright in the ST segment or T wave)
PR interval	None with the PVC because the ectopic beat originates in the ventricles
QRS duration	Usually 0.12 sec or greater; T wave is usually in the opposite direction of the QRS complex

Box 6.1	Common Causes of Premature Ventricular Complexes

- Acid–base imbalance
- Acute coronary syndromes
- Cardiomyopathy
- Digitalis toxicity
- Electrolyte imbalance (e.g., potassium, magnesium)
- Exercise
- Heart failure
- Hypoxia
- Increase in catecholamines and sympathetic tone (e.g., emotional stress, anxiety)
- Medications (e.g., sympathomimetic drugs)
- Normal variant
- Stimulants (e.g., caffeine, tobacco)
- Valvular heart disease
- Ventricular aneurysm

that a PVC that occurs during this period of the cardiac cycle will precipitate VT or VF. The term *R-on-T phenomenon* refers to the start of a ventricular tachydysrhythmia as a result of an improperly timed electrical impulse on the T wave (Spotts, 2011). The general characteristics of PVCs are shown in Table 6.1.

What Causes Them?

PVCs are common, occurring in healthy individuals with apparently normal hearts, as well as in individuals with structural heart disease. When cardiac monitoring extends over 24 hours or longer, PVCs may be seen in 50% of healthy individuals (Garan, 2016). PVCs can occur for no apparent cause, and the frequency with which they occur increases with age. PVCs can occur at rest or they can be associated with exercise. Common causes of PVCs are shown in Box 6.1.

What Do I Do About Them?

The signs and symptoms associated with PVCs vary and generally depend on their frequency. Depending on their frequency, PVCs may or may not affect cardiac output. Some patients experiencing PVCs are asymptomatic; others may experience palpitations (i.e., sensation of a racing heart, skipped beats, or flip-flops), weakness, lightheadedness, dizziness, fatigue, or a pounding sensation in the neck.

Treatment of PVCs depends on the cause, the patient's signs and symptoms, and the clinical situation. Most patients experiencing PVCs do not require treatment with antiarrhythmic medications; rather, treatment of PVCs focuses on the search for and treatment of potentially reversible causes. For example, provide reassurance to the patient who is complaining of palpitations while searching for possible triggers for his or her PVCs (e.g., excessive caffeine ingestion, nicotine use, emotional stress). In the setting of an acute coronary syndrome, treatment is directed at ensuring adequate oxygenation; relieving pain; and rapidly identifying and correcting hypoxia, heart failure, and electrolyte or acid–base abnormalities.

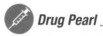 **Drug Pearl**

Antiarrhythmic Agents

When PVCs cause *serious* symptoms, antiarrhythmic medications (e.g., amiodarone, procainamide, lidocaine) are sometimes used to reduce the frequency with which they occur or to eliminate them. However, antiarrhythmics can cause a *proarrhythmic effect,* which means that they have the *potential* to cause serious adverse effects, more serious dysrhythmias, or both than those that they were intended to treat. For example, the treatment of occasional PVCs, which are not life threatening, may initiate a life-threatening sustained ventricular tachydysrhythmia.

VENTRICULAR ESCAPE BEATS OR RHYTHM

How Do I Recognize It?

[Objectives 3, 4, 5]

Remember that premature beats are *early,* and escape beats are *late.* We need to see at least two sinus beats in a row to establish the regularity of the underlying rhythm and to determine if a complex is early or late.

Although ventricular escape beats share some physical characteristics with PVCs (e.g., wide QRS complexes, T waves deflected in a direction opposite the QRS), they differ in some very important areas. A PVC appears *early*, before the next expected sinus beat. PVCs often reflect irritability in some area of the ventricles. A ventricular escape beat occurs after a pause in which a supraventricular pacemaker failed to fire; thus, the escape beat is *late*, appearing after the next expected sinus beat. A ventricular escape beat is a *protective* mechanism, safeguarding the heart from more extreme slowing or even **asystole**. Because it is protective, you would not want to administer any medication that would wipe out the escape beat.

Take a look at Fig. 6.12. In looking at this rhythm strip, one of the first things you notice is that the rhythm is irregular at a rate of about 60 beats/min, and there is a QRS complex that differs from the others. Although this beat looks interesting, let us first examine the rhythm strip systemically. There are upright P waves before beats 1, 2, 3, 5, and 6. Now we know that the underlying rhythm is sinus in origin. Next, let us examine the wide-QRS beat more closely and see what happened here. Look to the left of the wide-QRS beat and see if anything looks amiss. When you look closely at the T wave of beat 3, it has an extra protrusion or hump. If you take a moment to plot P waves across the strip, you will find that this extra hump is actually an early P wave that was not conducted. This is a nonconducted premature atrial complex (PAC). In plotting

the P waves, you should have noticed that the wide-QRS beat occurred *late*—after the next expected sinus beat. This late beat is an escape beat. Because the QRS associated with it is *wide*, it is a *ventricular* escape beat. A *junctional* escape beat is also late, but it usually has a *narrow* QRS. Notice that the T wave of this beat is deflected in a direction opposite that of its QRS complex. When you look at the PR intervals and ST segment, you will find that the PR interval is longer than normal, measuring about 0.24 second. For now, we will simply say that it is prolonged. We will explore the reasons for this and give it a name in the next chapter. ST-segment depression is also present. Our interpretation of this rhythm strip would be something like this: "Sinus rhythm with a prolonged PR interval, nonconducted PAC, ventricular escape beat, and ST-segment depression at 60 beats/min." My goodness! That was one complicated rhythm strip! The electrocardiogram (ECG) characteristics of ventricular escape beats are shown in Table 6.2.

An idioventricular rhythm (IVR), also called a *ventricular escape rhythm*, exists when three or more ventricular escape beats occur in a row at a rate of 20 to 40 beats/min. The QRS complexes seen in IVR are wide because the impulses begin in the ventricles, bypassing the normal conduction pathway. When the ventricular rate slows to less than 20 beats/min, some practitioners refer to the rhythm as an **agonal rhythm** or *dying heart*. An example of IVR is shown in Fig. 6.13, and the characteristics of this rhythm are described in Table 6.3.

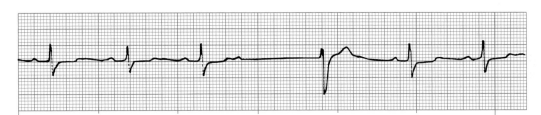

Fig. 6.12 Sinus rhythm with a prolonged PR interval, nonconducted premature atrial complex, ventricular escape beat, and ST-segment depression. (From Chou T, Ramaiah LS: *Electrocardiography in clinical practice: adult and pediatric,* ed 4, Philadelphia, 1996, Saunders.)

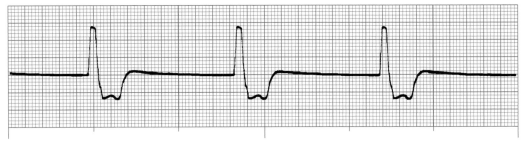

Fig. 6.13 Idioventricular rhythm. (From Aehlert B: *ECG study cards,* St. Louis, 2004, Mosby.)

TABLE 6.2	Characteristics of Ventricular Escape Beats
Rhythm	Irregular because of *late* beats; the ventricular escape beat occurs *after* the next expected sinus beat
Rate	Usually within normal range, but depends on the underlying rhythm
P waves	Usually absent or, with retrograde conduction to the atria, may appear after the QRS (usually upright in the ST segment or T wave)
PR interval	None with the ventricular escape beat because the ectopic beat originates in the ventricles
QRS duration	0.12 sec or greater; the T wave is frequently in the opposite direction of the QRS complex

TABLE 6.3	Characteristics of Idioventricular Rhythm
Rhythm	Ventricular rhythm is essentially regular
Rate	Ventricular rate 20 to 40 beats/min
P waves	Usually absent or, with retrograde conduction to the atria, may appear after the QRS (usually upright in the ST segment or T wave)
PR interval	None
QRS duration	0.12 sec or greater; the T wave is frequently in the opposite direction of the QRS complex

What Causes It?

A ventricular escape rhythm may occur under one of three circumstances: (1) the SA node and the AV junction fail to initiate an electrical impulse; (2) the SA node or AV junction discharge at a rate less than that of the intrinsic rate of the Purkinje fibers; or (3) the impulses generated by a supraventricular pacemaker site are blocked. A ventricular escape rhythm may also occur as a result of an acute coronary syndrome, digitalis toxicity, or metabolic imbalances.

What Do I Do About It?

[Objective 6]

Because the ventricular rate associated with IVR is slow (i.e., 20 to 40 beats/min) with a loss of atrial kick, the patient may experience serious signs and symptoms because of decreased cardiac output. If the patient has a pulse and is symptomatic

Box 6.2	Reversible Causes of Cardiac Emergencies

The 5 Hs and 5 Ts is a memory aid that can be used to recall the potentially reversible causes of cardiac emergencies, including cardiac arrest:

Five Hs and Five Ts

Hypovolemia	**T**amponade, cardiac
Hypoxia	**T**ension pneumothorax
Hypothermia	**T**hrombosis: lungs (massive pulmonary embolism)
Hypo-/hyperkalemia	**T**hrombosis: heart (acute coronary syndromes)
Hydrogen ion (acidosis)	**T**ablets/toxins: drug overdose

because of the slow rate, treatment should include application of a pulse oximeter and administration of supplemental oxygen if indicated. Establish intravenous (IV) access and obtain a 12-lead ECG. Because the ventricular rate is slow, IV atropine may be ordered. Reassess the patient's response and continue monitoring the patient. Transcutaneous pacing or a dopamine or epinephrine IV infusion may be tried if atropine is ineffective. Ventricular antiarrhythmic medications such as lidocaine should be avoided during the management of patients with this rhythm because they may abolish ventricular activity, possibly causing asystole in a patient with a ventricular escape rhythm.

If the patient is not breathing and has no pulse despite the appearance of organized electrical activity on the cardiac monitor, pulseless electrical activity (PEA) exists. The management of PEA should include cardiopulmonary resuscitation (CPR), giving oxygen, starting an IV, possible placement of an advanced airway, and an aggressive search for the underlying cause of the situation (Box 6.2).

ACCELERATED IDIOVENTRICULAR RHYTHM

How Do I Recognize It?

[Objective 7]

An **accelerated idioventricular rhythm (AIVR)** exists when three or more ventricular beats occur in a row at a rate of 41 to 100 beats/min (Fig. 6.14). Some cardiologists consider the ventricular rate range of AIVR to be 41 to 120 beats/min.

AIVR is usually considered a benign escape rhythm. It appears when the sinus rate slows and disappears when the sinus rate speeds up. Episodes of AIVR usually last a few seconds to 1 minute. Because AIVR usually begins and ends gradually, it is also called *nonparoxysmal VT*. Fusion beats are often seen at the onset and end of the rhythm. The ECG characteristics of AIVR are shown in Table 6.4.

What Causes It?

AIVR is usually considered a benign escape rhythm. It is often seen during the first 12 hours of an acute myocardial infarction (MI), and it is common after successful reperfusion therapy or after interventional coronary artery procedures

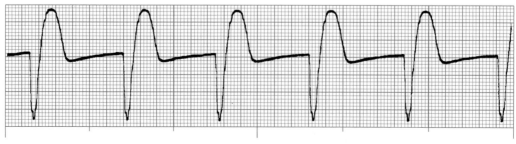

Fig. 6.14 Accelerated idioventricular rhythm. (From Aehlert B: *ECG study cards,* St. Louis, 2004, Mosby.)

(Goldberger et al, 2013). AIVR has been observed in patients with the following:

- Acute myocarditis
- Cocaine toxicity
- Digitalis toxicity
- Dilated cardiomyopathy
- Hypertensive heart disease
- Subarachnoid hemorrhage

What Do I Do About It?

AIVR generally requires no treatment because the rhythm is protective and often transient, spontaneously resolving on its own; however, possible dizziness, lightheadedness, or other signs of hemodynamic compromise may occur because of the loss of atrial kick. When treatment is indicated, apply a pulse oximeter and administer supplemental oxygen if indicated. Establish IV access and obtain a 12-lead ECG.

TABLE 6.4	Characteristics of Accelerated Idioventricular Rhythm
Rhythm	Ventricular rhythm is essentially regular
Rate	41 to 100 (41 to 120 per some cardiologists) beats/min
P waves	Usually absent or, with retrograde conduction to the atria, may appear after the QRS (usually upright in the ST segment or T wave)
PR interval	None
QRS duration	0.12 sec or greater; the T wave is frequently in the opposite direction of the QRS complex

IV atropine or atrial pacing may be ordered to suppress the AIVR (Chung et al, 2010; Olgin & Zipes, 2012). Reassess the patient's response and continue monitoring him or her.

VENTRICULAR TACHYCARDIA

Ventricular tachycardia (VT) exists when three or more sequential PVCs occur at a rate of more than 100 beats/min. VT may occur with or without pulses, and the patient may be stable or unstable with this rhythm.

How Do I Recognize It?

[Objective 8]

VT may occur as a short run that lasts less than 30 seconds and spontaneously ends (i.e., *nonsustained VT*) (Fig. 6.15). Episodes of nonsustained VT may be recorded in up to 3% of apparently healthy individuals with no identifiable heart disease (Garan, 2016). The frequency with which nonsustained VT occurs increases with age and with the presence and severity of underlying heart disease (Garan, 2016). In patients with heart disease, nonsustained VT is often a predictor of high risk for sustained VT or VF (Martin & Wharton, 2001).

Sustained VT persists for more than 30 seconds (Fig. 6.16). The rapid heart rate associated with sustained VT can cause a marked decrease in ventricular function and cardiac output, particularly in patients with underlying heart disease, resulting in acute heart failure, syncope, hypotension, or circulatory collapse within several seconds to minutes after the onset of VT (Garan, 2016).

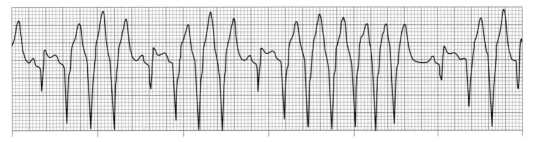

Fig. 6.15 Nonsustained ventricular tachycardia. (From Crawford MV, Spence MI: *Commonsense approach to coronary care,* rev ed 6, St. Louis, 1994, Mosby.)

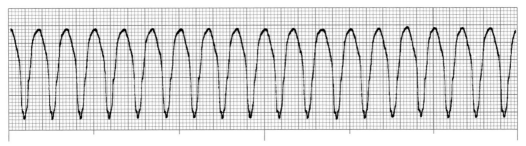

Fig. 6.16 If this rhythm lasts longer than 30 seconds, it is called *sustained ventricular tachycardia.* (From Aehlert B: *ECG study cards,* St. Louis, 2004, Mosby.)

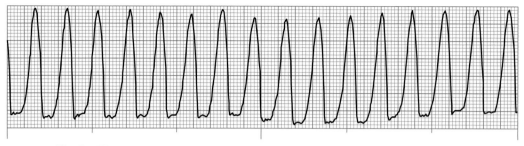

Fig. 6.17 Monomorphic ventricular tachycardia. (From Aehlert B: *ECG study cards,* St. Louis, 2004, Mosby.)

TABLE 6.5	Characteristics of Monomorphic Ventricular Tachycardia
Rhythm	Ventricular rhythm is essentially regular
Rate	101 to 250 (121 to 250 per some cardiologists) beats/min
P waves	Usually not seen; if present, they have no set relationship with the QRS complexes that appear between them at a rate different from that of the ventricular tachycardia
PR interval	None
QRS duration	0.12 sec or greater; often difficult to differentiate between the QRS and T wave

MONOMORPHIC VENTRICULAR TACHYCARDIA

[Objective 9]

Similar to PVCs, VT may originate from an ectopic focus in either ventricle. When the QRS complexes of VT are of the same shape and amplitude, the rhythm is called **monomorphic VT** (Fig. 6.17). Monomorphic VT with a ventricular rate of 150 to 300 beats/min is called *ventricular flutter* by some cardiologists (Olgin & Zipes, 2012). The ECG characteristics of monomorphic VT are shown in Table 6.5.

What Causes It?

Ventricular tachycardia may be the result of disorders of impulse formation, such as abnormal automaticity or triggered activity, or the result of disorders of conduction, such as reentry (Olgin & Zipes, 2012). Sustained monomorphic VT is often associated with underlying heart disease. When VT occurs in patients with underlying heart disease, the subsequent risk for sudden cardiac death is increased (Olgin & Zipes, 2012).

Possible causes of VT include the following:
- Acid–base imbalance
- Acute coronary syndromes
- Cardiomyopathy
- Cocaine abuse
- Digitalis toxicity
- Electrolyte imbalance (e.g., hypokalemia, hyperkalemia, hypomagnesemia)
- Mitral valve prolapse
- Trauma (e.g., myocardial contusion, invasive cardiac procedures)
- Tricyclic antidepressant overdose
- Valvular heart disease

What Do I Do About It?

Signs and symptoms associated with VT vary. A patient who has sustained monomorphic VT may be stable for long periods. However, if the ventricular rate is very fast or myocardial ischemia is present, monomorphic VT can degenerate to polymorphic VT or VF. Syncope or near-syncope may occur because of an abrupt onset of VT. The only warning symptom may be a brief period of lightheadedness.

During VT, the severity of the patient's symptoms is related to a number of factors, including how rapid the ventricular rate is, how long the tachycardia has been present, current medications, the presence and extent of underlying heart disease, and the presence and severity of peripheral vascular disease (Chung et al, 2010; Martin & Wharton, 2001). Signs and symptoms of hemodynamic instability related to VT may include the following:
- Acute altered mental status
- Acute heart failure
- Chest pain or discomfort
- Hypotension
- Pulmonary congestion
- Shock
- Shortness of breath

 ECG Pearl _____

Sustained VT does not always produce signs of hemodynamic instability.

Treatment is based on signs and symptoms and the type of VT. If the rhythm is monomorphic VT (and the patient's symptoms are caused by the tachycardia):
- CPR and defibrillation are used to treat the pulseless patient with VT.
- Stable but symptomatic patients are treated with oxygen (if indicated), IV access, and ventricular antiarrhythmics (e.g., procainamide, amiodarone, sotalol) to suppress the rhythm. Procainamide should be avoided if the patient has a prolonged QT interval or signs of heart failure. Sotalol should also be avoided if the patient has a prolonged QT interval.
- Unstable patients (usually a sustained heart rate of 150 beats/min or more) are treated with oxygen, IV access, and sedation (if the patient is awake and time permits) followed by synchronized cardioversion.

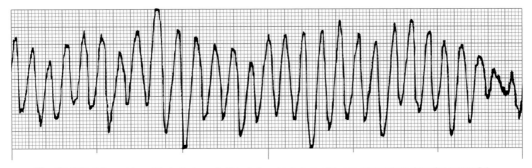

Fig. 6.18 Polymorphic ventricular tachycardia. This rhythm strip is from a 77-year-old man three days after myocardial infarction (MI). His chief complaint at the onset of this episode was chest pain. He had a past medical history of a previous MI and an abdominal aortic aneurysm repair. The patient was given a ventricular antiarrhythmic and defibrillated several times without success. Laboratory work revealed a serum potassium (K^+) level of 2.0. Intravenous K^+ was administered, and the patient converted to a sinus rhythm with the next defibrillation.

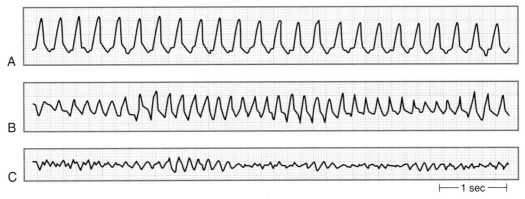

Fig. 6.19 Ventricular tachydysrhythmias. A, Rhythm strip showing monomorphic ventricular tachycardia. B, Example of polymorphic ventricular tachycardia. C, Example of ventricular fibrillation. All tracings are from lead V_1. (From Goldman L, Ausiello DA, Arend W, et al: *Cecil medicine,* ed 23, Philadelphia, 2007, Saunders.)

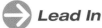 **Lead In** _____

Initiating Prompt Treatment for Possible Ventricular Tachycardia

A supraventricular tachycardia (SVT) with an intraventricular conduction delay may be difficult to distinguish from VT. Keep in mind that VT is considered a potentially life-threatening dysrhythmia. If you are unsure whether a regular, wide-QRS tachycardia is VT or SVT with an intraventricular conduction delay, treat the rhythm as VT until proven otherwise. Obtaining a 12-lead ECG may help differentiate VT from SVT, but do not delay treatment if the patient is symptomatic.

In all cases, an aggressive search must be made for the cause of the VT.

POLYMORPHIC VENTRICULAR TACHYCARDIA

[Objective 10]

With **polymorphic** VT (PMVT), the QRS complexes vary in shape and amplitude from beat to beat and appear to twist from upright to negative or negative to upright and back, resembling a spindle (Fig. 6.18). PMVT is a dysrhythmia of

TABLE 6.6	Characteristics of Polymorphic Ventricular Tachycardia
Rhythm	Ventricular rhythm may be regular or irregular
Rate	Ventricular rate 150 to 300 beats/min; typically 200 to 250 beats/min
P waves	None
PR interval	None
QRS duration	0.12 sec or more; there is a gradual alteration in the amplitude and direction of the QRS complexes; a typical cycle consists of 5 to 20 QRS complexes

intermediate severity between monomorphic VT and VF (Fig. 6.19). When PMVT is very fast, it may be difficult to distinguish from VF (Garan, 2016). The ECG characteristics of polymorphic VT are shown in Table 6.6.

What Causes It?

Several types of PMVT and their possible causes have been identified. Polymorphic VT that occurs in the presence of a long QT interval (typically 0.45 second or more and often 0.50 second or more) is called **torsades** de pointes (TdP). A long QT interval may be congenital, acquired (typically precipitated by antiarrhythmic drug use or hypokalemia, which are typically associated with bradycardia), or idiopathic (neither familial nor with an identifiable acquired cause). Polymorphic VT can occur in the presence of an abnormally short QT interval (typically less than 0.32 second). This type of polymorphic VT is called *short-QT PMVT*. Polymorphic VT that occurs in the presence of a normal QT interval is simply referred to as *polymorphic VT* or *normal-QT PMVT*.

What Do I Do About It?

The signs and symptoms associated with PMVT are usually related to the decreased cardiac output that occurs because of the fast ventricular rate. Signs of shock are often present. The patient may experience a syncopal episode or seizures. The rhythm may occasionally terminate spontaneously and recur after several seconds or minutes, or it may deteriorate to VF. The patient with sustained PMVT is rarely hemodynamically stable.

It is best to seek expert consultation when treating a patient with PMVT because of the diverse mechanisms of PMVT as there may or may not be clues as to its specific cause at the time of the patient's presentation. Treatment options vary and can be contradictory. For example, a medication that may be appropriate for the treatment of a patient with TdP may be contraindicated when treating a patient with another form of PMVT. In general, if the patient is symptomatic because of the tachycardia, treat ischemia (if it is present), correct electrolyte abnormalities, and discontinue any medications that the patient may be taking that prolong the QT interval. If the patient is stable, the use of IV amiodarone (if the QT interval is normal), magnesium, or beta-blockers may be effective, depending on the cause of the PMVT. If the patient is unstable or has no pulse, proceed with defibrillation as for VF.

VENTRICULAR FIBRILLATION

How Do I Recognize It?

[Objective 11]

Ventricular fibrillation (VF) is a chaotic rhythm that begins in the ventricles. In VF, there is no organized ventricular depolarization. The ventricular muscle quivers, and as a result, there is no effective myocardial contraction and no pulse. The resulting rhythm looks chaotic with deflections that vary in shape and amplitude. No normal-looking waveforms are visible. VF with waves that are 3 or more mm high is called *coarse VF* (Fig. 6.20). VF with low amplitude waves (i.e., less than 3 mm) is called *fine VF* (Fig. 6.21). Table 6.7 lists the ECG characteristics of VF, and Fig. 6.22 illustrates a comparison of ventricular dysrhythmias.

TABLE 6.7	Characteristics of Ventricular Fibrillation
Rhythm	Rapid and chaotic with no pattern or regularity
Rate	Cannot be determined because there are no discernible waves or complexes to measure
P waves	Not discernible
PR interval	Not discernible
QRS duration	Not discernible

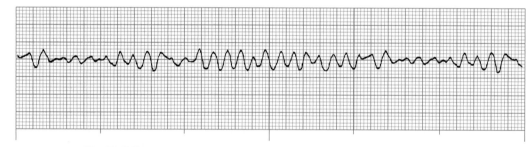

Fig. 6.20 Ventricular fibrillation (VF) with waves that are 3 mm high or more is called *coarse VF.*

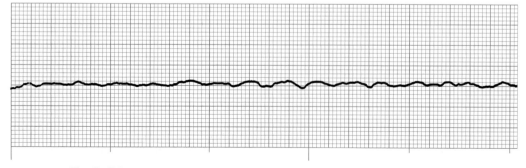

Fig. 6.21 Ventricular fibrillation (VF) with low-amplitude waves (i.e., less than 3 mm) is called *fine VF.*

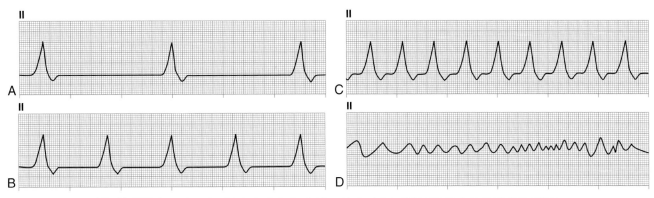

Fig. 6.22 Comparison of ventricular dysrhythmias. A, Idioventricular rhythm at 38 beats/min. B, Accelerated idioventricular rhythm at 75 beats/min. C, Monomorphic ventricular tachycardia at 150 beats/min. D, Coarse ventricular fibrillation. (From Grauer K: *A practical guide to ECG interpretation,* ed 2, St. Louis, 1998, Mosby.)

What Causes It?

Factors that increase the susceptibility of the myocardium to fibrillate include the following:

- Acute coronary syndromes
- Dysrhythmias
- Electrolyte imbalance
- Environmental factors (e.g., electrocution)
- Hypertrophy
- Increased sympathetic nervous system activity
- Proarrhythmic effect of antiarrhythmics and other medications
- Severe heart failure
- Vagal stimulation

What Do I Do About It?

The patient in VF is unresponsive, apneic, and pulseless. The priorities of care in cardiac arrest as a result of pulseless VT or VF are high-quality CPR and defibrillation. Use the mnemonic "the 5 Hs and 5 Ts" to recall possible reversible causes of pulseless VT or VF. Administer medications and perform additional interventions in accordance with current resuscitation guidelines. Cardiac arrest rhythms are shown in Box 6.3.

 CLINICAL CORRELATIONS

Because artifact can mimic VF, *always* check the patient's pulse before beginning treatment.

Box 6.3 Cardiac Arrest Rhythms

- Asystole
- Pulseless electrical activity (PEA)
- Ventricular fibrillation (VF)
- Pulseless ventricular tachycardia (VT)

VF and pulseless VT are *shockable* rhythms, which means that delivering a shock to the heart by means of a defibrillator may result in termination of the rhythm. Asystole and PEA are *nonshockable* rhythms.

DEFIBRILLATION
[Objective 12]

Defibrillation is the delivery of an electrical current across the heart muscle over a very brief period to terminate an abnormal heart rhythm. Defibrillation is also called *unsynchronized countershock* or *asynchronous countershock* because the delivery of current has no relationship to the cardiac cycle. The shock attempts to deliver a uniform electrical current of sufficient intensity to depolarize myocardial cells (including fibrillating cells) at the same time, thereby briefly stunning the heart. This provides an opportunity for the heart's natural pacemakers to resume normal activity. When the cells repolarize, the pacemaker with the highest degree of automaticity should assume responsibility for pacing the heart.

Manual defibrillation refers to the placement of paddles or pads on a patient's chest, the interpretation of the patient's cardiac rhythm by a trained health care professional, and the health care professional's decision to deliver a shock, if indicated. *Automated external defibrillation* refers to the placement of paddles or pads on a patient's chest and the interpretation of the patient's cardiac rhythm by an **automated external defibrillator (AED)**. The AED has a sophisticated computer system that analyzes a patient's heart rhythm using an algorithm to distinguish shockable rhythms from nonshockable rhythms and providing visual and auditory instructions to the rescuer to deliver an electrical shock, if a shock is indicated. Defibrillation is indicated in the treatment of pulseless monomorphic VT, sustained polymorphic VT, and VF.

ASYSTOLE (CARDIAC STANDSTILL)

How Do I Recognize It?
[Objective 13]

Asystole, also called *cardiac standstill,* is a total absence of atrial and ventricular electrical activity (Fig. 6.23). There is no atrial or ventricular rate or rhythm, no pulse, and no cardiac

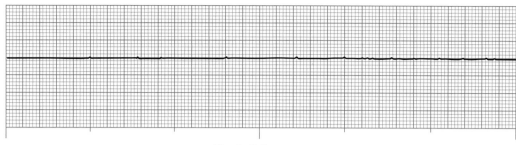

Fig. 6.23 Asystole.

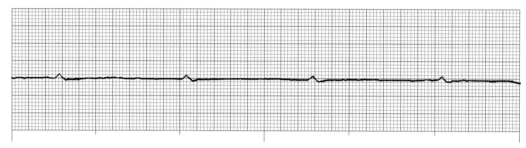

Fig. 6.24 P-wave asystole (also known as *ventricular standstill*).

TABLE 6.8	Characteristics of Asystole
Rhythm	Ventricular not discernible; atrial may be discernible
Rate	Ventricular not discernible, but atrial activity may be observed (i.e., P wave asystole)
P waves	Usually not discernible
PR interval	Not measurable
QRS duration	Absent

output. If atrial electrical activity is present, the rhythm is called *P wave asystole* or *ventricular standstill* (Fig. 6.24). The ECG characteristics of asystole are shown in Table 6.8.

What Causes It?

Use the mnemonic "the 5 Hs and 5 Ts" to recall possible reversible causes of asystole. In addition, ventricular asystole

may occur temporarily after termination of a tachycardia with medications, defibrillation, or synchronized cardioversion (Fig. 6.25).

What Do I Do About It?

When asystole is observed on a cardiac monitor, confirm that the patient is unresponsive and has no pulse, and then begin high-quality CPR. Additional care includes establishing vascular access, considering the possible causes of the arrest, and administering medications and performing additional interventions in accordance with current resuscitation guidelines. A summary of all ventricular rhythm characteristics appears in Table 6.9.

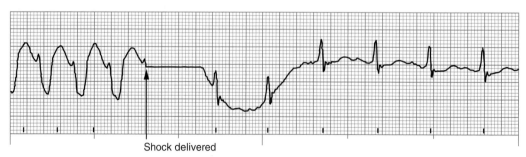

Shock delivered

Fig. 6.25 This rhythm strip is from a 62-year-old man complaining of palpitations. The patient's initial rhythm was monomorphic ventricular tachycardia. A synchronized shock was delivered, resulting in a sinus rhythm with a prolonged PR interval. Note the short period of asystole after the shock was delivered. (From Aehlert B: *ECG study cards,* St. Louis, 2004, Mosby.)

TABLE 6.9 Ventricular Rhythms: Summary of Characteristics

Characteristic	Premature Ventricular Complexes	Ventricular Escape Beat	Idioventricular Rhythm	Accelerated Idioventricular Rhythm
Rhythm	Irregular because of *early* beats	Irregular because of *late* beats	Essentially regular	Essentially regular
Rate (beats/min)	Usually within normal range, but depends on underlying rhythm	Usually within normal range, but depends on underlying rhythm	20 to 40	41 to 100; some experts consider the rate 41 to 120
P waves (lead II)	Usually absent or, with retrograde conduction to the atria, may appear after the QRS (usually upright in ST segment or T wave)	Usually absent or, with retrograde conduction to the atria, may appear after the QRS (usually upright in ST segment or T wave)	Usually absent or, with retrograde conduction to the atria, may appear after the QRS (usually upright in ST segment or T wave)	Usually absent or, with retrograde conduction to the atria, may appear after the QRS (usually upright in ST segment or T wave)
PR interval	None	None	None	None
QRS duration	Usually 0.12 sec or greater	0.12 sec or greater	0.12 sec or greater	0.12 sec or greater

Characteristic	Monomorphic Ventricular Tachycardia	Polymorphic Ventricular Tachycardia	Ventricular Fibrillation	Asystole
Rhythm	Usually regular	Irregular	Chaotic	None
Rate (beats/min)	101 to 250; some experts consider the rate 121 to 250	150 to 300	Not discernible	None
P waves (lead II)	May be present or absent; if present, they have no set relationship to the QRS complexes, appearing between the QRSs at a rate different from that of the ventricular tachycardia	Independent or none	Absent	Atrial activity may be observed (P-wave asystole)
PR interval	None	None	None	None
QRS duration	0.12 sec or greater	0.12 sec or greater	Not discernible	Absent

STOP & REVIEW

True/False

____**1.** TdP is a type of monomorphic VT.

____**2.** Uniform PVCs are unifocal, but multiform PVCs are not necessarily multifocal.

____**3.** An accelerated junctional or an accelerated ventricular rhythm is faster than its intrinsic rate but slower than 100 beats/min.

Multiple Choice

____**4.** How would you differentiate a junctional escape rhythm at 40 beats/min from an idioventricular rhythm at the same rate?

    a. It is impossible to differentiate a junctional escape rhythm from an idioventricular rhythm.

    b. The junctional escape rhythm will have a narrow QRS complex; the idioventricular rhythm will have a wide QRS complex.

    c. The rate (i.e., 40 beats/min) will indicate a junctional escape rhythm, not an idioventricular rhythm.

    d. The junctional escape rhythm will have a wide QRS complex; an idioventricular rhythm will have a narrow QRS complex.

____**5.** The term for three or more PVCs occurring in a row at a rate of more than 100/min is

    a. ventricular trigeminy.

    b. ventricular fibrillation.

    c. a run of VT.

    d. a run of ventricular escape beats.

Matching

a. Current
b. Fusion beat
c. AIVR
d. Compensatory pause
e. VT
f. Asystole
g. Monomorphic
h. Agonal rhythm
i. Defibrillation

j. Proarrhythmic
k. AV dissociation
l. Multiform
m. AED
n. Interpolated PVC
o. Polymorphic
p. R-on-T phenomenon
q. Idioventricular rhythm

____**6.** A dysrhythmia that is similar in appearance to an idioventricular rhythm but occurs at a rate of less than 20 beats/min

____**7.** Varying in shape

____**8.** A dysrhythmia that originates in the ventricles with a rate between 20 and 40 beats/min

____**9.** A machine with a sophisticated computer system that analyzes a patient's heart rhythm using an algorithm to distinguish shockable rhythms from nonshockable rhythms

____**10.** Antiarrhythmics can cause a(n) ___ effect, which means that they have the *potential* to cause serious adverse effects, more serious dysrhythmias, or both, than those that they were intended to treat.

____**11.** Any dysrhythmia in which the atria and the ventricles beat independently

____**12.** A PVC that occurs between two normally conducted QRS complexes and that does not disturb the next ventricular depolarization or sinoatrial node activity

____**13.** A total absence of atrial and ventricular electrical activity

____**14.** A beat that occurs because of the simultaneous activation of one cardiac chamber by two sites

____**15.** The flow of an electrical charge from one point to another

____**16.** A term used to describe PVCs that are different in appearance

____**17.** A dysrhythmia that originates in the ventricles with a rate between 41 and 100 beats/min

____**18.** The initiation of a ventricular tachydysrhythmia as a result of an improperly timed electrical impulse on the T wave

____**19.** Delivery of an electrical current across the heart muscle over a very brief period to terminate an abnormal heart rhythm

____**20.** A dysrhythmia that originates in the ventricles with a ventricular response greater than 100 beats/min

____**21.** Having the same shape

____**22.** This often follows a PVC and occurs because the sinoatrial node is usually not affected by the PVC

Short Answer

23. Explain the difference between a PVC and a ventricular escape beat.

_____

_____

_____

24. How do coarse and fine ventricular fibrillation differ?

_____

_____

_____

Ventricular Rhythms—Practice Rhythm Strips

Use the five steps of rhythm interpretation to interpret each of the following rhythm strips. All rhythms were recorded in lead II unless otherwise noted.

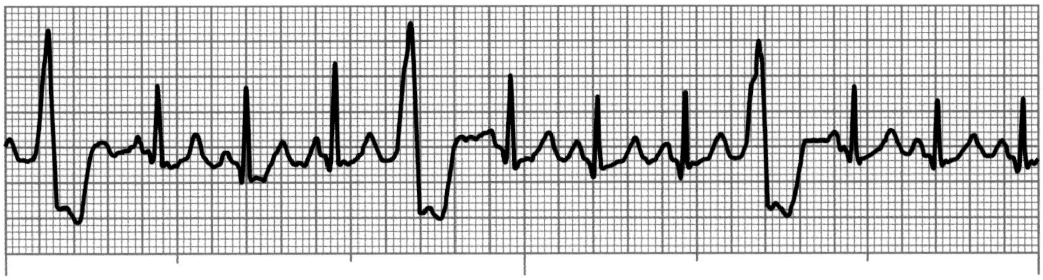

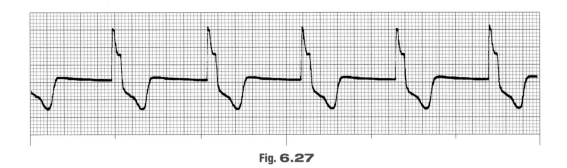

Fig. 6.26 (From Aehlert B: *ECG study cards,* St. Louis, 2004, Mosby.)

25. Fig. 6.26

Rhythm: _____ Rate: _____ P waves: _____

PR interval: _____ QRS duration: _____ QT interval: _____

Interpretation: _____

Fig. 6.27

26. Fig. 6.27

Rhythm: _____ Rate: _____ P waves: _____

PR interval: _____ QRS duration: _____ QT interval: _____

Interpretation: _____

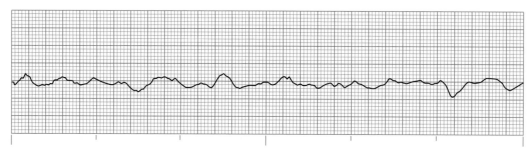

Fig. 6.28 (From Aehlert B: *ECG study cards*, St. Louis, 2004, Mosby.)

27. **Fig. 6.28**. This rhythm strip is from a 63-year-old man who collapsed on the kitchen floor. He is unresponsive, apneic, and pulseless. His past medical history includes a coronary artery bypass graft 8 years ago and pacemaker implantation 5 years ago.

Rhythm: _____ Rate: _____ P waves: _____

PR interval: _____ QRS duration: _____ QT interval: _____

Interpretation: _____

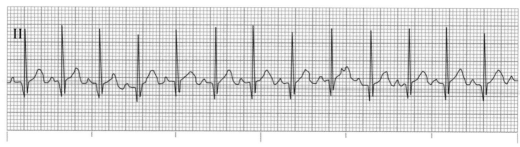

Fig. 6.29 (Modified from Aehlert B: *ECG study cards*, St. Louis, 2004, Mosby.)

28. **Fig. 6.29**. This rhythm strip is from a 1-month-old infant after a 3-minute seizure.

Rhythm: _____ Rate: _____ P waves: _____

PR interval: _____ QRS duration: _____ QT interval: _____

Interpretation: _____

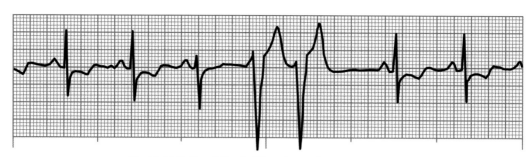

Fig. 6.30 (From Aehlert B: *ECG study cards*, St. Louis, 2004, Mosby.)

29. **Fig. 6.30**

Rhythm: _____ Rate: _____ P waves: _____

PR interval: _____ QRS duration: _____ QT interval: _____

Interpretation: _____

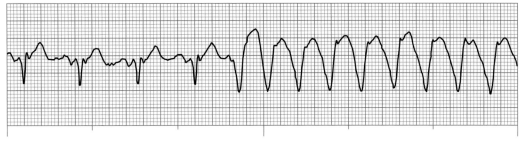

Fig. 6.31 (From Aehlert B: *ECG study cards,* St. Louis, 2004, Mosby.)

30. Fig. 6.31

Rhythm: _____ Rate: _____ P waves: _____

PR interval: _____ QRS duration: _____ QT interval: _____

Interpretation: _____

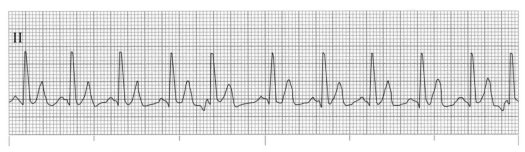

Fig. 6.32

31. Fig. 6.32

Rhythm: _____ Rate: _____ P waves: _____

PR interval: _____ QRS duration: _____ QT interval: _____

Interpretation: _____

Fig. 6.33 (Modified from Aehlert B: *ECG study cards,* St. Louis, 2004, Mosby.)

32. Fig. 6.33

Rhythm: _____ Rate: _____ P waves: _____

PR interval: _____ QRS duration: _____ QT interval: _____

Interpretation: _____

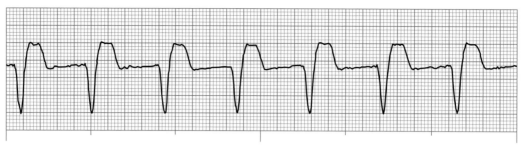

Fig. 6.34 (From Aehlert B: *ECG study cards,* St. Louis, 2004, Mosby.)

33. **Fig. 6.34.** This rhythm strip is from a 73-year-old woman complaining of chest pain.

Rhythm: _____ Rate: _____ P waves: _____

PR interval: _____ QRS duration: _____ QT interval: _____

Interpretation: _____

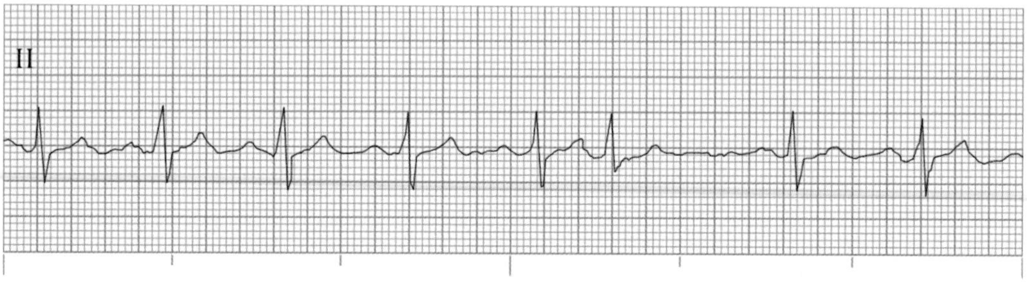

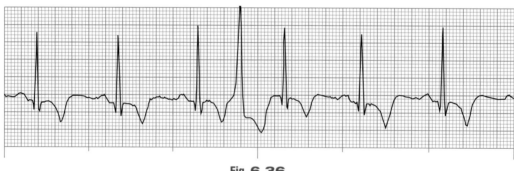

Fig. 6.35 (Modified from Aehlert B: *ECG study cards,* St. Louis, 2004, Mosby.)

34. **Fig. 6.35.** This rhythm strip is from a 25-year-old man with an altered level of responsiveness because of alcohol.

Rhythm: _____ Rate: _____ P waves: _____

PR interval: _____ QRS duration: _____ QT interval: _____

Interpretation: _____

Fig. 6.36

35. **Fig. 6.36**

Rhythm: _____ Rate: _____ P waves: _____

PR interval: _____ QRS duration: _____ QT interval: _____

Interpretation: _____

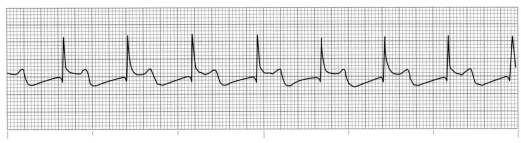

Fig. 6.37

36. **Fig. 6.37**

   Rhythm: _____ Rate: _____ P waves: _____

   PR interval: _____ QRS duration: _____ QT interval: _____

   Interpretation: _____

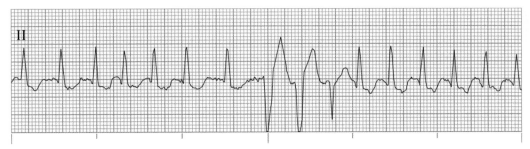

Fig. 6.38 (Modified from Aehlert B: *ECG study cards,* St. Louis, 2004, Mosby.)

37. **Fig. 6.38**

   Rhythm: _____ Rate: _____ P waves: _____

   PR interval: _____ QRS duration: _____ QT interval: _____

   Interpretation: _____

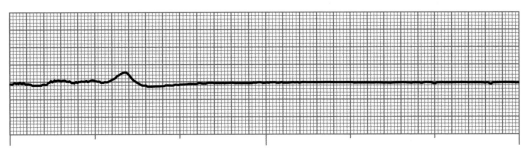

Fig. 6.39 (From Aehlert B: *ECG study cards,* St. Louis, 2004, Mosby.)

38. **Fig. 6.39**

   Rhythm: _____ Rate: _____ P waves: _____

   PR interval: _____ QRS duration: _____ QT interval: _____

   Interpretation: _____

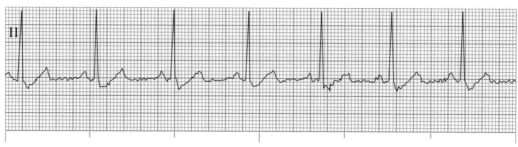

Fig. 6.40 (Modified from Aehlert B: *ECG study cards,* St. Louis, 2004, Mosby.)

39. **Fig. 6.40**. This rhythm strip is from a 47-year-old man with an altered level of responsiveness. His blood pressure is 118/86 mm Hg, and his blood sugar is 37 mg/dL.

Rhythm: _____ Rate: _____ P waves: _____

PR interval: _____ QRS duration: _____ QT interval: _____

Interpretation: _____

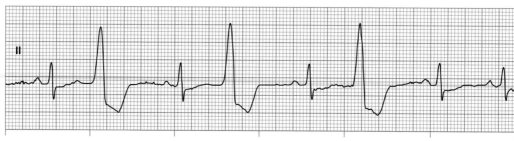

Fig. 6.41

40. **Fig. 6.41**. This rhythm strip is from a 69-year-old man who is complaining of substernal chest pain. He rates his discomfort as 9/10.

Rhythm: _____ Rate: _____ P waves: _____

PR interval: _____ QRS duration: _____ QT interval: _____

Interpretation: _____

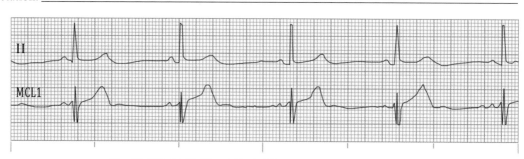

Fig. 6.42 (Modified from Aehlert B: *ECG study cards,* St. Louis, 2004, Mosby.)

41. **Fig. 6.42**. This rhythm strip is from a 68-year-old man with a head injury after a fall.

Rhythm: _____ Rate: _____ P waves: _____

PR interval: _____ QRS duration: _____ QT interval: _____

Interpretation: _____

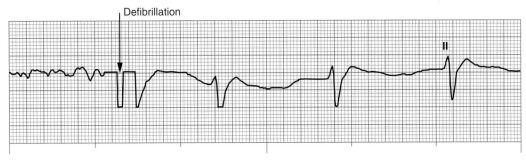

Fig. 6.43 (From Aehlert B: *ECG study cards,* St. Louis, 2004, Mosby.)

42. **Fig. 6.43**. This rhythm strip is from a 58-year-old man who was initially unresponsive, apneic, and pulseless.

Rhythm: _____ Rate: _____ P waves: _____

PR interval: _____ QRS duration: _____ QT interval: _____

Interpretation: _____

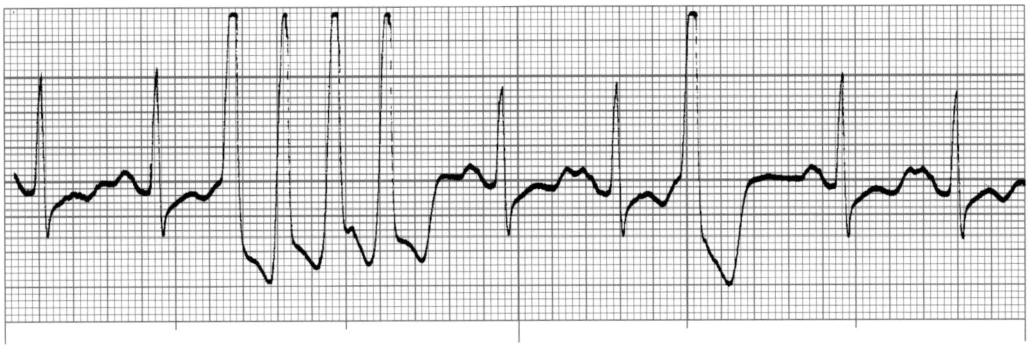

Fig. 6.44

43. **Fig. 6.44**

Rhythm: _____ Rate: _____ P waves: _____

PR interval: _____ QRS duration: _____ QT interval: _____

Interpretation: _____

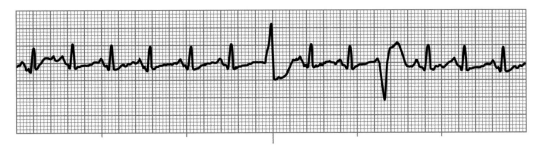

Fig. 6.45 (From Aehlert B: *ECG study cards,* St. Louis, 2004, Mosby.)

44. **Fig. 6.45**. This rhythm strip is from a 61-year-old woman who is complaining of shortness of breath.

Rhythm: _____ Rate: _____ P waves: _____

PR interval: _____ QRS duration: _____ QT interval: _____

Interpretation: _____

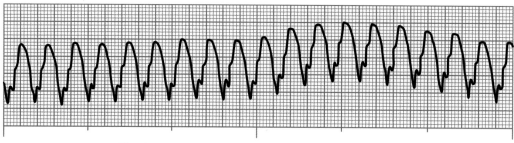

Fig. 6.46 (From Aehlert B: *ECG study cards,* St. Louis, 2004, Mosby.)

45. Fig. 6.46

Rhythm: _____ Rate: _____ P waves: _____

PR interval: _____ QRS duration: _____ QT interval: _____

Interpretation: _____

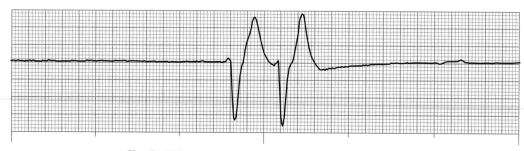

Fig. 6.47 (From Aehlert B: *ECG study cards,* St. Louis, 2004, Mosby.)

46. Fig. 6.47

Rhythm: _____ Rate: _____ P waves: _____

PR interval: _____ QRS duration: _____ QT interval: _____

Interpretation: _____

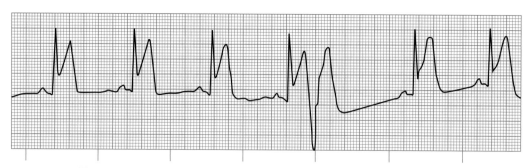

Fig. 6.48 (From Conover MB: *Understanding electrocardiography,* ed 7, St. Louis, 1995, Mosby.)

47. Fig. 6.48

Rhythm: _____ Rate: _____ P waves: _____

PR interval: _____ QRS duration: _____ QT interval: _____

Interpretation: _____

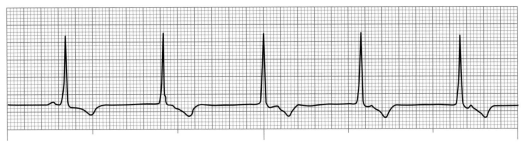

Fig. 6.49 (From Aehlert B: *ECG study cards,* St. Louis, 2004, Mosby.)

48. **Fig. 6.49**

Rhythm: _____ Rate: _____ P waves: _____

PR interval: _____ QRS duration: _____ QT interval: _____

Interpretation: _____

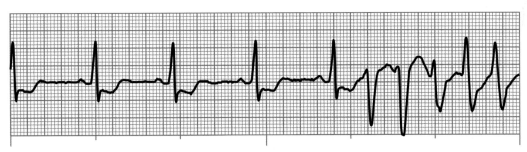

Fig. 6.50 (From Aehlert B: *ECG study cards,* St. Louis, 2004, Mosby.)

49. **Fig. 6.50**. This rhythm strip is from a 90-year-old unresponsive woman. She has a history of heart failure. Her medications include furosemide and albuterol.

Rhythm: _____ Rate: _____ P waves: _____

PR interval: _____ QRS duration: _____ QT interval: _____

Interpretation: _____

STOP & REVIEW / ANSWERS

1. F. TdP is a type of *polymorphic* VT that occurs in the presence of a long QT interval (typically 0.45 second or more and often 0.50 second or more).
OBJ: Describe the ECG characteristics, possible causes, signs and symptoms, and initial emergency care for PMVT.

2. T. Uniform PVCs are unifocal; that is, they arise from the same anatomic site. Multiform PVCs often, but do not always, arise from different anatomic sites; therefore, multiform PVCs are not necessarily multifocal. In general, multiform PVCs are considered more serious than uniform PVCs because they suggest a greater area of irritable myocardial tissue.
OBJ: Describe the ECG characteristics, possible causes, signs and symptoms, and initial emergency care for PVCs.

3. T. The intrinsic rate for an accelerated junctional rhythm is 61 to 100 beats/min. The intrinsic rate for an AIVR is 41 to 100 beats/min. Some cardiologists consider the ventricular rate range of AIVR to be 41 to 120 beats/min.
OBJ: Describe the ECG characteristics, possible causes, signs and symptoms, and initial emergency care for an AIVR.

4. B. The intrinsic rate of a junctional escape rhythm is 40 to 60 beats/min. A junctional escape rhythm has a narrow QRS complex. The intrinsic rate of an idioventricular rhythm is 20 to 40 beats/min. An idioventricular rhythm has a wide QRS complex.
OBJ: Describe the ECG characteristics, possible causes, signs and symptoms, and initial emergency care for an IVR.

5. C. Three or more sequential PVCs are termed a "run" or "burst," and three or more PVCs that occur in a row at a rate of more than 100 beats/min are considered a run of VT.
OBJ: Explain the terms *bigeminy*, *trigeminy*, *quadrigeminy*, and *run* as used to describe premature complexes.

6. H
7. O
8. Q
9. M
10. J
11. K
12. N
13. F
14. B
15. A
16. L
17. C
18. P
19. I
20. E
21. G
22. D

23. A PVC is premature and occurs before the next expected sinus beat. A ventricular escape beat is late, occurring after the next expected sinus beat.
OBJ: Explain the difference between PVCs and ventricular escape beats.

24. Coarse ventricular fibrillation (VF) is 3 mm or more in amplitude. Fine VF is less than 3 mm in amplitude.
OBJ: Describe the ECG characteristics, possible causes, signs and symptoms, and initial emergency care for VF.

Practice Rhythm Strip Answers

Note: Because of the distortion of ECGs that can occur during printing, a range of acceptable measurements is provided in the rhythm strip answers throughout this textbook.

25. **Fig. 6.26**
Rhythm: Irregular
Rate: 120 beats/min
P waves: Uniform and upright before each QRS (sinus beats)
PR interval: 0.12 to 0.16 second (sinus beats)
QRS duration: 0.06 to 0.08 second (sinus beats)
QT interval: 0.32 to 0.34 second (sinus beats)
Interpretation: Sinus tachycardia at 120 beats/min with ventricular quadrigeminy

26. **Fig. 6.27**
Rhythm: Regular
Rate: 55 beats/min
P waves: None visible
PR interval: None
QRS duration: 0.12 to 0.14 second
QT interval: 0.44 second
Interpretation: AIVR at 55 beats/min

27. **Fig. 6.28**
Rhythm: Irregular
Rate: None
P waves: None
PR interval: None
QRS duration: None
QT interval: None
Interpretation: Coarse ventricular fibrillation

28. **Fig. 6.29**
Rhythm: Regular
Rate: 125 beats/min (within normal limits for age)
P waves: Upright before each QRS; most are smooth and rounded; a few are pointed
PR interval: 0.14 to 0.16 second
QRS duration: 0.06 to 0.08 second
QT interval: 0.24 second
Interpretation: Sinus rhythm at 125 beats/min

29. Fig. 6.30
Rhythm: Irregular
Rate: 70 beats/min
P waves: Upright before sinus beats and the fusion beat
PR interval: 0.16 second (sinus beats)
QRS duration: 0.06 to 0.08 second (sinus beats)
QT interval: 0.32 to 0.36 second (sinus beats)
Interpretation: Sinus rhythm at 70 beats/min with a fusion beat, a pair of PVCs, ST-segment depression, and inverted T waves

30. Fig. 6.31
Rhythm: Irregular; two rhythms are present
Rate: 90 beats/min (sinus beats); 160 beats/min (VT) (because two rhythms are present, a rate for each should be documented)
P waves: Upright in sinus beats; none visible with VT
PR interval: 0.16 second (sinus beats)
QRS duration: 0.10 second (sinus beats); 0.14 second (VT)
QT interval: 0.32 to 0.36 second (sinus beats)
Interpretation: Sinus rhythm at 90 beats/min, a fusion beat, and then monomorphic VT at 160 beats/min

31. Fig. 6.32
Rhythm: Irregular; two rhythms are present
Rate: 60 beats/min (sinus beats); 300 to 375 beats/min (VT)
P waves: Upright in sinus beats; one is notched; none visible with VT
PR interval: 0.16 second (sinus beats)
QRS duration: 0.08 to 0.10 second (sinus beats); 0.12 second (VT)
QT interval: 0.40 second (sinus beats)
Interpretation: Sinus rhythm at 60 beats/min to PMVT at 300 to 375 beats/min

32. Fig. 6.33
Rhythm: Irregular
Rate: 110 beats/min
P waves: Upright with sinus beats; early and inverted in beats 5 and 11
PR interval: 0.12 to 0.16 second
QRS duration: 0.08 to 0.10 second (sinus beats)
QT interval: 0.32 second (sinus beats)
Interpretation: Sinus tachycardia at 110 beats/min with two premature junctional complexes

33. Fig. 6.34
Rhythm: Regular
Rate: 68 beats/min
P waves: None visible
PR interval: None
QRS duration: 0.12 second
QT interval: 0.32 to 0.38 sec (difficult to clearly identify end of T waves)
Interpretation: AIVR at 68 beats/min; artifact is present

34. Fig. 6.35
Rhythm: Irregular
Rate: 80 beats/min
P waves: Upright with sinus beats; early with beat 6, distorting the T wave of beat 5
PR interval: 0.18 to 0.20 second
QRS duration: 0.10 second
QT interval: 0.32 to 0.34 second
Interpretation: Sinus rhythm at 80 beats/min with a premature atrial complex

35. Fig. 6.36
Rhythm: Irregular
Rate: 70 beats/min
P waves: Upright before sinus beats; none visible with beat 4
PR interval: 0.20 to 0.22 second
QRS duration: 0.10 second
QT interval: 0.40 to 0.44 second
Interpretation: Sinus rhythm at 70 beats/min with an interpolated PVC and inverted T waves

36. Fig. 6.37
Rhythm: Regular
Rate: 79 beats/min
P waves: None visible
PR interval: None
QRS duration: 0.08 second
QT interval: 0.32 second
Interpretation: Accelerated junctional rhythm at 79 beats/min with ST-segment elevation

37. Fig. 6.38
Rhythm: Irregular to regular
Rate: 143 to 167 beats/min (atrial beats); 150 beats/min with beats 11 through 16
P waves: None visible
PR interval: None
QRS duration: 0.08 second (atrial beats)
QT interval: 0.20 to 0.24 second
Interpretation: Atrial fibrillation (AFib) at 143 to 167 beats/min with two ventricular complexes and a fusion beat, changing to supraventricular tachycardia (SVT) at 150 beats/min; ST-segment depression is present

38. Fig. 6.39
Rhythm: None
Rate: None
P waves: None
PR interval: None
QRS duration: None
QT interval: None
Interpretation: Asystole

39. **Fig. 6.40**
    Rhythm: Irregular
    Rate: 70 beats/min
    P waves: Uniform and upright before each QRS
    PR interval: 0.16 second
    QRS duration: 0.06 to 0.08 second
    QT interval: 0.40 second
    Interpretation: Sinus arrhythmia at 70 beats/min with ST-segment depression; artifact is present

40. **Fig. 6.41**
    Rhythm: Irregular
    Rate: 80 beats/min
    P waves: Uniform and upright with sinus beats; none with beats 2, 4, and 6
    PR interval: 0.16 to 0.20 second (sinus beats)
    QRS duration: 0.10 second (sinus beats)
    QT interval: 0.40 second (sinus beats)
    Interpretation: Sinus rhythm at 80 beats/min with uniform PVCs

41. **Fig. 6.42**
    Rhythm: Regular
    Rate: 47 beats/min
    P waves: Uniform and upright before each QRS
    PR interval: 0.14 to 0.16 second
    QRS duration: 0.06 to 0.08 second
    QT interval: 0.44 second
    Interpretation: Sinus bradycardia at 47 beats/min; U waves are visible in lead MCL$_1$

42. **Fig. 6.43**
    Rhythm: Irregular
    Rate: None to 40 beats/min
    P waves: None visible
    PR interval: None
    QRS duration: 0.16 second
    QT interval: 0.36 second
    Interpretation: Ventricular fibrillation, a shock (defibrillation), idioventricular rhythm at 40 beats/min

43. **Fig. 6.44**
    Rhythm: Irregular
    Rate: Sinus rate 88 beats/min; overall rate about 110 beats/min
    P waves: Upright with sinus beats but some are notched
    PR interval: 0.20 second (sinus beats)
    QRS duration: 0.08 second (sinus beats)
    QT interval: 0.36 second (sinus beats)
    Interpretation: Sinus rhythm at 88 beats/min with a run of VT and a PVC, ST-segment depression, and inverted T waves

44. **Fig. 6.45**
    Rhythm: Irregular
    Rate: 130 beats/min
    P waves: Upright before each QRS (sinus beats); none visible with beats 7 and 10
    PR interval: 0.12 second (sinus beats)

QRS duration: 0.06 second (sinus beats)
QT interval: Unable to determine because T waves are not visible
Interpretation: Sinus tachycardia at 130 beats/min with multiform PVCs

45. **Fig. 6.46**
    Rhythm: Regular
    Rate: 188 beats/min
    P waves: None visible
    PR interval: None
    QRS duration: 0.14 to 0.18 second
    QT interval: Unable to determine
    Interpretation: Monomorphic VT at 188 beats/min

46. **Fig. 6.47**
    Rhythm: Irregular
    Rate: Two ventricular complexes to none
    P waves: One visible on the far right of the strip; otherwise none
    PR interval: None
    QRS duration: 0.14 second to none
    QT interval: 0.48 second to none
    Interpretation: Agonal rhythm/asystole

47. **Fig. 6.48**
    Rhythm: Irregular
    Rate: 70 beats/min
    P waves: Upright before each QRS (sinus beats); none visible with beat 5
    PR interval: 0.16 to 0.18 second (sinus beats)
    QRS duration: 0.08 to 0.10 second (sinus beats)
    QT interval: 0.28 second (sinus beats)
    Interpretation: Sinus rhythm at 70 beats/min with an R-on-T PVC and ST-segment elevation

48. **Fig. 6.49**
    Rhythm: Regular
    Rate: 52 beats/min
    P waves: Upright before QRS in beat 1; none visible with remaining beats
    PR interval: 0.14 sec (sinus beat)
    QRS duration: 0.06 to 0.08 second
    QT interval: 0.44 second
    Interpretation: Sinus beat to junctional rhythm at 52 beats/min; inverted T waves

49. **Fig. 6.50**
    Rhythm: Irregular
    Rate: 65 beats/min (sinus beats) to 167 to 214 beats/min (PMVT)
    P waves: Upright before each QRS (sinus beats); none visible with PMVT
    PR interval: 0.16 second (sinus beats)
    QRS duration: 0.10 to 0.12 second (sinus beats)
    QT interval: 0.32 second (sinus beats)
    Interpretation: Sinus rhythm at 65 beats/min with ST-segment depression to PMVT at 167 to 214 beats/min

REFERENCES

Berger, M. G., Rubenstein, J. C., & Roth, J. A. (2016). Cardiac arrhythmias. In I. J. Benjamin, R. C. Griggs, E. J. Wing, & J. G. Fitz (Eds.), *Andreoli and Carpenter's Cecil essentials of medicine* (9th ed.) (pp. 110–135). Philadelphia: Saunders.

Chung, E. H., Sheahan, R. G., & Mounsey, J. P. (2010). Ventricular tachycardia. In M. S. Runge (Ed.), *Netter's cardiology* (2nd ed.) (pp. 241–249). Philadelphia: Saunders.

Crawford, M. V., & Spence, M. I. (1995). Electrical complications in coronary artery disease: Arrhythmias. In *Common sense approach to coronary care* (6th ed.) (p. 220). St. Louis: Mosby.

Garan, H. (2016). Ventricular arrhythmias. In L. Goldman & A. I. Schafer (Eds.), *Goldman-Cecil medicine* (25th ed.) (pp. 367–373). Philadelphia: Saunders.

Goldberger, A. L., Goldberger, Z. D., & Shvilkin, A. (2013). Ventricular arrhythmias. In *Clinical electrocardiography: A simplified approach* (8th ed.) (pp. 145–158). Philadelphia: Saunders.

Martin, D., & Wharton, J. M. (2001). Sustained monomorphic ventricular tachycardia. In P. J. Podrid & P. R. Kowey (Eds.), *Cardiac arrhythmia: Mechanisms, diagnosis, and management* (2nd ed.) (pp. 573–601). Philadelphia: Lippincott Williams & Wilkins.

Olgin, J., & Zipes, D. P. (2012). Specific arrhythmias: Diagnosis and treatment. In R. O. Bonow, D. L. Mann, D. P. Zipes, & P. Libby (Eds.), *Braunwald's heart disease: A textbook of cardiovascular medicine* (9th ed.) (pp. 771–824). Philadelphia: Saunders.

Spotts, V. (2011). Temporary transcutaneous (external) pacing. In D. L. Lynn-McHale Wiegand (Ed.), *AACN procedure manual for critical care* (6th ed.) (pp. 413–420). St. Louis: Saunders.

Atrioventricular Blocks

7

LEARNING OBJECTIVES

After reading this chapter, you should be able to:

1. Describe the electrocardiogram (ECG) characteristics, possible causes, signs and symptoms, and emergency management for first-degree atrioventricular (AV) block.
2. Describe the ECG characteristics, possible causes, signs and symptoms, and emergency management for second-degree AV block type I.
3. Describe the ECG characteristics, possible causes, signs and symptoms, and emergency management for second-degree AV block type II.
4. Describe 2:1 AV block and advanced second-degree AV block.
5. Describe the ECG characteristics, possible causes, signs and symptoms, and emergency management for third-degree AV block.

KEY TERM

atrioventricular (AV) block: A delay or interruption in impulse conduction from the atria to the ventricles that occurs because of a transient or permanent anatomic or functional impairment in the conduction system

INTRODUCTION

You have learned that the atrioventricular (AV) node and AV bundle have many important functions (Fig. 7.1). First, a supraventricular impulse that enters the AV node is normally delayed, thereby allowing the atrial chambers to contract and empty blood into the ventricles before the next ventricular contraction begins. Second, the healthy AV node is able to filter some of the supraventricular impulses coming to it, thereby protecting the ventricles from excessively rapid rates. Third, the AV bundle has pacemaker cells that have an intrinsic rate of 40 to 60 beats/min and can function as an escape pacemaker if the sinoatrial (SA) node fails.

Depolarization and repolarization are slow in the AV node, which makes this area vulnerable to blocks in conduction. When impulse conduction from the atria to the ventricles is delayed or interrupted because of a transient or permanent anatomic or functional impairment in the conduction system, the resulting dysrhythmia is called an **AV block** (Issa et al, 2012).

When analyzing a rhythm strip, you can assess PR intervals to detect AV conduction disturbances. Remember that the PR interval is made up of the P wave and the PR segment. The normal PR interval measures 0.12 to 0.20 second.

AV block is classified into (1) first-degree AV block, (2) second-degree AV block, and (3) third-degree AV block (Fig. 7.2). With first-degree AV block, impulses from the SA node to the ventricles are *delayed*; they are not blocked. With second-degree AV blocks, there is an *intermittent* disturbance in the conduction of impulses between the atria and the ventricles. With third-degree AV block, there is a *complete* block in the conduction of impulses between the atria and the ventricles.

First-degree AV block usually occurs because of a conduction delay within the AV node. Second- and third-degree AV blocks can occur at the level of the AV node, the bundle of His, or the bundle branches. AV blocks located at the bundle of His or bundle branches are called *infranodal* or *subnodal AV blocks.*

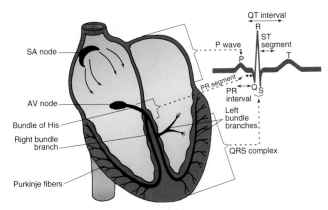

Fig. 7.1 Interruptions in impulse transmission between the atria and ventricles can be detected by assessing PR intervals. *AV,* Atrioventricular; *SA,* sinoatrial. (From Ignatavicius DD, Workman LM: *Medical-surgical nursing: patient-centered collaborative care,* ed 8, Philadelphia, 2016, Saunders.)

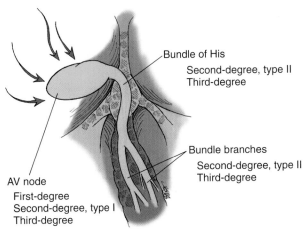

Fig. 7.2 Common locations of atrioventricular (AV) blocks.

AV blocks that occur at the level of the AV node have a tremendous advantage because there is usually a reliable junctional pacemaker available that can fire at 40 to 60 beats/min. However, when an AV block occurs below the AV junction, the only available pacemaker may be a slow ventricular one, firing at 20 to 40 beats/min. Not only are ventricular pacemakers slow, but they are also prone to long pauses, making them less than reliable. Therefore, AV blocks at the level of the AV node usually have a more effective and reliable escape pacemaker than do AV blocks at the bundle of His or below.

CLINICAL CORRELATIONS

The clinical significance of an AV block depends on the following:
- The degree of the block
- The rate of the escape pacemaker (junctional versus ventricular)
- The patient's response to that ventricular rate

FIRST-DEGREE ATRIOVENTRICULAR BLOCK

[Objective 1]

With a first-degree AV block, all components of the cardiac cycle are usually within normal limits, with the exception of the PR interval. This is because electrical impulses travel normally from the SA node through the atria, but there is a delay in impulse conduction, usually at the level of the AV node (Fig. 7.3). Despite its name, the SA node impulse is not blocked during a first-degree AV block; rather, each sinus impulse is *delayed* for the same period before it is conducted to the ventricles. The terms *AV delay* and *delayed AV conduction* have been suggested as alternative names for first-degree AV block. Delayed AV conduction results in a PR interval that is longer than normal (i.e., more than 0.20 second in duration in adults) and constant before each QRS complex. Despite the prolonged PR interval, each P wave is followed by a QRS complex (i.e., there is a 1:1 relationship of P waves to QRS complexes).

When the QRS complex associated with a first-degree AV block is narrow, the conduction abnormality is usually within the AV node (Hamdan, 2010). When the QRS complex associated with a first-degree AV block is wide, the conduction abnormality may be located in the AV node, the bundle of His, or the bundle branches (Issa et al, 2012).

→ *Lead In*

Not all AV blocks have a 1:1 relationship of P wave to QRS complex. When inspecting a rhythm strip, be sure to determine both atrial and ventricular regularity, identify P waves, assess the PR interval, and determine if the QRS complex is narrow or wide.

How Do I Recognize It?

Let's look at the rhythm shown in Fig. 7.4. The ventricular rhythm is regular at a rate of 88 beats/min. Each QRS complex is preceded by an upright P wave. The atrial rhythm is also regular at a rate of 88 beats/min. On the basis of these findings, we now know that the underlying rhythm is a sinus rhythm at 88 beats/min. The QRS duration is within normal limits; however, the PR interval measures 0.28 second, which is longer than normal, and the interval is consistent before each QRS. The 1:1 relationship of P wave to QRS complex and a longer than normal PR interval fit the criteria for a first-degree AV block.

First-degree AV block is not a dysrhythmia itself; rather, it is a condition that describes the prolonged (but constant) PR interval that is seen on the rhythm strip. Our interpretation of the rhythm strip in Fig. 7.4 must include a description of the underlying rhythm, the ventricular rate, and then a description of anything that appears amiss. In this case, we will identify the rhythm as sinus rhythm at 88 beats/min with a first-degree AV block and ST-segment

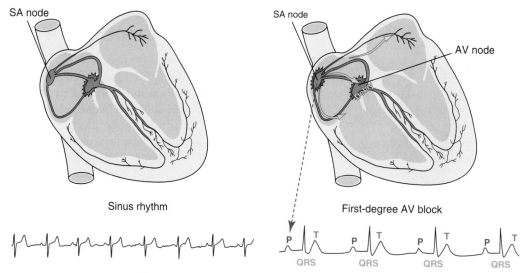

Fig. 7.3 First-degree atrioventricular (AV) block. *SA,* Sinoatrial.

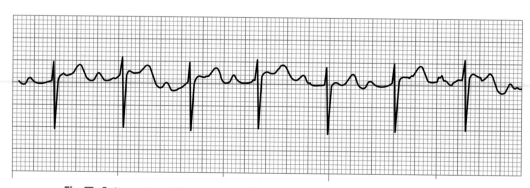

Fig. 7.4 Sinus rhythm at 88 beats/min with a first-degree atrioventricular block and ST-segment elevation.

TABLE 7.1	Characteristics of First-Degree Atrioventricular Block
Rhythm	Regular
Rate	Usually within normal range, but depends on underlying rhythm
P waves	Normal in size and shape; one positive (upright) P wave before each QRS
PR interval	Prolonged (i.e., more than 0.20 sec) but constant
QRS duration	Usually 0.11 sec or less unless abnormally conducted

elevation (STE). The characteristics of first-degree AV block are shown in Table 7.1.

What Causes It?

First-degree AV block may be a normal finding in individuals with no history of cardiac disease, especially in athletes. In some people, mild prolongation of the PR interval may be

a normal variant, especially with sinus bradycardia during rest or sleep. First-degree AV block may also occur because of the following:

- Acute myocardial infarction
- Acute myocarditis or endocarditis
- Cardiomyopathy
- Degenerative fibrosis and sclerosis of the conduction system
- Drug effect
- Hyperkalemia
- Increased vagal tone (e.g., carotid massage, inferior infarction, vomiting)
- Ischemia or injury to the AV node or AV bundle
- Rheumatic heart disease
- Valvular heart disease

 Drug Pearl

Agents that can cause AV blocks include amiodarone, beta-blockers, digoxin, diltiazem, procainamide, and verapamil.

What Do I Do About It?

Patients with first-degree AV block are often asymptomatic; however, marked first-degree AV block can cause symptoms even in the absence of higher degrees of AV block (Barold, 1996). First-degree AV block that occurs with acute myocardial infarction (MI) should be monitored closely to detect progression to higher-degree AV block (Blank et al, 2014). If first-degree AV block accompanies a symptomatic bradycardia, treat the bradycardia.

SECOND-DEGREE ATRIOVENTRICULAR BLOCKS

The term *second-degree AV block* is used when one or more, but not all, sinus impulses are blocked from reaching the ventricles. Because the SA node is generating impulses in a normal manner, each P wave will occur at a regular interval across the rhythm strip (i.e., all P waves will plot through on time), although not every P wave will be followed by a QRS complex. This suggests that the atria are being depolarized normally, but not every impulse is being conducted to the ventricles (i.e., intermittent conduction). As a result, more P waves than QRS complexes are seen on the electrocardiogram (ECG).

Second-degree AV block is classified as type I or type II, depending on the behavior of the PR intervals associated with the dysrhythmia. The type I or type II designation is used to describe the *ECG pattern* of the PR intervals and should not be used to describe the anatomic site (i.e., location) of the AV block (Issa et al, 2012). At least two consecutively conducted PR intervals must be observed to determine their pattern.

SECOND-DEGREE ATRIOVENTRICULAR BLOCK TYPE I

[Objective 2]

Second-degree AV block type I is also known as *type I block*, *Mobitz I*, or *Wenckebach* (Fig. 7.5). *Wenckebach phenomenon* is a progressive lengthening of conduction time in any cardiac conduction tissue that eventually results in the dropping of a beat or a reversion to the initial conduction time. With type I AV block, atrial impulses arrive earlier and earlier during the relative refractory period of the AV node, resulting in longer and longer conduction delays and PR intervals, until an impulse arrives during the absolute refractory period and fails to conduct (Issa et al, 2012). The nonconducted impulse appears on the ECG as a P wave with no QRS complex after it.

The following features are associated with classic Wenckebach phenomenon (Blank et al, 2014):

- Progressive prolongation of the PR intervals; the greatest increase in the duration of the PR interval is noted in the second beat of a cycle

- Gradual shortening of R to R intervals
- A P wave not followed by a QRS complex
- A pause with an R to R interval less than the sum of two P to P intervals
- The first conducted atrial impulse after the pause shows a shorter or normal PR interval

It is generally recognized that all of the classic Wenckebach features are found in perhaps fewer than 50% of cases (Latcu & Nadir, 2010). For example, the second conducted PR interval after a blocked impulse may fail to show the greatest increase in length; instead, the PR interval may actually shorten and then lengthen in the middle of a grouped beating pattern (Barold & Hayes, 2001). Alternately, the duration of the PR intervals may show no obvious change in the middle or for a few beats just before the end of a group (Barold & Hayes, 2001).

When a second-degree AV block type I occurs with a narrow QRS complex, the conduction delay and site of block is almost always within the AV node (Issa et al, 2012). When a second-degree AV block type I occurs with a wide QRS complex, the site of block may be in the AV node, but it is more likely to lie within or below the His-Purkinje system (Blank et al, 2014).

How Do I Recognize It?

Second-degree AV block type I is characterized by a repeating pattern that consists of conducted P waves (i.e., each P wave is followed by a QRS) and then a P wave that is not conducted (i.e., the P wave is not followed by a QRS). In second-degree AV block type I, any P to QRS ratio may be seen. For example, an AV conduction ratio of 3:2 means that for every three P waves, two are followed by QRS complexes. Four conducted P waves to three QRS complexes results in 4:3 conduction, five conducted P waves to four QRS complexes results in 5:4 conduction, and so on. The P wave that is not conducted ends a *group* of beats. Because QRS complexes are periodically absent, the ventricular rhythm is irregular. The cycle then begins again. The repetition of this cyclic pattern is called *grouped beating*. It is important to note that this pattern of grouped beats occurs in fewer than 50% of patients with second-degree AV block type I (Olgin & Zipes, 2012).

Let's look at the example of this type of AV block in Fig. 7.6. For the purposes of our discussion, consider first labeling the QRS complexes on this rhythm strip 1 through 6. You can quickly see that the ventricular rhythm is irregular with an overall rate of about 60 beats/min. Now look to the left of each QRS and label each P wave in the rhythm strip. Place your calipers or a piece of paper on two P waves and begin moving from the left side of the strip to the right to see if the P waves occur on time. You will find that there is an extra P wave after beat 3. The extra P wave occurs on time, but there is no QRS after it. The remainder of the P waves occur on time. The atrial rhythm is regular with a rate of about 68 beats/min.

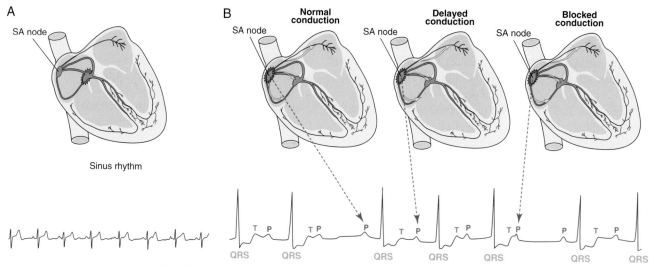

Fig. **7.5** A, Sinus rhythm. B, Second-degree atrioventricular block type I. *SA,* Sinoatrial.

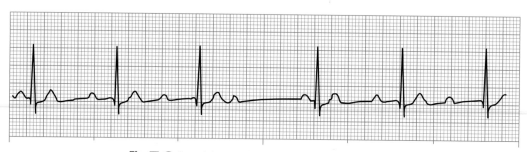

Fig. **7.6** Second-degree atrioventricular block type I at 60 beats/min.

Although we are discussing AV blocks in this chapter, how do you know that the extra P wave with no QRS after it isn't a nonconducted premature atrial complex (PAC)? Well, the difference is in the timing of the P waves. If you have not been plotting P waves when analyzing rhythm strips until now, it is *very* important that you do so when identifying AV blocks. In second- and third-degree AV blocks, there are more P waves than QRS complexes, and the P waves occur *on time.* This happens because the problem in second- and third-degree AV blocks is not within the SA node. The problem occurs somewhere in the conduction system *below* the SA node. Therefore, the sinus fires regularly—as it is supposed to. The P wave that occurs after beat 3 is not a nonconducted PAC because all of the P waves are on time. By definition, the P wave of a nonconducted *premature* atrial complex is early.

The duration of the QRS complexes in Fig. 7.6 is within normal limits. Now, look closely at the PR intervals and determine if a pattern exists. To do this, we need to see at least two PQRST cycles in a row that do not contain extra waveforms. Beats 1, 2, and 3 allow us to do this because there is one P wave before each QRS. When you compare the PR intervals of these beats, the PR interval of beat 1 is short. The PR interval of beat 2 is longer than that of beat 1, and the PR interval of beat 3 is longer than that of the first two beats. The PR intervals of beats 1 through 3 can be described as

lengthening. The blocked sinus impulse appears on the ECG as a P wave with no QRS after it (i.e., a dropped beat). The cycle begins again after the dropped beat. The PR interval of the first conducted beat *after* the blocked sinus impulse (i.e., beat 4) is shorter than the PR interval of the conducted beat *before* the blocked beat (i.e., beat 3). This finding is an important one in identifying second-degree AV block type I. We would interpret this rhythm strip as second-degree AV block type I at 60 beats/min. The ECG characteristics of second-degree AV block type I are shown in Table 7.2.

What Causes It?

Remember that the right coronary artery (RCA) supplies the AV node in 90% of the population. The RCA also supplies the inferior wall of the left ventricle and the right ventricle in most individuals. Blockage of the RCA, resulting in an inferior MI or right ventricular infarction, can result in conduction delays such as first-degree AV block and second-degree AV block type I. Second-degree AV block type I can also occur in athletes, probably related to an increase in resting vagal tone (Olgin & Zipes, 2012), and in healthy individuals during sleep. Other possible causes of this dysrhythmia include aortic valve disease, atrial septal defect, medications (e.g., beta-blockers, digoxin, diltiazem, verapamil), mitral valve prolapse, and rheumatic heart disease.

TABLE **7.2**	Characteristics of Second-Degree Atrioventricular Block Type I
Rhythm	Ventricular irregular; atrial regular (i.e., P waves plot through on time); grouped beating may be present
Rate	Atrial rate is greater than the ventricular rate
P waves	Normal in size and shape; some P waves are not followed by a QRS complex (i.e., more P waves than QRS complexes)
PR interval	Lengthens with each cycle (although lengthening may be very slight) until a P wave appears without a QRS complex; the PR interval after a nonconducted P wave is shorter than the interval preceding the nonconducted beat
QRS duration	Usually 0.11 sec or less; complexes are periodically dropped

What Do I Do About It?

The patient with type I AV block is usually asymptomatic because the ventricular rate often remains nearly normal, and cardiac output is not significantly affected. When it is associated with an acute inferior wall MI, this dysrhythmia is usually transient and resolves within 48 to 72 hours as the effects of parasympathetic stimulation disappear.

If the heart rate is slow and serious signs and symptoms occur because of the slow rate, treatment should include applying a pulse oximeter and administering oxygen (if indicated), obtaining the patient's vital signs, and establishing intravenous (IV) access. A 12-lead ECG should be obtained. Atropine, administered intravenously, is the drug of choice. Reassess the patient's response and continue monitoring him or her. When this rhythm occurs in conjunction with acute MI, the patient should be observed closely for increasing AV block.

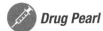 *Drug Pearl* _____

If the patient with an AV block is symptomatic and the dysrhythmia is a result of medications, these agents should be withheld.

SECOND-DEGREE ATRIOVENTRICULAR BLOCK TYPE II

[Objective 3]

Second-degree AV block type II is also called *type II block* or *Mobitz II AV block*. The site of block in second-degree AV block type II is almost always below the AV node, occurring in the bundle of His about 30% of the time and within the bundle branches in the remainder (Issa et al, 2012). Although second-degree AV block type II is less common than type I, type II is more serious and is a cause for concern because it has a greater potential to progress to a third-degree AV block.

How Do I Recognize It?

As it is with second-degree AV block type I, there are more P waves than QRS complexes with second-degree AV block type II, and the P waves occur on time. The PR interval with type II block can be normal or prolonged, but it is constant for the conducted beats. Most important, the PR intervals before and after a blocked sinus impulse (i.e., P wave) are *constant*.

Let's look at Fig. 7.7. You can see right away that the ventricular rhythm is irregular at an overall rate of about 70 beats/min. You can quickly see that there are more P waves than QRS complexes in this rhythm strip. Use your calipers or paper to plot the P waves and see whether they occur on time. Indeed, they occur regularly at a rate of about 94 beats/min, although not every P wave is followed by a QRS complex. Each P wave occurs at a regular interval across the rhythm strip (i.e., all P waves plot through on time) because the SA node is generating impulses in a normal manner. Impulses generated by the SA node are conducted to the ventricles until a sinus impulse is suddenly blocked—appearing on the ECG as a P wave with no QRS after it (i.e., a dropped beat); this results in an irregular ventricular rhythm. Looking at the QRS complexes in Fig. 7.7, you can see that they are slightly wider than normal, measuring about 0.12 second.

Now look closely at each of the PR intervals and compare them. Are they the same or different? In this rhythm strip, the PR intervals are the same, and then a P wave suddenly appears with no QRS after it. When the PR intervals measure the same, we say that they are *constant* or *fixed*. This is an important difference between second-degree AV block type

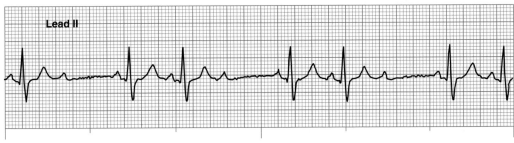

Fig. 7.7 Second-degree atrioventricular block type II at 70 beats/min. (From Aehlert B: *ECG study cards*, St. Louis, 2004, Mosby.)

TABLE **7.3**	Characteristics of Second-Degree Atrioventricular Block Type II
Rhythm	Ventricular irregular; atrial regular (i.e., P waves plot through on time)
Rate	Atrial rate is greater than the ventricular rate; ventricular rate is often slow
P waves	Normal in size and shape; some P waves are not followed by a QRS complex (i.e., more P waves than QRS complexes)
PR interval	Within normal limits or prolonged but constant for the conducted beats; the PR intervals before and after a blocked P wave are constant
QRS duration	Within normal limits if the block occurs above or within the bundle of His; greater than 0.11 sec if the block occurs below the bundle of His; complexes are periodically absent after P waves

I and second-degree AV block type II. In second-degree AV block type II, the PR interval may be within normal limits or prolonged, but it is constant for the conducted beats. Most important, the PR intervals before and after a blocked sinus impulse (i.e., P wave) are *constant.*

Our interpretation of the rhythm in Fig. 7.7 is second-degree AV block type II at 70 beats/min. The ECG characteristics of second-degree AV block type II are shown in Table 7.3.

What Causes It?

You will recall that the site of block in second-degree AV block type II is almost always below the AV node, occurring in the bundle branches about 70% of the time (Issa et al, 2012). Because a branch of the left coronary artery supplies the bundle branches and the anterior wall of the left ventricle, disease of the left coronary artery or an anterior MI is often associated with conduction defects that occur within the bundle branches. Second-degree AV block type II may also occur because of acute myocarditis, aortic valve disease, cardiomyopathy, fibrosis of the conduction system, or rheumatic heart disease.

What Do I Do About It?

The patient's response to this rhythm is usually related to the ventricular rate. If the ventricular rate is within normal limits, the patient may be asymptomatic. More commonly, the ventricular rate is significantly slowed and serious signs and symptoms result because of the slow rate and decreased cardiac output. The greater the number is of nonconducted beats, the greater the impact is on the cardiac output.

Because second-degree AV block type II may abruptly progress to third-degree AV block, the patient should be closely monitored for increasing AV block. If the heart rate is slow and serious signs and symptoms occur because of the slow rate, treatment should include applying a pulse oximeter, obtaining the patient's vital signs, administering oxygen (if indicated), and establishing IV access. A 12-lead ECG should be obtained and a cardiology consult should be sought. Temporary or permanent pacing may be necessary. Continue monitoring the patient and observe closely for increasing AV block.

2:1 ATRIOVENTRICULAR BLOCK

How Do I Recognize It?
[Objective 4]

Before we discuss 2:1 AV block, let's review a few very important points regarding second-degree AV blocks. So far you have learned how important it is to plot P waves to make sure that they occur on time. If there are more P waves than QRS complexes and the P waves occur on time, you know that you have some type of AV block. The ventricular rhythm is irregular with both second-degree AV block type I and type II. The QRS complex with a second-degree AV block type I is usually narrow; it is usually wide with a second-degree AV block type II, although exceptions exist with both types of second-degree blocks.

You have also learned that there are differences in the PR interval patterns with second-degree AV block type I and type II, and that these differences are important in differentiating between type I and type II AV block. To compare PR intervals, we must see at least two PQRST cycles in a row. More important, we must look at the PR interval of the conducted beat *after* a dropped QRS complex and compare it with the PR interval of the last conducted beat *before* the dropped QRS. With this information, you can then begin to differentiate what type of second-degree AV block it is. For example, if the PR interval after a dropped QRS complex is shorter than the PR interval before the dropped complex, a pattern consistent with second-degree AV block type I is present. If the PR interval after a dropped QRS complex is the same as the PR interval before the dropped complex, a pattern consistent with second-degree AV block type II exists.

With second-degree AV block in the form of 2:1 AV block, there is one conducted P wave followed by a blocked P wave; thus, two P waves occur for every one QRS complex (i.e., 2:1 conduction). Because there are no two PQRST cycles in a row from which to compare PR intervals, 2:1 AV block cannot be conclusively classified as type I or type II. To determine the type of block with certainty, it is necessary to continue close ECG monitoring of the patient until the conduction ratio of P waves to QRS complexes changes to 3:2, 4:3, and so on, which would enable PR interval comparison.

If the QRS complex measures 0.11 second or less, the block is likely to be located within the AV node and a form of second-degree AV block type I (Fig. 7.8). A 2:1 AV block

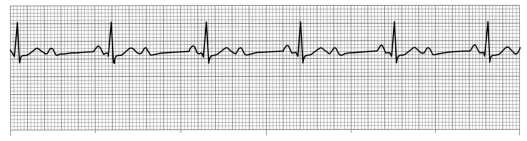

Fig. 7.8 2:1 atrioventricular block with narrow QRS complexes.

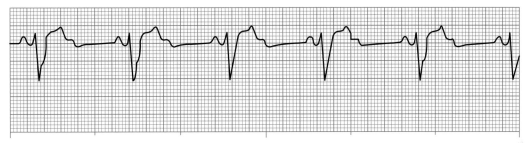

Fig. 7.9 2:1 atrioventricular block with wide QRS complexes.

TABLE 7.4	Characteristics of Second-Degree 2:1 Atrioventricular Block
Rhythm	Ventricular regular; atrial regular (P waves plot through on time)
Rate	Atrial rate is twice the ventricular rate
P waves	Normal in size and shape; every other P wave is not followed by a QRS complex (i.e., more P waves than QRS complexes)
PR interval	Constant
QRS duration	May be narrow or wide; complexes are absent after every other P wave

associated with a wide QRS complex (i.e., more than 0.11 second) is usually associated with a block below the AV node; thus, it is usually a type II block (Fig. 7.9). The ECG characteristics of 2:1 AV block are shown in Table 7.4. The causes and emergency management for 2:1 AV block are those of type I or type II block previously described.

ADVANCED SECOND-DEGREE ATRIOVENTRICULAR BLOCK

[Objective 4]

The term *advanced* or *high-grade* second-degree AV block may be used to describe three or more consecutive P waves that are not conducted. For example, with 3:1 AV block, every third P wave is conducted (i.e., followed by a QRS complex); with 4:1 AV block, every fourth P wave is conducted (Fig. 7.10).

As is the case with 2:1 AV block, advanced second-degree AV block cannot be conclusively classified as type I or type II because there are no two PQRST cycles in a row from which to compare PR intervals. Monitoring of the patient's ECG for changes in P wave to QRS conduction ratios to enable PR interval comparison is essential. Because of the frequency with which impulses from the SA node to the Purkinje fibers are blocked, the presence of advanced AV block is a cause for concern, and the development of third-degree AV block should be anticipated.

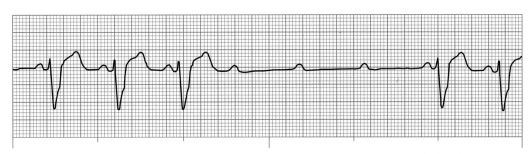

Fig. 7.10 An example of advanced second-degree atrioventricular block. (From Aehlert B: *ECG study cards,* St. Louis, 2004, Mosby.)

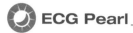

A Quick Look at P Waves and Atrioventricular (AV) Blocks

AV Block	P Wave Conduction
First degree	All P waves conducted but delayed; slowed conduction
Second degree	Some P waves conducted, others blocked; intermittent conduction
Third degree	No P waves conducted; absent conduction

THIRD-DEGREE ATRIOVENTRICULAR BLOCK

Second-degree AV blocks are types of *incomplete* blocks because at least some of the impulses from the SA node are conducted to the ventricles. With third-degree AV block, there is a *complete* block in conduction of impulses between the atria and the ventricles.

How Do I Recognize It?

[Objective 5]

With third-degree AV block, the site of block may occur at the level of the AV node, the bundle of His, or distal to the bundle of His (Fig. 7.11). A secondary pacemaker (either junctional or ventricular) stimulates the ventricles; therefore, the QRS may be narrow or wide, depending on the location of the escape pacemaker and the condition of the intraventricular conduction system.

Let's look at the rhythm strip in Fig. 7.12. Determine the ventricular rhythm and then calculate the ventricular rate. You will find that the ventricular rhythm is regular and the ventricular rate is 29 beats/min. Next, locate the P waves. In locating P waves, it often helps to place your calipers, or to make marks on a piece of paper, on two clearly identifiable P waves and then move the calipers (or paper) left and right across the strip, marking the remaining P waves as you go. For example, it would be a good idea to mark P waves 2 and 3 first in this rhythm strip because they are readily seen; then move to the left, identifying P wave 1, and then move to the right, identifying P waves 4 through 7. P wave 4 is hidden in the T wave following the second QRS complex. When all of the P waves have been identified, determine their regularity and then determine their rate. You will find that the P waves occur regularly and that the atrial rate is 68 beats/min. So far, because you have more P waves than QRS complexes and the P waves occur on time, you know that you have some type of AV block. To determine which one, you must look closely at the PR intervals. As you can see, there is no true PR interval because the atria and ventricles are beating independently of each other. The ECG characteristics

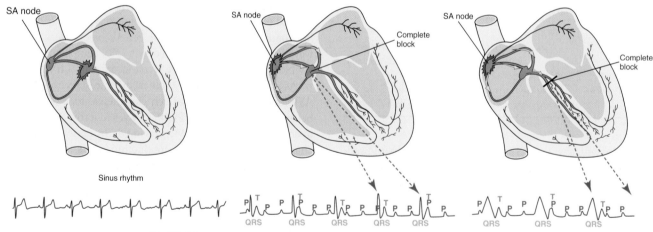

Fig. 7.11 A comparison of sinus rhythm and third-degree atrioventricular block. *SA*, Sinoatrial.

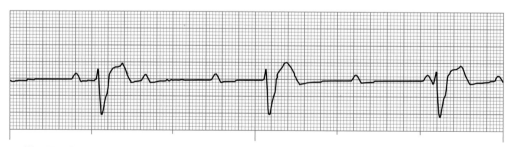

Fig. 7.12 Third-degree atrioventricular block at 29 beats/min with a wide QRS. (From Aehlert B: *ECG study cards,* St. Louis, 2004, Mosby.)

TABLE **7.5**	Characteristics of Third-Degree Atrioventricular Block
Rhythm	Ventricular regular; atrial regular (P waves plot through); no relationship between the atrial and ventricular rhythms (i.e., atrioventricular dissociation is present)
Rate	The ventricular rate is determined by the origin of the escape pacemaker; the atrial rate is greater than (and independent of) the ventricular rate
P waves	Normal in size and shape; some P waves are not followed by a QRS complex (i.e., more P waves than QRS complexes)
PR interval	None; the atria and the ventricles beat independently of each other, so there is no true PR interval
QRS duration	Narrow or wide, depending on the location of the escape pacemaker and the condition of the intraventricular conduction system

discussed so far and the fact that there is no true PR interval fit the criteria for a third-degree AV block. The QRS is wide, measuring 0.16 second, and the QT interval measures 0.36 to 0.38 second. Our interpretation of the dysrhythmia in Fig. 7.12 is third-degree AV block at 29 beats/min with a wide QRS. The ECG characteristics of third-degree AV block are shown in Table 7.5.

What Causes It?

Causes of third-degree AV block include the following:
- Acute MI
- Acute myocarditis
- Congenital heart disease
- Drug effect
- Fibrosis of the conduction system
- Increased parasympathetic tone

Third-degree AV block associated with an inferior MI is thought to be the result of a block above the bundle of His. It often occurs after progression from first-degree AV block or second-degree AV block type I. The resulting rhythm is usually stable because the escape pacemaker is usually junctional (i.e., narrow QRS complexes) with a ventricular rate of more than 40 beats/min. Third-degree AV block that is associated with an anterior or an anteroseptal MI is often preceded by second-degree AV block type II or an intraventricular conduction delay (i.e., right or left bundle branch block) (Issa et al, 2012). The resulting rhythm is usually unstable because the escape pacemaker is usually ventricular (i.e., wide QRS complexes) with a ventricular rate of less than 40 beats/min. In the setting of an acute anterior MI, the development of third-degree AV block is associated with a higher risk of ventricular tachycardia and ventricular fibrillation, hypotension, pulmonary edema, and in-hospital mortality (Issa et al, 2012).

What Do I Do About It?

The patient's signs and symptoms will depend on the origin of the escape pacemaker (i.e., junctional versus ventricular) and the patient's response to a slower ventricular rate. Possible rate-related signs and symptoms include dizziness, lightheadedness, generalized weakness, seizures, and *Adams-Stokes syndrome* (which is also known as *Stokes-Adams attacks*). Adams-Stokes syndrome is sudden, recurring episodes of loss of consciousness caused by the transient interruption of cardiac output by incomplete or complete heart block; the ventricular rate is inadequate to maintain cerebral perfusion and results in a syncopal episode.

If the patient is symptomatic as a result of the slow rate, treatment should include applying a pulse oximeter and administering oxygen (if indicated), obtaining the patient's vital signs, establishing IV access, and obtaining a 12-lead ECG. IV administration of atropine may be tried. If the disruption in AV nodal conduction is caused by increased parasympathetic tone, the administration of atropine may be effective in reversing excess vagal tone and improving AV node conduction. Other interventions that may be used in the treatment of third-degree AV block include epinephrine or dopamine IV infusions, or transcutaneous pacing. Frequent patient reassessment is essential. Most patients with third-degree AV block have an indication for permanent pacemaker placement.

Examples of most of the AV blocks discussed in this chapter appear in Fig. 7.13. A summary of AV block characteristics is given in Table 7.6.

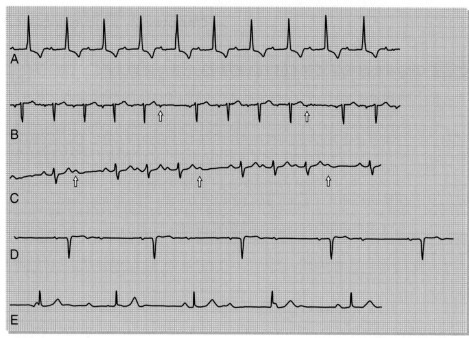

Fig. 7.13 Atrioventricular (AV) blocks. A, First-degree AV block; the PR interval is constant and more than 0.20 second. B, Second-degree AV block type I. The PR intervals after the nonconducted P waves *(arrows)* are shorter than the interval preceding the nonconducted beat. C, Second-degree AV block type II. Nonconducted P waves are seen *(arrows)*. The PR intervals before and after the nonconducted P waves are constant. D, 2:1 AV block during which every other P wave is conducted. E, Third-degree AV block with AV dissociation and a junctional escape rhythm. (From Andreoli TE, Griggs R, Wing W, Fitz JG: *Andreoli and Carpenter's Cecil essentials of medicine,* ed 9, Philadelphia, 2016, Saunders.)

TABLE 7.6   **Atrioventricular Blocks: Summary of Characteristics**

Characteristic	First-Degree Block	Second-Degree Block Type I	Second-Degree Block Type II	Second-Degree 2:1 AV Block	Third-Degree Block
Rhythm	Atrial regular, ventricular regular	Atrial regular, ventricular irregular	Atrial regular, ventricular irregular	Atrial regular, ventricular regular	Atrial regular, ventricular regular
Rate	Usually within normal range, but depends on underlying rhythm	Atrial rate greater than ventricular rate; both often within normal limits	Atrial rate greater than ventricular rate; ventricular rate often slow	Atrial rate greater than ventricular rate	Atrial rate greater than ventricular rate; ventricular rate determined by origin of escape rhythm
P waves (lead II)	Normal; one P wave precedes each QRS	Normal in size and shape; some P waves are not followed by a QRS complex (i.e., more Ps than QRSs)	Normal in size and shape; some P waves are not followed by a QRS complex (i.e., more Ps than QRSs)	Normal in size and shape; every other P wave is not followed by a QRS complex (i.e., more Ps than QRSs)	Normal in size and shape; some P waves are not followed by a QRS complex (i.e., more Ps than QRSs)
PR interval (PRI)	Greater than 0.20 sec and constant	Lengthening; the PRI after the nonconducted beat is shorter than the interval preceding the nonconducted beat	Within normal limits or prolonged but constant for the conducted beats; the PRIs before and after a blocked sinus impulse (i.e., P wave) are constant	Constant	None; the atria and ventricles beat independently of each other, so there is no true PRI
QRS duration	Usually 0.11 sec or less unless an intraventricular conduction delay exists	Usually 0.11 sec or less and is periodically dropped	Within normal limits if the block occurs above or within the bundle of His; greater than 0.11 sec if the block occurs below the bundle of His; periodically absent after P waves	Narrow or wide depending on location of escape pacemaker and condition of intraventricular conduction system; absent after every other P wave	Narrow or wide depending on location of escape pacemaker and condition of intraventricular conduction system

AV, Atrioventricular.

STOP & REVIEW

True/False

Indicate whether the statement is true or false.

_____ **1.** During a first-degree AV block, the PR intervals are completely variable because the atria and ventricles beat independently of each other.

_____ **2.** Second-degree AV blocks are examples of *incomplete* AV blocks.

_____ **3.** The site of block in second-degree AV block type II is limited to the bundle branches.

_____ **4.** With second-degree AV block type II, the PR intervals before and after a blocked sinus impulse (i.e., P wave) are constant.

Multiple Choice

Identify the choice that best completes the statement or answers the question.

_____ **5.** Which of the following dysrhythmias may be a normal finding in individuals with no history of cardiac disease, especially in athletes?
 a. Atrial fibrillation
 b. First-degree AV block
 c. Third-degree AV block
 d. Ventricular tachycardia

_____ **6.** An ECG rhythm strip shows a regular ventricular rhythm at a rate of 128 beats/min, one upright P wave before each QRS, a regular atrial rate, a constant PR interval of 0.24 second, and a QRS duration of 0.08 second. This rhythm is
 a. third-degree AV block.
 b. second-degree AV block type I.
 c. sinus tachycardia with first-degree AV block.
 d. junctional tachycardia with first-degree AV block.

_____ **7.** Third-degree AV block is characterized by
 a. irregular P to P intervals.
 b. irregular R to R intervals.
 c. regular P to P intervals and regular R to R intervals.
 d. regular P to P intervals and irregular R to R intervals.

_____ **8.** An ECG rhythm strip reveals second-degree 2:1 AV block. Which of the following statements is correct regarding this rhythm?
 a. The ventricular rate is twice the atrial rate.
 b. The presence of constant PR intervals allows classification of the block as type I or type II.
 c. The PR intervals are generally progressive until a P wave appears without a QRS after it.
 d. This rhythm is characterized by P waves that are normal in size and shape, but every other P wave is not followed by a QRS.

_____ **9.** The term *second-degree AV block type I* is the same as
 a. Mobitz II.
 b. AV dissociation.
 c. Mobitz I or Wenckebach.
 d. Wolff-Parkinson-White pattern.

_____ **10.** Which of the following dysrhythmias is more commonly seen with an inferior wall myocardial infarction?
 a. Sinus arrhythmia
 b. Second-degree AV block type I
 c. Second-degree AV block type II
 d. Third-degree AV block with a wide QRS

_____ **11.** An ECG rhythm strip reveals an irregular ventricular rhythm at a rate of 28 to 40 beats/min, more P waves than QRS complexes, regular P-P intervals, a constant PR interval of 0.16 second, and a QRS duration of 0.14 second. This rhythm is
 a. 2:1 AV block.
 b. third-degree AV block.
 c. second-degree AV block type I.
 d. second-degree AV block type II.

_____ **12.** Of the following, which dysrhythmia has the greatest potential for sudden, third-degree AV block?
 a. Sinus bradycardia
 b. Junctional escape rhythm
 c. Second-degree AV block type I
 d. Second-degree AV block type II

_____ **13.** The difference between second-degree type I and type II AV block is that with
 a. type I the P waves occur irregularly.
 b. type I the ventricular rhythm is regular.
 c. type II the QRS duration is consistently more than 0.12 sec in duration.
 d. type II the PR intervals before and after a blocked P wave are constant.

_____ **14.** With a third-degree AV block, the PR interval
 a. shortens.
 b. is absent.
 c. is inconstant.
 d. remains constant.

_____ **15.** An ECG rhythm strip reveals an irregular ventricular rhythm at a rate of 46 to 54 beats/min, more P waves than QRS complexes with regular P-P intervals, PR intervals after nonconducted P waves are shorter than the interval preceding the nonconducted beats, and a QRS duration of 0.08 second. This rhythm is
 a. 2:1 AV block.
 b. third-degree AV block.
 c. second-degree AV block type I.
 d. second-degree AV block type II.

Matching

Match the terms below with their descriptions by placing the letter of each correct answer in the space provided.

a. Regular

b. Third-degree AV block

c. PRI pattern in second-degree AV block type I

d. First-degree AV block

e. PRI pattern in second-degree AV block type II

f. Irregular

_____ 16. Ventricular rhythm pattern in second-degree AV block types I and II

_____ 17. The PRI after the nonconducted P wave is shorter than the interval preceding the nonconducted beat

_____ 18. AV block characterized by a PR interval greater than 0.20 sec and one P wave for each QRS complex

_____ 19. Ventricular rhythm pattern in 2:1 and third-degree AV block

_____ 20. The PRIs before and after a blocked P wave are constant

_____ 21. AV block characterized by regular P-P intervals, regular R-R intervals, and a PR interval with no consistent value or pattern

Short Answer

22. Indicate the ECG criteria for the following dysrhythmias.

	Second-Degree AV Block Type I	**Third-Degree AV Block**
Ventricular rhythm	_____	_____
PR interval	_____	_____
QRS width	_____	_____

23. Indicate the ECG criteria for the following dysrhythmias.

	Second-Degree AV Block Type II	**2:1 AV Block**
Ventricular rhythm	_____	_____
PR interval	_____	_____
QRS width	_____	_____

AV Blocks—Practice Rhythm Strips

Use the five steps of rhythm interpretation to interpret each of the following rhythm strips. All rhythms were recorded in lead II unless otherwise noted.

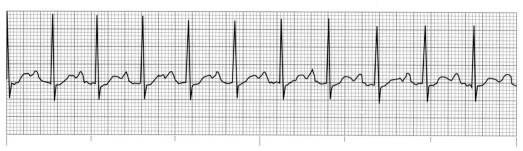

Fig. 7.14 (From Aehlert B: *ECG study cards,* St. Louis, 2004, Mosby.)

24. Fig. 7.14

Rhythm: _____ Rate: _____ P waves: _____

PR interval: _____ QRS duration: _____ QT interval: _____

Interpretation: _____

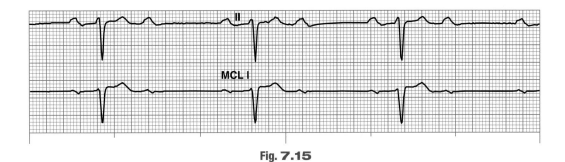

Fig. 7.15

25. **Fig. 7.15**

Rhythm: _____ Rate: _____ P waves: _____

PR interval: _____ QRS duration: _____ QT interval: _____

Interpretation: _____

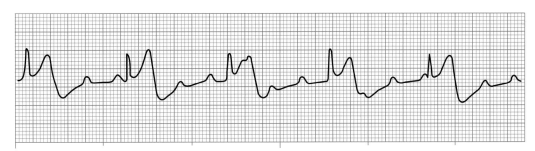

Fig. 7.16

26. **Fig. 7.16**

Rhythm: _____ Rate: _____ P waves: _____

PR interval: _____ QRS duration: _____ QT interval: _____

Interpretation: _____

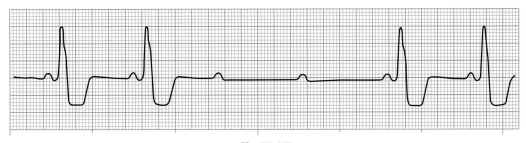

Fig. 7.17

27. **Fig. 7.17**

Rhythm: _____ Rate: _____ P waves: _____

PR interval: _____ QRS duration: _____ QT interval: _____

Interpretation: _____

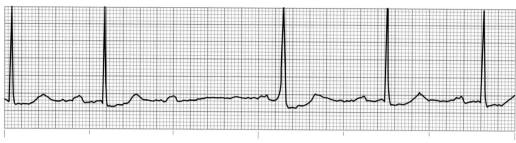

Fig. 7.18 (From Phillips RE, Feeney MK: *The cardiac rhythms: a systematic approach to interpretation,* ed 3, Philadelphia, 1990, Saunders.)

28. **Fig. 7.18**

Rhythm: _____ Rate: _____ P waves: _____

PR interval: _____ QRS duration: _____ QT interval: _____

Interpretation: _____

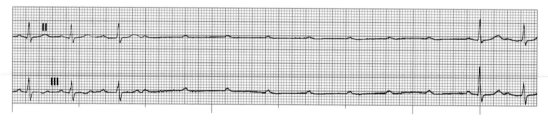

Fig. 7.19

29. **Fig. 7.19**

Rhythm: _____ Rate: _____ P waves: _____

PR interval: _____ QRS duration: _____ QT interval: _____

Interpretation: _____

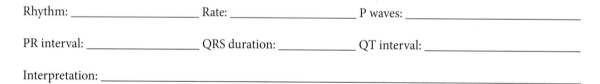

Fig. 7.20 (From Aehlert B: *ECG study cards,* St. Louis, 2004, Mosby.)

30. **Fig. 7.20**

Rhythm: _____ Rate: _____ P waves: _____

PR interval: _____ QRS duration: _____ QT interval: _____

Interpretation: _____

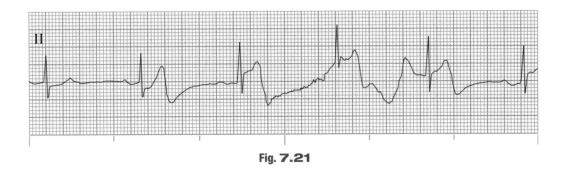

Fig. 7.21

31. Fig. 7.21. This rhythm strip was recorded as a 58-year-old man began complaining of a sudden onset of chest pain.

Rhythm: _____ Rate: _____ P waves: _____

PR interval: _____ QRS duration: _____ QT interval: _____

Interpretation: _____

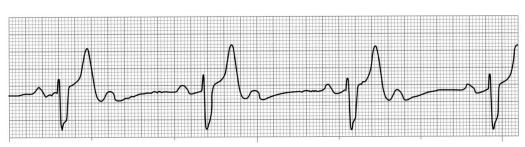

Fig. 7.22

32. Fig. 7.22. This rhythm strip is from a 77-year-old woman who stated that she felt fine. She stopped at a blood pressure machine in Walmart, and the machine would not read her pulse rate. She later went to her physician's office and then to the emergency department.

Rhythm: _____ Rate: _____ P waves: _____

PR interval: _____ QRS duration: _____ QT interval: _____

Interpretation: _____

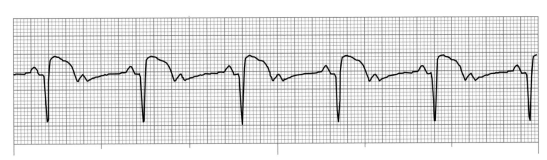

Fig. 7.23 (From Aehlert B: *ECG study cards,* St. Louis, 2004, Mosby.)

33. Fig. 7.23

Rhythm: _____ Rate: _____ P waves: _____

PR interval: _____ QRS duration: _____ QT interval: _____

Interpretation: _____

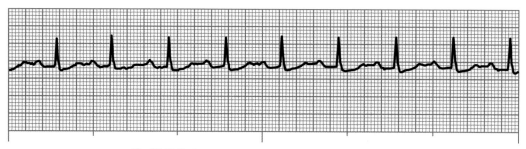

Fig. 7.24 (From Aehlert B: *ECG study cards*, St. Louis, 2004, Mosby.)

34. Fig. 7.24. This rhythm strip is from a 97-year-old woman after a fall.

Rhythm: _____ Rate: _____ P waves: _____

PR interval: _____ QRS duration: _____ QT interval: _____

Interpretation: _____

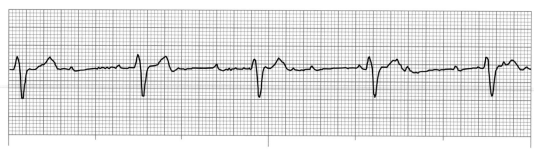

Fig. 7.25 (From Aehlert B: *ECG study cards*, St. Louis, 2004, Mosby.)

35. Fig. 7.25

Rhythm: _____ Rate: _____ P waves: _____

PR interval: _____ QRS duration: _____ QT interval: _____

Interpretation: _____

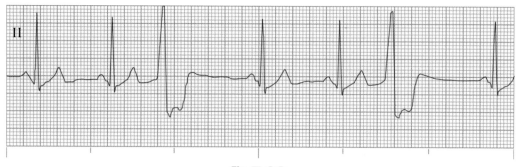

Fig. 7.26

36. Fig. 7.26

Rhythm: _____ Rate: _____ P waves: _____

PR interval: _____ QRS duration: _____ QT interval: _____

Interpretation: _____

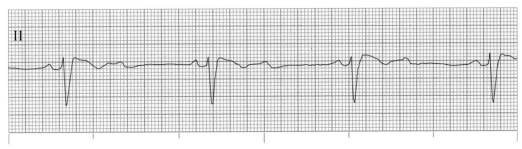

Fig. 7.27 (Modified from Aehlert B: *ECG study cards,* St. Louis, 2004, Mosby.)

37. Fig. 7.27. This rhythm strip is from an 86-year-old woman complaining of dizziness.

Rhythm: _____ Rate: _____ P waves: _____

PR interval: _____ QRS duration: _____ QT interval: _____

Interpretation: _____

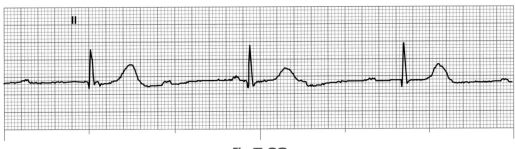

Fig. 7.28

38. Fig. 7.28

Rhythm: _____ Rate: _____ P waves: _____

PR interval: _____ QRS duration: _____ QT interval: _____

Interpretation: _____

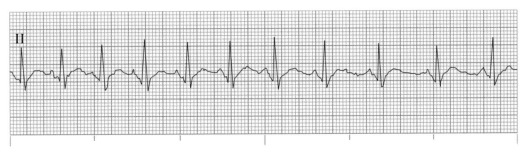

Fig. 7.29 (Modified from Aehlert B: *ECG study cards,* St. Louis, 2004, Mosby.)

39. Fig. 7.29. This rhythm strip is from a 25-year-old asymptomatic paramedic student.

Rhythm: _____ Rate: _____ P waves: _____

PR interval: _____ QRS duration: _____ QT interval: _____

Interpretation: _____

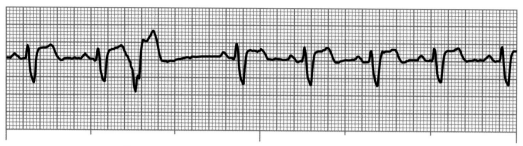

Fig. 7.30 (From Aehlert B: *ECG study cards,* St. Louis, 2004, Mosby.)

40. **Fig. 7.30.** This rhythm strip is from an asymptomatic 56-year-old man.

Rhythm: _____ Rate: _____ P waves: _____

PR interval: _____ QRS duration: _____ QT interval: _____

Interpretation: _____

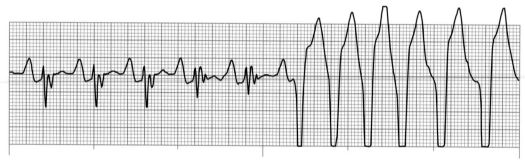

Fig. 7.31 (From Aehlert B: *ECG study cards,* St. Louis, 2004, Mosby.)

41. **Fig. 7.31**

Rhythm: _____ Rate: _____ P waves: _____

PR interval: _____ QRS duration: _____ QT interval: _____

Interpretation: _____

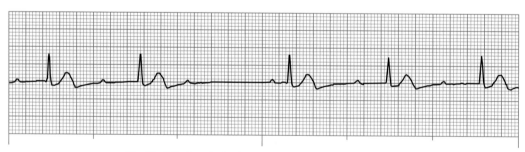

Fig. 7.32 (From Aehlert B: *ECG study cards,* St. Louis, 2004, Mosby.)

42. **Fig. 7.32**

Rhythm: _____ Rate: _____ P waves: _____

PR interval: _____ QRS duration: _____ QT interval: _____

Interpretation: _____

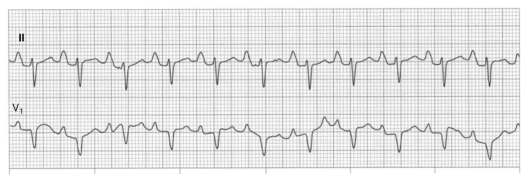

Fig. 7.33

43. **Fig. 7.33**. These rhythm strips are from a 26-year-old man with end-stage cardiomyopathy. His condition was apparently the result of chronic methamphetamine use.

Rhythm: _____ Rate: _____ P waves: _____

PR interval: _____ QRS duration: _____ QT interval: _____

Interpretation: _____

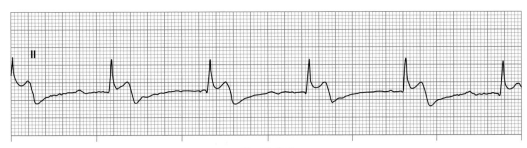

Fig. 7.34

44. **Fig. 7.34**. This rhythm strip is from a 51-year-old man complaining of dull chest pain that began about 2 hours earlier. He rates his discomfort as 6/10. His blood pressure is 70/48 mm Hg. His skin is cool, pale, and diaphoretic.

Rhythm: _____ Rate: _____ P waves: _____

PR interval: _____ QRS duration: _____ QT interval: _____

Interpretation: _____

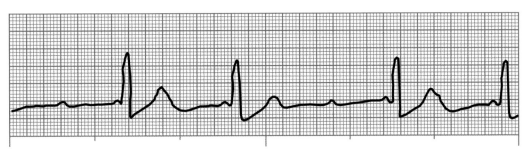

Fig. 7.35 (From Aehlert B: *ECG study cards*, St. Louis, 2004, Mosby.)

45. **Fig. 7.35**. This rhythm strip is from a 62-year-old woman who experienced a syncopal episode.

Rhythm: _____ Rate: _____ P waves: _____

PR interval: _____ QRS duration: _____ QT interval: _____

Interpretation: _____

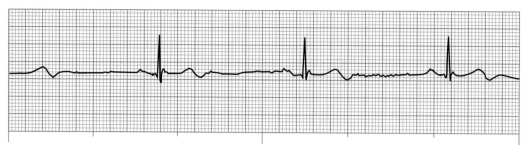

Fig. 7.36 (From Aehlert B: *ECG study cards,* St. Louis, 2004, Mosby.)

46. **Fig. 7.36**. This rhythm strip is from a 66-year-old woman with abdominal pain and weakness that began suddenly while she was eating breakfast.

Rhythm: _____   Rate: _____   P waves: _____

PR interval: _____   QRS duration: _____   QT interval: _____

Interpretation: _____

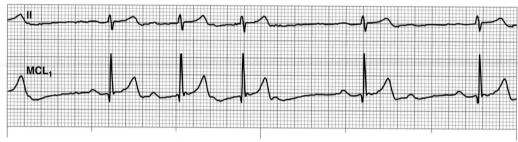

Fig. 7.37 (From Aehlert B: *ECG study cards,* St. Louis, 2004, Mosby.)

47. **Fig. 7.37**

Rhythm: _____   Rate: _____   P waves: _____

PR interval: _____   QRS duration: _____   QT interval: _____

Interpretation: _____

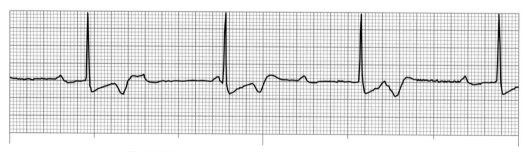

Fig. 7.38 (From Aehlert B: *ECG study cards,* St. Louis, 2004, Mosby.)

48. **Fig. 7.38**

Rhythm: _____   Rate: _____   P waves: _____

PR interval: _____   QRS duration: _____   QT interval: _____

Interpretation: _____

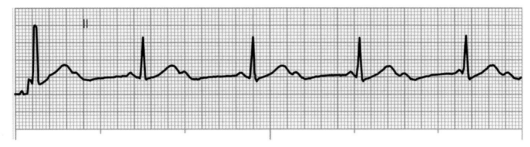

Fig. 7.39 (From Aehlert B: *ECG study cards,* St. Louis, 2004, Mosby.)

49. Fig. 7.39

Rhythm: _____ Rate: _____ P waves: _____

PR interval: _____ QRS duration: _____ QT interval: _____

Interpretation: _____

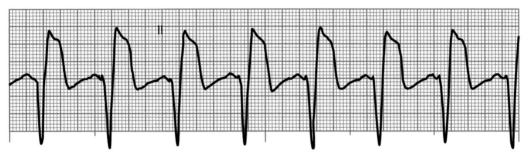

Fig. 7.40 (From Aehlert B: *ECG study cards,* St. Louis, 2004, Mosby.)

50. Fig. 7.40 This rhythm strip is from a 78-year-old woman complaining of left upper quadrant abdominal pain.

Rhythm: _____ Rate: _____ P waves: _____

PR interval: _____ QRS duration: _____ QT interval: _____

Interpretation: _____

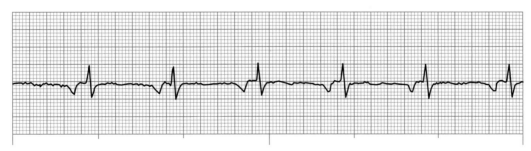

Fig. 7.41 (From Aehlert B: *ECG study cards,* St. Louis, 2004, Mosby.)

51. Fig. 7.41

Rhythm: _____ Rate: _____ P waves: _____

PR interval: _____ QRS duration: _____ QT interval: _____

Interpretation: _____

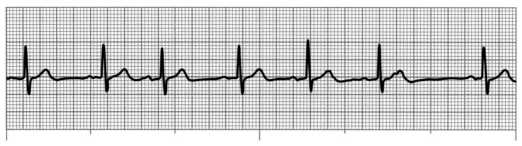

Fig. 7.42 (From Aehlert B: *ECG study cards,* St. Louis, 2004, Mosby.)

52. Fig. 7.42

Rhythm: _____ Rate: _____ P waves: _____

PR interval: _____ QRS duration: _____ QT interval: _____

Interpretation: _____

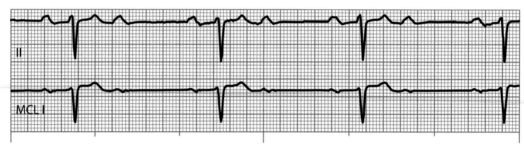

Fig. 7.43 (From Aehlert B: *ECG study cards,* St. Louis, 2004, Mosby.)

53. Fig. 7.43

Rhythm: _____ Rate: _____ P waves: _____

PR interval: _____ QRS duration: _____ QT interval: _____

Interpretation: _____

STOP & REVIEW / ANSWERS

1. F. With a first-degree AV block, there is a 1:1 relationship between P waves and QRS complexes. The PR intervals are prolonged (i.e., more than 0.20 second) but constant.
OBJ: Describe the ECG characteristics, possible causes, signs and symptoms, and emergency management for first-degree AV block.

2. T. Second-degree AV blocks are types of *incomplete* blocks because at least some of the impulses from the SA node are conducted to the ventricles. With third-degree AV block, there is a *complete* block in conduction of impulses between the atria and the ventricles.
OBJ: Describe the ECG characteristics, possible causes, signs and symptoms, and emergency management for third-degree AV block.

3. F. The conduction delay in second-degree AV block type II occurs below the AV node, within the His-Purkinje system. About 70% of the time, the block occurs below the bundle of His, which usually produces a wide QRS (i.e., more than 0.11 second in duration). About 30% of the time, the block occurs in the bundle of His, which is associated with a narrow QRS.
OBJ: Describe the ECG characteristics, possible causes, signs and symptoms, and emergency management for second-degree AV block type II.

4. T. With second-degree AV block type II, the PR intervals are within normal limits or prolonged but constant for the conducted beats, and the PR intervals before and after a blocked sinus impulse (i.e., P wave) are constant.
OBJ: Describe the ECG characteristics, possible causes, signs and symptoms, and emergency management for second-degree AV block type II.

5. B. First-degree AV block may be a normal finding in individuals with no history of cardiac disease, especially in athletes. In some people, mild prolongation of the PR interval may be a normal variant, especially with sinus bradycardia during rest or sleep. Second-degree AV block type I can also occur in athletes, probably related to an increase in resting vagal tone, and in healthy individuals during sleep.
OBJ: Describe the ECG characteristics, possible causes, signs and symptoms, and emergency management for first-degree AV block.

6. C. A sinus tachycardia is present when there is a 1:1 relationship between P waves and QRS complexes and the ventricular rate is faster than 100 beats/min. A first-degree AV block is present when there is a 1:1 relationship between P waves and QRS complexes and the PR interval is prolonged (i.e., more than 0.20 second) and constant.
OBJ: Describe the ECG characteristics, possible causes, signs and symptoms, and emergency management for first-degree AV block.

7. C. Third-degree AV block is characterized by regular P to P intervals (i.e., a regular atrial rhythm) and regular R to R intervals (i.e., a regular ventricular rhythm); however, there is no relationship between the atrial and ventricular rhythms.
OBJ: Describe the ECG characteristics, possible causes, signs and symptoms, and emergency management for third-degree AV block.

8. D. Second-degree 2:1 AV block is characterized by P waves that are normal in size and shape, but every other P wave is not followed by a QRS. The atrial rate is twice the ventricular rate. Because there are no two PQRST cycles in a row from which to compare PR intervals, 2:1 AV block cannot be conclusively classified as type I or type II. To determine the type of block with certainty, it is necessary to continue close ECG monitoring of the patient until the conduction ratio of P waves to QRS complexes changes to 3:2, 4:3, and so on, which would enable PR interval comparison.
OBJ: Describe 2:1 AV block and advanced second-degree AV block.

9. C. Second-degree AV block type I is also known as *type I block*, *Mobitz I*, or *Wenckebach*.
OBJ: Describe the ECG characteristics, possible causes, signs and symptoms, and emergency management for second-degree AV block type I.

10. B. Remember that the right coronary artery (RCA) supplies the AV node in 90% of the population. The RCA also supplies the inferior wall of the left ventricle and the right ventricle in most individuals. Blockage of the RCA, resulting in an inferior myocardial infarction or right ventricular infarction, can also result in conduction delays such as first-degree AV block and second-degree AV block type I.
OBJ: Describe the ECG characteristics, possible causes, signs and symptoms, and emergency management for second-degree AV block type I.

11. D. With second-degree AV block type II, the ventricular rhythm is irregular. There are more P waves than QRS complexes, and the P-P interval is regular. P waves are normal in size and shape, but some P waves are not followed by a QRS complex. The PR interval may be within normal limits or prolonged, but it is constant for the conducted beats; the PR intervals before and after a blocked P wave are constant. The QRS duration is within normal limits if the block occurs above or within the bundle of His; it is greater than 0.11 second if the block occurs below the bundle of His. QRS complexes are periodically absent after P waves.
OBJ: Describe the ECG characteristics, possible causes, signs and symptoms, and emergency management for second-degree AV block type II.

12. D. Although second-degree AV block type II is less common than second-degree AV block type I, type II is more serious and is a cause for concern because it has a greater potential to progress to a third-degree AV block.

OBJ: Describe the ECG characteristics, possible causes, signs and symptoms, and emergency management for second-degree AV block type II.

13. D. With both second-degree type I and type II AV blocks, P waves occur regularly and the ventricular rhythm is irregular. With second-degree type II, the QRS duration is within normal limits if the block occurs above or within the bundle of His and it is greater than 0.11 second if the block occurs below the bundle of His. QRS complexes are periodically absent after P waves. With second-degree AV block type II, the PR intervals before and after a blocked P wave are constant; with second-degree AV block type I, the PR interval after a nonconducted P wave is shorter than the interval preceding the nonconducted beat.

OBJ: Describe the ECG characteristics, possible causes, signs and symptoms, and emergency management for second-degree AV block type II.

14. B. Third-degree AV block is characterized by regular P-P intervals (i.e., a regular atrial rhythm) and regular R-R intervals (i.e., a regular ventricular rhythm); however, because there is no relationship between the atrial and ventricular rhythms, there is no true PR interval.

OBJ: Describe the ECG characteristics, possible causes, signs and symptoms, and emergency management for third-degree AV block.

15. C. With second-degree AV block type I, the ventricular rhythm is irregular. There are more P waves than QRS complexes, and the P-P interval is regular. P waves are normal in size and shape, but some P waves are not followed by a QRS complex. The PR intervals are inconstant. The PRI after a nonconducted P wave is shorter than the interval preceding the nonconducted beat. The QRS duration is usually 0.11 second or less, and QRS complexes are periodically dropped.

OBJ: Describe the ECG characteristics, possible causes, signs and symptoms, and emergency management for second-degree AV block type I.

16. F
17. C
18. D
19. A
20. E
21. B
22.

	Second-Degree AV Block Type I	Third-Degree AV Block
Ventricular rhythm	**Irregular**	**Regular**
PR interval	**Inconstant; generally progressive**	**None**
QRS width	**Usually narrow**	**Narrow or wide**

OBJ: Describe the ECG characteristics, possible causes, signs and symptoms, and emergency management for second-degree AV block type I and third-degree AV block.

23.

	Second-Degree AV Block Type II	2:1 AV Block
Ventricular rhythm	**Irregular**	**Regular**
PR interval	**Constant**	**Constant**
QRS width	**Narrow or wide**	**Narrow or wide**

OBJ: Describe 2:1 AV block and advanced second-degree AV block.

Practice Rhythm Strip Answers

Note: Because of the distortion of ECGs that can occur during printing, a range of acceptable measurements is provided in the rhythm strip answers throughout this textbook.

24. **Fig. 7.14**
Rhythm: Regular
Rate: 107 beats/min
P waves: Upright before each QRS; 1:1 relationship
PR interval: 0.24 second
QRS duration: 0.06 to 0.08 second
QT interval: 0.28 to 0.32 second
Interpretation: Sinus tachycardia at 107 beats/min with first-degree AV block

25. **Fig. 7.15**
Rhythm: Regular
Rate: Ventricular 34 beats/min; atrial 65 beats/min
P waves: Upright before each QRS; 2:1 relationship
PR interval: 0.32 second
QRS duration: 0.12 to 0.14 second
QT interval: 0.40 second
Interpretation: 2:1 AV block at 34 beats/min with a wide QRS

26. **Fig. 7.16**
Rhythm: Regular
Rate: Ventricular 50 beats/min; atrial 167 beats/min
P waves: Upright; more Ps than QRSs; no relationship to QRSs
PR interval: None
QRS duration: 0.06 second
QT interval: 0.32 second
Interpretation: Third-degree AV block at 50 beats/min with STE

27. **Fig. 7.17**
Rhythm: Ventricular irregular; atrial regular
Rate: Ventricular about 40 beats/min; atrial 60 beats/min
P waves: Upright; more Ps than QRSs
PR interval: 0.16 second
QRS duration: 0.12 second
QT interval: Unable to determine because T waves are not visible
Interpretation: Advanced second-degree AV block at 40 beats/min with a wide QRS and ST-segment depression

28. **Fig. 7.18**
Rhythm: Ventricular irregular; atrial regular
Rate: Ventricular about 50 beats/min; atrial 56 beats/min
P waves: Upright; more Ps than QRSs
PR interval: Lengthening
QRS duration: 0.06 to 0.08 second
QT interval: 0.48 to 0.52 second
Interpretation: Second-degree AV block type I at 50 beats/min with ST-segment depression and a prolonged QT interval

29. **Fig. 7.19**
Rhythm: Ventricular irregular; atrial regular
Rate: Ventricular ranges from less than 20 to 94 beats/min; atrial 94 beats/min
P waves: Upright; more Ps than QRSs
PR interval: Lengthening
QRS duration: 0.06 to 0.08 second
QT interval: 0.36 second
Interpretation: Second-degree AV block type I with a ventricular response ranging from less than 20 to 94 beats/min; note the absence of ventricular activity for slightly more than 5 seconds

30. **Fig. 7.20**
Rhythm: Irregular
Rate: 40 beats/min
P waves: Upright before the QRS of beats 1, 2 and 4, none visible in beat 3
PR interval: 0.36 second
QRS duration: 0.06 second
QT interval: 036 to 0.40 second
Interpretation: Sinus bradycardia at 40 beats/min with first-degree AV block and a premature junctional complex

31. **Fig. 7.21**
Rhythm: Regular
Rate: 54 beats/min
P waves: Upright but artifact obscures visibility with some beats
PR interval: 0.20 to 0.24 second
QRS duration: 0.06 to 0.08 second
QT interval: 0.28 to 0.32 second
Interpretation: Sinus bradycardia at 54 beats/min with first-degree AV block and STE; artifact is present

32. **Fig. 7.22**
Rhythm: Regular
Rate: Ventricular 36 beats/min; atrial 68 beats/min
P waves: Upright; 2:1 relationship
PR interval: 0.28 second
QRS duration: 0.14 to 0.16 second
QT interval: 0.44 second
Interpretation: 2:1 AV block at 36 beats/min with a wide QRS and STE

33. **Fig. 7.23**
Rhythm: Regular
Rate: Ventricular 56 beats/min; atrial 107 beats/min
P waves: Upright; 2:1 relationship
PR interval: 0.16 second
QRS duration: 0.04 to 0.06 second
QT interval: 0.36 second (estimated; difficult to determine because T waves are not clearly visible)
Interpretation: 2:1 AV block at 56 beats/min with STE

34. **Fig. 7.24**
Rhythm: Regular
Rate: 88 beats/min
P waves: Upright before each QRS
PR interval: 0.24 second
QRS duration: 0.06 second
QT interval: 0.32 second
Interpretation: Sinus rhythm at 88 beats/min with first-degree AV block and ST-segment depression

35. **Fig. 7.25**
Rhythm: Regular
Rate: Ventricular 45 beats/min; atrial 115 beats/min
P waves: Upright; more Ps than QRSs
PR interval: None
QRS duration: 0.14 to 0.16 second
QT interval: 0.40 to 0.44 second
Interpretation: Third-degree AV block at 45 beats/min

36. **Fig. 7.26**
Rhythm: Irregular
Rate: 70 beats/min
P waves: Sinus P waves; none with early beats
PR interval: 0.14 to 0.16 second (sinus beats)
QRS duration: 0.08 to 0.10 second (sinus beats)
QT interval: 0.36 to 0.38 second (sinus beats)
Interpretation: Sinus rhythm at 70 beats/min with uniform PVCs and ST-segment depression

37. **Fig. 7.27**
Rhythm: Regular
Rate: Ventricular rate 35 beats/min; atrial rate 70 beats/min
P waves: Upright before each QRS; 2:1 relationship
PR interval: 0.20 second
QRS duration: 0.12 to 0.14 second
QT interval: 0.48 to 0.52 second
Interpretation: 2:1 AV block at 35 beats/min with a wide QRS and a prolonged QT interval

38. **Fig. 7.28**
Rhythm: Essentially regular
Rate: Ventricular 32 beats/min; atrial 71 beats/min
P waves: Upright; more Ps than QRSs
PR interval: None
QRS duration: 0.10 second
QT interval: 0.52 second
Interpretation: Third-degree AV block at 32 beats/min with a prolonged QT interval

39. **Fig. 7.29**
Rhythm: Irregular
Rate: 110 beats/min
P waves: Upright before each QRS; artifact is present
PR interval: 0.12 to 0.16 second
QRS duration: 0.10 second
QT interval: 0.28 to 0.30 second
Interpretation: Sinus tachyarrhythmia at 110 beats/min

40. **Fig. 7.30**
Rhythm: Irregular
Rate: 80 beats/min
P waves: Upright before each QRS; none with early ventricular beat
PR interval: 0.16 to 0.18 second (sinus beats)
QRS duration: 0.12 to 0.16 second (sinus beats)
QT interval: 0.32 to 0.36 second (sinus beats)
Interpretation: Sinus rhythm at 80 beats/min with a wide QRS, an R-on-T premature ventricular complex, and STE

41. **Fig. 7.31**
Rhythm: Irregular
Rate: 100 beats/min (sinus beats); 150 beats/min (ventricular tachycardia [VT])
P waves: Sinus P waves; none with ventricular beats
PR interval: 0.24 second (sinus beats)
QRS duration: 0.08 second (sinus beats)
QT interval: 0.28 to 0.30 second (sinus beats)
Interpretation: Sinus rhythm at 100 beats/min with first-degree AV block to monomorphic VT at 150 beats/min

42. **Fig. 7.32**
Rhythm: Ventricular irregular; atrial regular
Rate: Ventricular 50 beats/min; atrial 60 beats/min
P waves: Upright; more Ps than QRSs
PR interval: Lengthening

QRS duration: 0.06 to 0.08 second
QT interval: 0.32 second
Interpretation: Second-degree AV block type I at 50 beats/min

43. **Fig. 7.33**
Rhythm: Regular
Rate: 111 beats/min
P waves: Tall and upright before each QRS
PR interval: 0.20 second (borderline first-degree AV block)
QRS duration: 0.08 to 0.10 second
QT interval: 0.28 second
Interpretation: Sinus tachycardia at 111 beats/min; tall P waves

44. **Fig. 7.34**
Rhythm: Ventricular regular; atrial slightly irregular
Rate: Ventricular 52 beats/min; atrial 71 beats/min
P waves: Upright; more Ps than QRSs
PR interval: None
QRS duration: 0.08 to 0.10 second
QT interval: 0.24 to 0.28 second
Interpretation: Third-degree AV block at 52 beats/min with STE

45. **Fig. 7.35**
Rhythm: Ventricular irregular; atrial regular
Rate: Ventricular 40 beats/min; atrial 100 beats/min
P waves: Upright; more Ps than QRSs
PR interval: 0.14 second
QRS duration: 0.10 to 0.12 second
QT interval: 0.48 to 0.52 second (prolonged)
Interpretation: Second-degree AV block type II at 40 beats/min with ST-segment depression and a prolonged QT interval

46. **Fig. 7.36**
Rhythm: Regular
Rate: 37 beats/min
P waves: Upright; 1:1 relationship
PR interval: 0.22 to 0.24 second
QRS duration: 0.06 to 0.08 second
QT interval: 0.44 to 0.48 second (slightly prolonged)
Interpretation: Sinus bradycardia at 37 beats/min with first-degree AV block and a slightly prolonged QT interval

47. **Fig. 7.37**
Rhythm: Ventricular irregular; atrial regular
Rate: Ventricular 50 beats/min; atrial 83 beats/min
P waves: Upright; more Ps than QRSs
PR interval: Lengthening
QRS duration: 0.08 second
QT interval: 0.32 second
Interpretation: Second-degree AV block type I at 50 beats/min; although the complexes on the right side of the rhythm strip show 2:1 conduction, comparison of the PR intervals of beats 1 through 3 enables a diagnosis of second-degree type I AV block

48. **Fig. 7.38**
Rhythm: Ventricular regular; atrial regular
Rate: Ventricular 38 beats/min; atrial 63 beats/min
P waves: Upright; more Ps than QRSs
PR interval: None
QRS duration: 0.06 second
QT interval: 0.52 second (prolonged)
Interpretation: Third-degree AV block at 38 beats/min with ST-segment depression, inverted T waves, and a prolonged QT interval

49. **Fig. 7.39**
Rhythm: Ventricular regular; atrial regular
Rate: Ventricular 47 beats/min; atrial 92 beats/min
P waves: Upright; more Ps than QRSs; 2:1 relationship
PR interval: 0.12 to 0.16 second
QRS duration: 0.06 to 0.08 second
QT interval: 0.44 second
Interpretation: 2:1 AV block at 47 beats/min

50. **Fig. 7.40**
Rhythm: Regular
Rate: 75 beats/min
P waves: Low amplitude, but upright before each QRS
PR interval: 0.16 second
QRS duration: 0.10 to 0.12 second
QT interval: 0.32 to 0.36 second (estimated; difficult to determine because the ends of the T waves are not clearly visible)
Interpretation: Sinus rhythm at 75 beats/min with STE

51. **Fig. 7.41**
Rhythm: Regular
Rate: 62 beats/min
P waves: Inverted before each QRS
PR interval: 0.14 to 0.16 second
QRS duration: 0.08 to 0.10 second
QT interval: Unable to determine
Interpretation: Accelerated junctional rhythm at 62 beats/min

52. **Fig. 7.42**
Rhythm: Irregular
Rate: 70 beats/min
P waves: Upright before each QRS; the P wave of beat 3 is early; an early P wave with no QRS after it distorts the T wave of beat 6
PR interval: 0.20 second (sinus beats)
QRS duration: 0.08 second (sinus beats)
QT interval: 0.32 second (sinus beats)
Interpretation: Sinus rhythm at 70 beats/min with a PAC and a nonconducted PAC

53. **Fig. 7.43**
Rhythm: Ventricular regular; atrial regular
Rate: Ventricular 36 beats/min; atrial 70 beats/min
P waves: Upright; more Ps than QRSs; 2:1 relationship
PR interval: 0.32 second
QRS duration: 0.10 to 0.12 second
QT interval: 0.36 to 0.40 second
Interpretation: 2:1 AV block at 36 beats/min

REFERENCES

Barold, S. S. (1996). Indications for permanent cardiac pacing in first-degree AV block: class I, II, or III? *PACE, 19*(5), 745–751.

Barold, S. S., & Hayes, D. L. (2001). Second-degree atrioventricular block: a reappraisal. *Mayo Clin Proc, 76*(1), 44–57.

Blank, A. C., Loh, P., & Vos, M. A. (2014). Atrioventricular block. In D. P. Zipes & J. Jalife (Eds.), *Cardiac electrophysiology: From cell to bedside* (6th ed.) (pp. 1043–1049). Philadelphia: Saunders.

Hamdan, M. H. (2010). Cardiac arrhythmias. In T. E. Andreoli, I. J. Benjamin, R. C. Griggs, & E. J. Wing (Eds.), *Andreoli and Carpenter's Cecil essentials of medicine* (8th ed.) (pp. 118–144). Philadelphia: Saunders.

Issa, Z. F., Miller, J. M., & Zipes, D. P. (2012). Atrioventricular conduction abnormalities. In *Clinical arrhythmology and electrophysiology: A companion to Braunwald's Heart Disease* (2nd ed.) (pp. 175–193). Philadelphia: Saunders.

Latcu, D.-G., & Nadir, S. (2010). Atrioventricular and intraventricular conduction disorders. In M. H. Crawford, J. P. DiMarco, & W. J. Paulus (Eds.), *Cardiology* (3rd ed.) (pp. 725–739). Philadelphia: Elsevier.

Olgin, J., & Zipes, D. P. (2012). Specific arrhythmias: diagnosis and treatment. In R. O. Bonow, D. L. Mann, D. P. Zipes, & P. Libby (Eds.), *Braunwald's heart disease: A textbook of cardiovascular medicine* (9th ed.) (pp. 771–824). Philadelphia: Saunders.

Pacemaker Rhythms

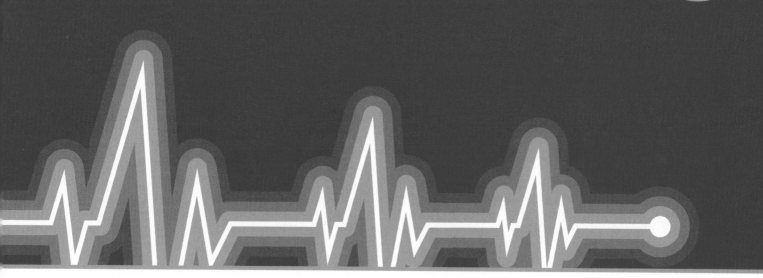

LEARNING OBJECTIVES

After reading this chapter, you should be able to:

1. Identify the components of a pacemaker system.
2. Discuss the terms *triggering, inhibition, pacing, capture, electrical capture, mechanical capture,* and *sensitivity.*
3. Describe the appearance of a typical pacemaker spike on the electrocardiogram (ECG).
4. Describe the appearance of the waveform on the ECG produced as a result of atrial pacing and ventricular pacing.
5. Explain the differences between single-chamber and dual-chamber pacemakers and between fixed-rate and demand pacemakers.
6. List three types of pacemaker malfunction.
7. Describe how to analyze pacemaker function on the ECG.

KEY TERMS

atrioventricular (AV) interval: In dual-chamber pacing, the length of time between an atrial sensed or atrial paced event and the delivery of a ventricular pacing stimulus; analogous to the PR interval of intrinsic waveforms; also called the *artificial* or *electronic PR interval*

base rate: Rate at which the pacemaker's pulse generator initiates impulses when no intrinsic activity is detected; expressed in pulses per minute (ppm)

capture: The successful conduction of an artificial pacemaker's impulse through the myocardium, resulting in depolarization

demand pacemaker: Pacemaker that discharges only when the patient's heart rate drops below the preset rate for the pacemaker; also known as a *synchronous* or *noncompetitive pacemaker*

dual-chamber pacemaker: Pacemaker that stimulates the atrium and ventricle; dual-chamber pacing is also called *physiologic pacing*

escape interval: Time measured between a sensed cardiac event and the next pacemaker output

failure to capture: A pacemaker malfunction that occurs when the artificial pacemaker stimulus is unable to depolarize the myocardium

failure to pace: A pacemaker malfunction that occurs when the pacemaker fails to deliver an electrical stimulus at its programmed time; also referred to as *failure to fire* or *failure of pulse generation*

fixed-rate pacemaker: Pacemaker that continuously discharges at a preset rate regardless of the patient's intrinsic activity; also known as an *asynchronous pacemaker*

inhibition: Pacemaker response in which the output pulse is suppressed when an intrinsic event is sensed

oversensing: A pacemaker malfunction that results from inappropriate sensing of extraneous electrical signals

paced interval: Period between two consecutive paced events in the same cardiac chamber; also known as the *automatic interval*

pacemaker: A battery-powered device that delivers an electrical current to the heart to stimulate depolarization

sensitivity: The extent to which an artificial pacemaker recognizes intrinsic cardiac electrical activity

threshold: The minimum amount of voltage (i.e., milliamperes) needed to obtain consistent capture

undersensing: A pacemaker malfunction that occurs when the artificial pacemaker fails to recognize spontaneous myocardial depolarization

PACEMAKER SYSTEMS

[Objectives 1, 2]

A cardiac **pacemaker** is a battery-powered device that delivers an electrical current to the heart to stimulate depolarization. A pacemaker system consists of a *pulse generator* (i.e., the power source) and pacing leads. The pulse generator houses a battery and electronic circuitry. The circuitry works like a computer, converting energy from the battery into electrical pulses. Whereas a lithium battery is usually the power source for implanted pacemakers and implantable cardioverter-defibrillators (ICDs), a 9-volt alkaline battery is usually used to power a temporary external pulse generator. A *pacing lead* is an insulated wire that is used to carry an electrical impulse from the pulse generator to the patient's heart. It also carries information about the heart's electrical activity back to the pacemaker. The pacemaker responds to the information received either by sending a pacing impulse to the heart (i.e., *triggering*) or by not sending a pacing impulse to the heart (i.e., **inhibition**).

An artificial pacemaker can be external (a temporary intervention) or implanted. An external pacemaker may be used to control transient disturbances in heart rate or conduction that result from drug toxicity or that occurs during a myocardial infarction (MI) or after cardiac surgery when increased vagal tone is often present. Patients who have chronic dysrhythmias that are unresponsive to medication therapy and that result in decreased cardiac output may require the surgical implantation of a permanent pacemaker or an ICD.

Permanent Pacemakers and Implantable Cardioverter-Defibrillators

A permanent pacemaker is used to treat disorders of the sinoatrial (SA) node (e.g., bradycardias), disorders of the atrioventricular (AV) conduction pathways (e.g., second-degree AV block type II, third-degree AV block), or both, that produce signs and symptoms as a result of inadequate cardiac output (Box 8.1). The pacemaker's pulse generator is usually implanted under local anesthesia into the subcutaneous tissue of the anterior chest just below the right or left clavicle (Fig. 8.1). The patient's handedness, occupation, and hobbies determine whether the pacemaker is implanted on the right or left side.   .

Box **8.1**	Clinical Indications of Decreased Cardiac Output
• Acutely altered mental status • Dizziness • Exercise intolerance • Fainting • Fatigue • Heart failure	• Lightheadedness • Palpitations • Pulsations in the neck • Seizures • Shortness of breath • Tightness in the chest

An ICD is a programmable device that can deliver a range of therapies (also called *tiered therapy*), including defibrillation, antitachycardia pacing (i.e., *overdrive pacing*), synchronized cardioversion, and bradycardia pacing, depending on the dysrhythmia detected and how the device is programmed (Fig. 8.2). A physician determines the appropriate ICD therapies for each patient.

 Did You Know?

During overdrive pacing, the pacemaker is set to pace at a rate faster than the rate of the tachycardia. After a few seconds, the pacemaker is stopped to allow the return of the heart's intrinsic pacemaker.

When ICDs were initially introduced, they were surgically placed subcutaneously in the left upper quadrant of the patient's abdomen. With improvements in technology, ICDs are now small enough to be surgically placed in the pectoral area. ICDs were initially used for patients with one or more sudden cardiac arrests or drug-refractory ventricular fibrillation or sustained ventricular tachycardia. Today, ICDs are also used for patients who have experienced an extensive MI resulting in decreased cardiac output, patients who have a history of MI with recurrent episodes of unexplained syncope, and children with congenital long-QT syndrome, among other conditions.

The circuitry of pacemakers and ICDs is housed in a hermetically sealed case made of titanium that is airtight and impermeable to fluid. Pacemakers and ICDs store information about the activities of the patient's heart, as well as information about the device itself (e.g., number of dysrhythmia episodes; provoking rhythm; dates of pacing, defibrillation, or both). The stored information is periodically retrieved and reviewed by the patient's physician and, if necessary, changes in the device's settings are made. Lithium batteries are almost exclusively used in modern pacemakers and ICDs. Battery life depends on the number of times therapies

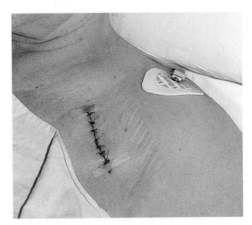

Fig. 8.1 Site of implantation of a permanent pacemaker or implantable cardioverter-defibrillator. The pacemaker is usually implanted in the left pectoral region, but it may be placed elsewhere if necessary. (From Forbes C, Jackson W: *Color atlas and text of clinical medicine,* St. Louis, 2003, Mosby.)

ICD: Tiered Therapy

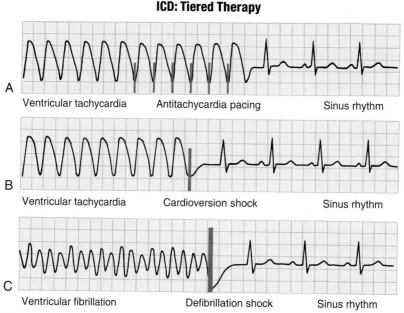

Fig. 8.2 Tiered (staged) dysrhythmia therapy and implantable cardioverter-defibrillators (ICDs). These devices are capable of automatically delivering staged therapy in treating ventricular tachycardia (VT) or ventricular fibrillation (VF), including anti-tachycardia pacing A, or cardioversion shocks B, for VT and defibrillation shocks C, for VF. (From Goldberger AL, Goldberger ZD, Shvilkin A: *Goldberger's clinical electrocardiography: a simplified approach,* ed 8, Philadelphia, 2013, Saunders.)

are delivered, the frequency of pacing, and the number of cardiac chambers paced.

Complications of permanent pacing associated with the implantation procedure include bleeding, local tissue reaction, pneumothorax, cardiac dysrhythmias, air embolism, and thrombosis. Long-term complications of permanent pacing may include infection, electrode displacement, heart failure, fracture of the pacing lead, pacemaker-induced dysrhythmias, externalization of the pacemaker generator, and perforation of the right ventricle with or without pericardial tamponade.

Temporary Pacemakers

The pulse generator of a temporary pacemaker is located externally. Temporary pacing can be accomplished through transvenous, epicardial, or transcutaneous means.

TRANSVENOUS PACING

Transvenous pacemakers stimulate the endocardium of the right atrium or ventricle (or both) by means of an electrode introduced into a central vein, such as the subclavian, femoral, brachial, internal jugular, or external jugular vein. Complications of temporary transvenous pacing include bleeding; infection; pneumothorax; cardiac dysrhythmias; MI; lead displacement; fracture of the pacing lead; hematoma at the insertion site; perforation of the right ventricle with or without pericardial tamponade; and perforation of the inferior vena cava, pulmonary artery, or coronary arteries because of improper placement of the pacing lead.

EPICARDIAL PACING

Epicardial pacing is the placement of pacing leads directly onto or through the epicardium. Epicardial leads may be used when a patient is undergoing cardiac surgery and the outer surface of the heart is easy to reach.

TRANSCUTANEOUS PACING

Transcutaneous pacing (TCP), also called *temporary external pacing* or *noninvasive pacing*, is the use of electrical stimulation through pacing pads positioned on a patient's torso to stimulate contraction of the heart. TCP is indicated for significant bradycardias that are unresponsive to atropine therapy or when atropine is not immediately available or indicated. It may also be used as a bridge until transvenous pacing can be accomplished or the cause of the bradycardia is reversed (e.g., drug overdose, hyperkalemia). *Standby pacing* refers to the application of the pacing pads to the patient's chest in anticipation of possible use, but pacing is not yet needed. For example, standby pacing is often warranted when second-degree AV block type II or third-degree AV block is present in the setting of acute MI.

TCP requires attaching two pacing electrodes to the skin surface of the patient's outer chest wall. The electrical signal exits from the negative terminal on the machine (and subsequently the negative electrode) and passes through the chest wall to the heart. The range of output current of a transcutaneous pacemaker varies depending on the manufacturer (Fig. 8.3).

The primary limitation of TCP is patient discomfort that is proportional to the intensity of skeletal muscle contraction

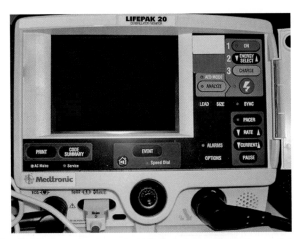

Fig. 8.3 An example of a monitor/defibrillator that provides cardiac monitoring, defibrillation, cardioversion, and transcutaneous pacing. (Copyright ©2016 Medtronic. All rights reserved. Used with the permission of Medtronic.)

Fig. 8.4 Example of a temporary unipolar pacing lead. (Copyright ©2016 Medtronic. All rights reserved. Used with the permission of Medtronic.)

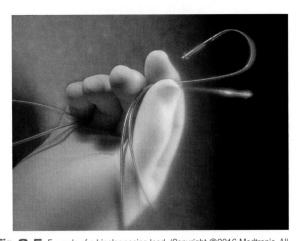

Fig. 8.5 Example of a bipolar pacing lead. (Copyright ©2016 Medtronic. All rights reserved. Used with the permission of Medtronic.)

and the direct electrical stimulation of cutaneous nerves. Because TCP is uncomfortable, the administration of sedatives or analgesics is usually necessary in responsive patients. Temporary transvenous pacing is indicated when prolonged TCP is needed.

Possible complications of TCP include the following:

- Coughing
- Skin burns
- Interference with sensing from patient agitation or muscle contractions
- Discomfort as a result of the electrical stimulation of the skin and muscles
- Failure to recognize that the pacemaker is not capturing
- Tissue damage, including third-degree burns, with improper or prolonged TCP
- When pacing is prolonged, pacing **threshold** changes, thereby leading to capture failure

Pacing Lead Systems

[Objectives 2, 3]

Pacemaker lead systems may consist of single, double, or multiple leads. The exposed portion of the pacing lead—that is, the *electrode*—is placed in direct contact with the heart. Pacing, also called *pacemaker firing*, occurs when the pacemaker's pulse generator delivers energy (milliamperes [mA]) through the pacing electrode to the myocardium. Evidence of pacing can be seen as a vertical line or spike on the electrocardiogram (ECG). **Capture** is the successful conduction of an artificial pacemaker's impulse through the myocardium, resulting in depolarization. Capture is obtained after the pacemaker electrode is properly positioned in the heart; with one-to-one capture, each pacing stimulus results in depolarization of the appropriate chamber. On the ECG, evidence of *electrical capture* can be seen as a pacemaker spike followed by an atrial or a ventricular complex, depending on the cardiac chamber that is being paced. *Mechanical capture* is assessed by palpating the patient's pulse or by observing

right atrial pressure, left atrial pressure, or pulmonary artery or arterial pressure waveforms.

A unipolar electrode has one pacing electrode that is located at its distal tip (Fig. 8.4). The negative electrode is in contact with the cardiac tissue, and the pulse generator (located outside the heart) functions as the positive electrode. The pacemaker spike produced by a unipolar lead system is often large because of the distance between the positive and negative electrode. Unipolar leads are less commonly used than bipolar lead systems because of the potential for pacing the chest wall muscles and the susceptibility of the unipolar leads to electromagnetic interference.

A bipolar lead system contains a positive and negative electrode at the distal tip of the pacing lead wire (Fig. 8.5). Most temporary transvenous pacemakers use a bipolar lead system. A permanent pacemaker may have either a bipolar or a unipolar lead system. The pacemaker spike produced by a bipolar lead system is smaller than that of a unipolar system because of the shorter distance between the positive and negative electrodes (Fig. 8.6).

Bipolar spike

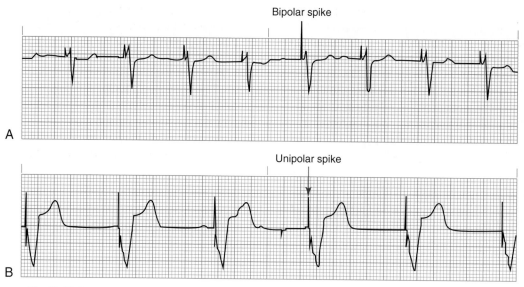

Unipolar spike

Fig. 8.6 Bipolar and unipolar pacing. A, Pacemaker spike produced by a bipolar lead system. B, Pacemaker spike produced by a unipolar lead system. (From Urden LD, Stacy KM, Lough ME: *Critical care nursing*, ed 8, St. Louis, 2018, Mosby.)

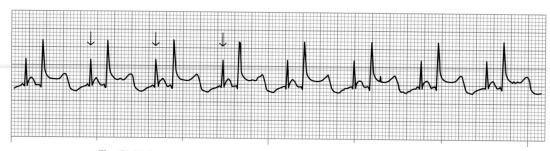

Fig. 8.7 Electrocardiogram of a single-chamber pacemaker with atrial pacing spikes *(arrows)*.

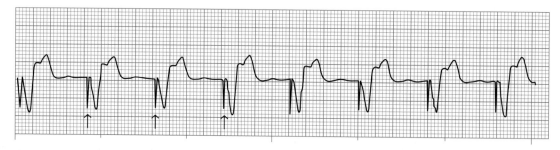

Fig. 8.8 Electrocardiogram of a single-chamber pacemaker with ventricular pacing spikes *(arrows)*.

PACING CHAMBERS AND MODES

A pacemaker system may be single or dual chamber.

Single-Chamber Pacemakers

[Objectives 4, 5]

A pacemaker that paces a single heart chamber, either the atrium or ventricle, has one lead placed in the heart. Atrial pacing is achieved by placing the pacing electrode in the right atrium. Stimulation of the atria produces a pacemaker

spike on the ECG followed by a P wave (Fig. 8.7). Atrial pacing may be used when the SA node is diseased or damaged, but conduction through the AV junction and ventricles is normal. This type of pacemaker is ineffective if an AV block develops because it cannot pace the ventricles.

Ventricular pacing is accomplished by placing the pacing electrode in the right ventricle. Stimulation of the ventricles produces a pacemaker spike on the ECG followed by a wide QRS, resembling a ventricular ectopic beat (Fig. 8.8). The QRS complex is wide because a paced impulse does not follow the normal conduction pathway in the heart. A single-chamber ventricular pacemaker can pace the ventricles but it cannot coordinate pacing with the patient's intrinsic atrial rate. This results in asynchronous contraction of the atrium and ventricle (i.e., AV asynchrony). Because of this loss of AV synchrony, a ventricular demand pacemaker is rarely used in patients with an intact SA node. Conversely, a ventricular demand pacemaker may be used for patients with chronic atrial fibrillation.

Dual-Chamber Pacemakers

[Objectives 4, 5]

A **dual-chamber pacemaker** uses two leads: One lead is placed in the right atrium and the other in the right ventricle (Fig. 8.9). Dual-chamber pacing is also called *physiologic pacing*. A dual-chamber pacemaker stimulates the right atrium and right ventricle sequentially (stimulating first the atrium and then the ventricle), mimicking normal cardiac physiology and thus preserving the atrial contribution to ventricular filling (i.e., atrial kick).

When spontaneous atrial depolarization does not occur within a preset interval, the atrial pulse generator fires and stimulates atrial depolarization at a preset rate. The pacemaker is programmed to wait—simulating the normal delay in conduction through the AV node (i.e., the PR interval). The artificial or electronic PR interval is referred to as an **atrioventricular (AV) interval** (Fig. 8.10). If spontaneous

ventricular depolarization does not occur within a preset interval, the pacemaker fires and stimulates ventricular depolarization at a preset rate.

Biventricular Pacemakers

A *biventricular pacemaker* has three leads—one lead for each ventricle and one lead for the right atrium. This device uses cardiac resynchronization therapy to restore normal simultaneous ventricular contraction for patients with heart failure, thereby improving cardiac output and exercise tolerance.

Fixed-Rate Pacemakers

[Objective 5]

A **fixed-rate pacemaker**, also known as an *asynchronous pacemaker*, continuously discharges at a preset rate (usually 70 to 80 impulses/min) regardless of the patient's heart rate or metabolic demands. An advantage of the fixed-rate pacemaker is its simple circuitry, reducing the risk of pacemaker failure; however, this type of pacemaker does not sense the patient's own cardiac rhythm. This may result in competition between the patient's cardiac rhythm and that of the pacemaker. Ventricular tachycardia or ventricular fibrillation may be induced if the pacemaker were to fire during the T wave (i.e., the vulnerable period) of a preceding patient beat. Fixed-rate pacemakers are not often used today.

Demand Pacemakers

[Objective 5]

A **demand pacemaker**, also known as a *synchronous* or *noncompetitive pacemaker*, discharges only when the patient's heart rate drops below the pacemaker's **base rate**. For example, if the demand pacemaker was preset at a base rate of 70 impulses/min, it would sense the patient's heart rate and allow electrical impulses to flow from the pacemaker through the pacing lead to stimulate the heart only when the rate falls below 70 beats/min. Demand pacemakers can be programmable or nonprogrammable. The voltage level and impulse rate are preset at the time of manufacture in nonprogrammable pacemakers.

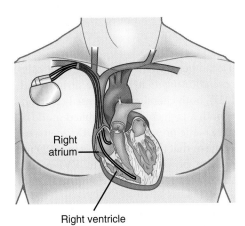

Fig. 8.9 Pacing leads in both the atrium and the ventricle enable a dual-chamber pacemaker to sense and pace in both heart chambers. (From Lewis SL, Bucher L, Heitkemper MM, Harding MM: *Medical-surgical nursing: assessment and management of clinical problems,* ed 10, St. Louis, 2017, Elsevier.)

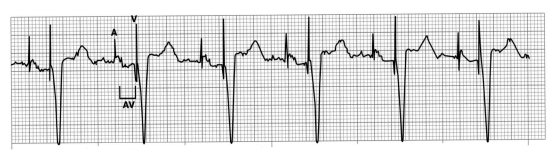

Fig. 8.10 Electrocardiogram of a dual-chamber pacemaker with atrial pacing spikes (A) and ventricular pacing spikes (V). *AV,* Atrioventricular interval.

TABLE 8.1	Revised NASPE/BPEG Generic Code for Antibradycardia Pacing				
Position	I	II	III	IV	V
Category	Chamber(s) Paced	Chamber(s) Sensed	Response to Sensing	Rate Modulation	Multisite Pacing
Manufacturer's designation only	O = None A = Atrium V = Ventricle D = Dual (A + V) S = Single (A or V)	O = None A = Atrium V = Ventricle D = Dual (A + V) S = Single (A or V)	O = None T = Triggered I = Inhibited D = Dual (T + I)	O = None R = Rate modulation	O = None A = Atrium V = Ventricle D = Dual (A + V)

NASPE/BPEG, North American Society of Pacing and Electrophysiology/British Pacing and Electrophysiology Group.
From Bernstein A, Daubert J, Fletcher R, Hayes D, et al. The revised NASPE/BPEG generic code for antibradycardia, adaptive-rate, and multisite pacing. North American Society of Pacing and Electrophysiology/British Pacing and Electrophysiology Group, *Pacing Clin Electrophysiol* 2002;25(2):260-264.

Pacemaker Codes

[Objective 5]

Pacemaker codes are used to assist in identifying a pacemaker's preprogrammed pacing, sensing, and response functions (Table 8.1). The *first letter* of the code identifies the heart chamber (or chambers) paced (stimulated). A pacemaker used to pace only a single chamber is represented by either A (atrial) or V (ventricular). A pacemaker capable of pacing in both chambers is represented by D (dual). The *second letter* identifies the chamber of the heart where patient-initiated (i.e., intrinsic) electrical activity is sensed by the pacemaker. The *third letter* indicates how the pacemaker will respond when it senses patient-initiated electrical activity. The *fourth letter* identifies the availability of rate modulation (i.e., the pacemaker's ability to adapt its rate to meet the body's needs caused by increased physical activity and then increase or decrease the pacing rate accordingly). A pacemaker's rate modulation capability may also be referred to as *rate responsiveness* or *rate adaptation.* The *fifth letter* denotes multisite pacing (i.e., biventricular pacing or more than one pacing site in one ventricle). Although the use of all five letters is sometimes needed for completeness, the first three letters are *always* required (Bernstein et al, 2002).

The ventricular demand (VVI) pacemaker is a common type of pacemaker. With this device, the pacemaker electrode is placed in the right ventricle (V); the ventricle is sensed (V) and the pacemaker is inhibited (I) when spontaneous ventricular depolarization occurs within a preset interval. When spontaneous ventricular depolarization does not occur within this preset interval, the pacemaker fires and stimulates ventricular depolarization at a preset rate (Fig. 8.11). P waves can appear anywhere in the cardiac cycle and have no relationship with the QRS complexes because a ventricular demand pacemaker does not sense or pace atrial activity. A disadvantage of ventricular demand pacing is its fixed rate, regardless of the patient's level of physical activity.

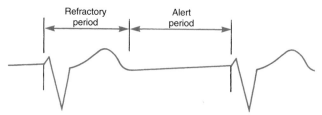

Fig. 8.11 During the refractory period, a ventricular demand pacemaker does not sense any electrical activity. The refractory period is followed by the alert period. If no QRS complex is sensed by the end of the alert period, the pacemaker fires and stimulates ventricular depolarization at a preset rate. (From Goldberger AL: *Clinical electrocardiography: a simplified approach,* ed 7, St. Louis, 2006, Mosby.)

A dual-chamber pacemaker may also be called a *DDD pacemaker,* indicating that both the atrium and ventricle are paced (D), both chambers are sensed (D), and the pacemaker has both a triggered and inhibited mode of response (D) (Fig. 8.12). The presence of a DDD pacemaker does not necessarily mean that the pacemaker is in DDD mode. DDD pacemakers can be programmed to VVI mode, depending on patient need (e.g., the development of chronic atrial fibrillation).

A defibrillator code was developed in 1993, and it is used to describe the capabilities and operation of ICDs (Table 8.2).

PACEMAKER MALFUNCTION

Problems that can occur with pacing include failure to pace, failure to capture, and failure to sense (e.g., undersensing, oversensing).

Failure to Pace

[Objective 6]

Failure to pace, also referred to as *failure to fire* or *failure of pulse generation,* is a pacemaker malfunction that occurs when the pacemaker fails to deliver an electrical stimulus at its programmed time. Failure to pace is recognized on

Dual-Chamber (DDD) Pacemaker Functions

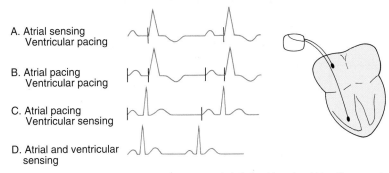

A. Atrial sensing
    Ventricular pacing

B. Atrial pacing
    Ventricular pacing

C. Atrial pacing
    Ventricular sensing

D. Atrial and ventricular
    sensing

Fig. 8.12 A dual-chamber (DDD) pacemaker senses and paces in both the atria and ventricles. The pacemaker emits a stimulus (spike) whenever an intrinsic P wave or QRS complex is not sensed within some programmed time interval. (From Goldberger AL: *Clinical electrocardiography: a simplified approach,* ed 7, St. Louis, 2006, Mosby.)

TABLE 8.2	NASPE/BPEG Defibrillator Codes		
Position I	**Position II**	**Position III**	**Position IV**
Shock Chamber	**Antitachycardia Pacing Chamber**	**Tachycardia Detection**	**Antibradycardia Pacing Chamber**
O = None	O = None	E = Electrogram	O = None
A = Atrium	A = Atrium	H = Hemodynamic	A = Atrium
V = Ventricle	V = Ventricle		V = Ventricle
D = Dual (A + V)	D = Dual (A + V)		D = Dual (A + V)

NASPE/BPEG, North American Society of Pacing and Electrophysiology/British Pacing and Electrophysiology Group.
From Bernstein AD, Camm AJ, Fisher JD, Fletcher RD, et al. North American Society of Pacing and Electrophysiology policy statement: The NASPE/BPEG defibrillator code, *Pacing Clin Electrophysiol* 1993;16:1776-1780.

Failure to pace

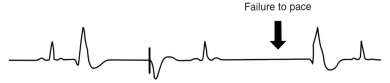

Fig. 8.13 Failure to pace. (From Lynn-McHale Wiegand DJ, editor: *AACN procedure manual for critical care,* ed 6, Philadelphia, 2011, Saunders.)

the ECG as an absence of pacemaker spikes, even though the patient's intrinsic rate is less than that of the pacemaker, and a return of the underlying rhythm for which pacing was initiated (Fig. 8.13). Patient signs and symptoms may include bradycardia, chest discomfort, hypotension, and syncope.

Causes of failure to pace are listed in Box 8.2. Treatment may include adjusting the sensitivity setting, replacing the pulse generator battery, replacing the pacing lead, replacing the pulse generator unit, tightening connections between the pacing lead and pulse generator, or removing the source of electromagnetic interference.

Failure to Capture

[Objective 6]
Failure to capture is the inability of the artificial pacemaker stimulus to depolarize the myocardium and is recognized on the ECG by visible pacemaker spikes not followed by P waves (if the electrode is located in the atrium) or QRS

Box 8.2	Causes of Failure to Pace

- Battery failure
- Fracture of the pacing lead wire
- Displacement of the electrode tip
- Pulse generator failure
- Broken or loose connection between the pacing lead and the pulse generator
- Electromagnetic interference
- Sensitivity set too high

complexes (if the electrode is located in the right ventricle) (Fig. 8.14). Patient signs and symptoms may include bradycardia, fatigue, and hypotension.

Causes of failure to capture are shown in Box 8.3. If the problem is a result of low output energy, slowly increasing the output setting (mA) until capture occurs may resolve the problem. With transvenous pacing, repositioning the patient to the left side may promote the contact of a transvenous pacing lead with the endocardium and septum.

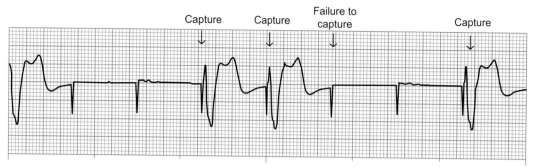

Fig. 8.14 Failure to capture.

- Displacement of pacing lead wire (common cause)
- Output energy (i.e., mA) set too low (common cause)
- Battery failure
- Fracture of the pacing lead wire
- Edema or scar tissue formation at the electrode tip
- Increased stimulation threshold as a result of medications or electrolyte imbalance

Failure to Sense

[Objective 6]

Sensitivity is the extent to which an artificial pacemaker recognizes intrinsic cardiac electrical activity. **Undersensing** occurs when the artificial pacemaker fails to recognize spontaneous myocardial depolarization and it is recognized on the ECG by pacemaker spikes that occur within P waves, pacemaker spikes that follow too closely behind the patient's QRS complexes, or pacemaker spikes that appear within T waves (Fig. 8.15). Because pacemaker spikes occur when they should not, this type of pacemaker malfunction may result in pacemaker spikes that fall on T waves (i.e., R-on-T phenomenon), competition between the pacemaker and the patient's own cardiac rhythm, or both. The patient may complain of palpitations or skipped beats.

Causes of failure to sense are shown in Box 8.4. Treatment may include increasing the sensitivity setting, replacing the pulse generator battery, or replacing or repositioning the pacing lead.

Oversensing is a pacemaker malfunction that results from inappropriate sensing of extraneous electrical signals. Atrial sensing pacemakers may inappropriately sense ventricular activity; ventricular sensing pacemakers may misidentify a tall, peaked intrinsic T wave as a QRS complex. Oversensing is recognized on the ECG as pacemaker spikes at a rate slower than the pacemaker's preset rate or no paced beats even though the pacemaker's preset rate is greater than the patient's intrinsic rate (Fig. 8.16). Treatment includes adjustment of the pacemaker's sensitivity setting or possible insertion of a bipolar lead if oversensing is caused by unipolar lead dysfunction.

ANALYZING PACEMAKER FUNCTION ON THE ECG

[Objective 7]

To practice analyzing pacemaker function on the ECG, let's look at Fig. 8.17. The first step in our analysis of this rhythm strip should include identification of the patient's underlying rhythm and its rate, if possible. Fig. 8.17 provides a look at the patient's rhythm from two leads, and six QRS complexes are visible in each lead. Each QRS complex is preceded by one upright P wave. Based on this information, we know that the underlying rhythm is sinus in origin. The atrial and ventricular rates are regular at 65 beats/min.

Next, let's look for evidence of paced activity (i.e., atrial pacer spikes, ventricular pacer spikes, or both) and evaluate the paced interval. The **paced interval**, also called the *automatic interval*, is the period between two consecutive paced events in the same cardiac chamber. Measure the distance between two consecutively paced atrial beats using calipers or paper when atrial pacer spikes are present. Because there is no pacemaker spike before any of the P waves in this rhythm strip, there is no evidence of paced atrial activity; however, a pacer spike is clearly visible before each QRS complex.

Because paced ventricular activity is present, we must evaluate the rate and regularity of the ventricular paced interval by measuring the distance between two consecutively paced ventricular beats. The ventricular paced interval is regular at 65 pulses/min. If both atrial and ventricular pacemaker spikes were present, you would know that this patient had a dual-chamber pacemaker. Because only wide-QRS complexes are present and each QRS is preceded by a pacemaker spike, it is reasonable to conclude that this patient has a ventricular pacemaker. Next, compare the escape interval with the paced interval measured earlier. The **escape interval** is the time measured between a sensed cardiac event and the next pacemaker output. The paced interval and escape interval should measure the same. In Fig. 8.17, the paced interval and the escape interval are the same.

Next, analyze the rhythm strip for failure to pace, failure to capture, and failure to sense. Remember that with failure to pace, the ECG will reveal an absence of pacemaker spikes at their programmed time. Because the pacer

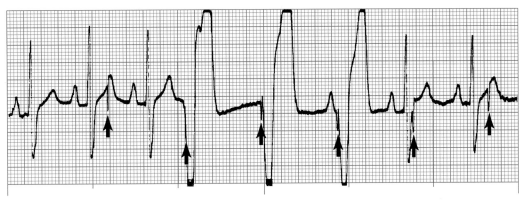

Fig. 8.15 Undersensing.

Box **8.4**	**Causes of Failure to Sense**

- Displacement of the electrode tip (most common cause)
- Battery failure
- Fracture of the pacing lead wire
- Decreased P wave or QRS voltage
- Circuitry dysfunction (e.g., pulse generator unable to process the QRS signal)
- Increased sensing threshold from antiarrhythmic medications
- Severe electrolyte disturbances
- Myocardial perforation

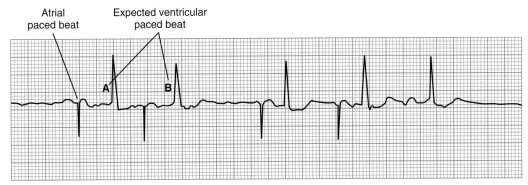

Fig. 8.16 Ventricular oversensing and possibly ventricular pulse generation failure. Ventricular spike expected at 150 msec. Ventricular spike and corresponding ventricular depolarization did not occur at points *A* and *B*. Also, atrial timing reset by oversensed ventricular activity resulted in erratic atrial pacing (suspicious for fracture of ventricular lead). (From Lynn-McHale Wiegand DJ, editor: *AACN procedure manual for critical care,* ed 6, Philadelphia, 2011, Saunders.)

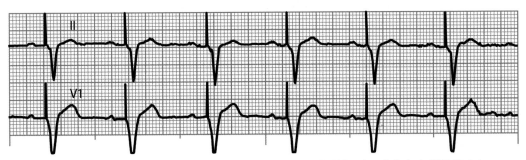

Fig. 8.17 Practice strip, analyzing pacemaker function. (From Aehlert B: *ECG study cards,* St. Louis, 2004, Mosby.)

spikes in Fig. 8.17 occur regularly, we know that failure to pace is not present. When failure to capture occurs, pacer spikes appear regularly but the waveforms after them are periodically absent (i.e., P waves are periodically absent if the pacing electrode is in the atrium, QRS complexes are periodically absent if the pacing electrode is in the ventricle). Because there is a 1:1 relationship between pacemaker spikes and QRS complexes in this rhythm strip, we know that 100% ventricular capture is present. When failure to sense exists, unexpected paced beats or unexpected pacer spikes are present (i.e., undersensing), or prolonged pauses are present (i.e., oversensing). Evaluation of the waveforms and pacer spikes in Fig. 8.17 reveals that there are no unexpected beats, there are no unexpected pacer spikes, and there are no prolonged pauses; thus, failure to sense is not present.

Before we complete our interpretation, we should briefly discuss what looks like ST-segment elevation in this rhythm strip. The QRS complexes are negatively deflected (i.e., a QS configuration), and the ST segments and T waves are in the opposite direction of the last portion of the QRS complex. As you have learned, these findings are common in ventricular rhythms and in left bundle branch block (LBBB). A ventricular paced beat can be thought of as a manmade LBBB. Consider that when LBBB occurs,

the electrical impulse travels down the right bundle branch and depolarizes the right ventricle, and the impulse spreads through the myocardium to depolarize the left ventricle. Pacemakers are most often introduced into the right ventricle. When a pacemaker fires, it sends its impulse into the right ventricle, which depolarizes, and the impulse is spread through the myocardium to depolarize the left ventricle. Therefore, just as with LBBB, ventricular paced rhythms may exhibit ST-segment elevation that is not the result of any infarct-related causes because ventricular depolarization is abnormal.

 ECG Pearl

Careful correlation of the patient's ECG, his or her clinical presentation, and the results of other diagnostic studies is essential.

In summary, we will identify the rhythm strip in Fig. 8.17 as a sinus rhythm with a ventricular pacemaker and 100% capture and a paced interval of 65 pulses/min. If the patient's intrinsic rate were different from that of the pacemaker, we would include the paced rate in pulses per minute and the patient's heart rate in beats per minute in our rhythm description.

STOP & REVIEW

Matching

Match the terms below with their descriptions by placing the letter of each correct answer in the space provided.

a. AV interval
b. Oversensing
c. Dual chamber
d. Inhibition
e. Demand
f. Failure to capture
g. Base rate
h. Pacemaker spike

i. Failure to pace
j. Rate modulation
k. Pulse generator
l. Undersensing
m. Threshold
n. Paced interval
o. Fixed rate

_____ 1. A vertical line on the ECG that indicates the pacemaker has discharged
_____ 2. A pacemaker malfunction that occurs when the artificial pacemaker fails to recognize spontaneous myocardial depolarization
_____ 3. A pacemaker malfunction that occurs when the artificial pacemaker stimulus is unable to depolarize the myocardium
_____ 4. The period between two consecutive paced events in the same cardiac chamber
_____ 5. This type of pacemaker stimulates the atrium and ventricle
_____ 6. In dual-chamber pacing, the length of time between an atrial sensed or atrial paced event and the delivery of a ventricular pacing stimulus; an artificial or electronic PR interval
_____ 7. This type of pacemaker discharges only when the patient's heart rate drops below the preset rate for the pacemaker
_____ 8. Ability of a pacemaker to increase the pacing rate in response to physical activity or metabolic demand
_____ 9. This type of pacemaker continuously discharges at a preset rate regardless of the patient's intrinsic activity
_____ 10. A pacemaker malfunction that results from inappropriate sensing of extraneous electrical signals
_____ 11. Power source that houses the battery and circuitry for regulating a pacemaker
_____ 12. The rate at which the pacemaker's pulse generator initiates impulses when no intrinsic activity is detected; expressed in pulses per minute
_____ 13. The minimum amount of voltage (i.e., milliamperes) needed to obtain consistent capture
_____ 14. Pacemaker response in which the output pulse is suppressed when an intrinsic event is sensed
_____ 15. A pacemaker malfunction that occurs when the pacemaker fails to deliver an electrical stimulus at its programmed time

Pacemaker Rhythms—Practice Rhythm Strips

For each of the following rhythm strips, identify the patient's underlying rhythm (if possible); determine the presence of atrial paced activity, ventricular paced activity, or both; and then analyze the rhythm strip for pacemaker malfunction. All rhythm strips were recorded in lead II unless otherwise noted.

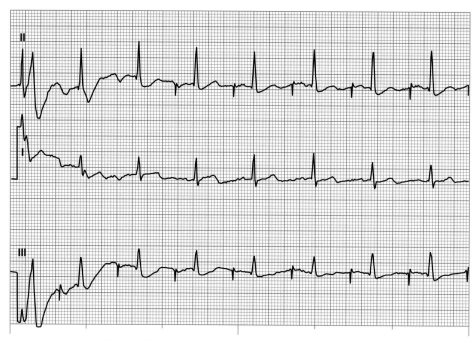

Fig. 8.18   (From Aehlert B: *ECG study cards,* St. Louis, 2004, Mosby.)

16. **Fig. 8.18**. These rhythm strips are from a 52-year-old man with syncope.

Atrial paced activity? _____ Ventricular paced activity? _____

Pacemaker malfunction? _____ Interpretation: _____

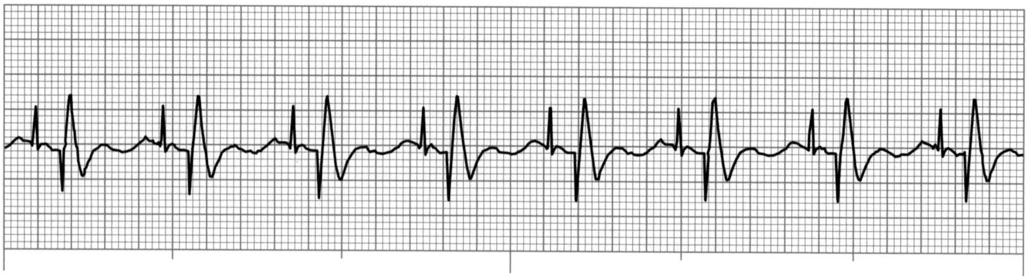

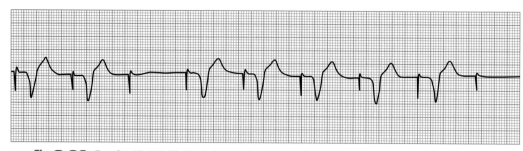

Fig. 8.19   (From Aehlert B: *ECG study cards,* St. Louis, 2004, Mosby.)

17. **Fig. 8.19**

Atrial paced activity? _____ Ventricular paced activity? _____

Pacemaker malfunction? _____ Interpretation: _____

Fig. 8.20   (From Sole ML, Klein DG, Moseley MJ: *Introduction to critical care nursing,* ed 5, Philadelphia, 2008, Saunders.)

18. **Fig. 8.20**

Atrial paced activity? _____ Ventricular paced activity? _____

Pacemaker malfunction? _____ Interpretation: _____

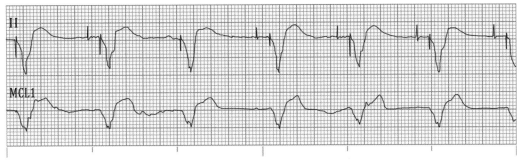

Fig. 8.21 (Modified from Aehlert B: *ECG study cards,* St. Louis, 2004, Mosby.)

19. **Fig. 8.21.** These rhythm strips are from a 63-year-old man complaining of epigastric pain.

    Atrial paced activity? _____ Ventricular paced activity? _____

    Pacemaker malfunction? _____ Interpretation: _____

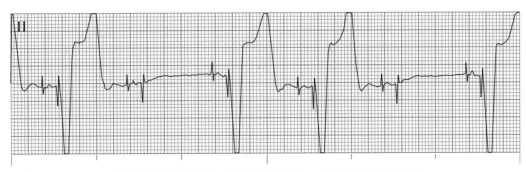

Fig. 8.22 (Modified from Aehlert B: *ECG study cards,* St. Louis, 2004, Mosby.)

20. **Fig. 8.22.** This rhythm strip is from a 97-year-old man with chest pain.

    Atrial paced activity? _____ Ventricular paced activity? _____

    Pacemaker malfunction? _____ Interpretation: _____

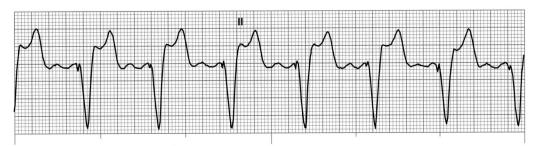

Fig. 8.23 (From Aehlert B: *ECG study cards,* St. Louis, 2004, Mosby.)

21. **Fig. 8.23**

    Atrial paced activity? _____ Ventricular paced activity? _____

    Pacemaker malfunction? _____ Interpretation: _____

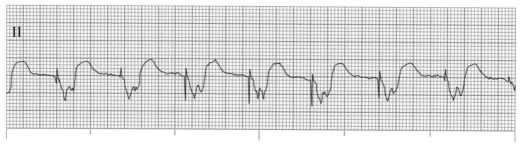

Fig. 8.24 (Modified from Aehlert B: *ECG study cards,* St. Louis, 2004, Mosby.)

22. **Fig. 8.24**

Atrial paced activity? _____ Ventricular paced activity? _____

Pacemaker malfunction? _____ Interpretation: _____

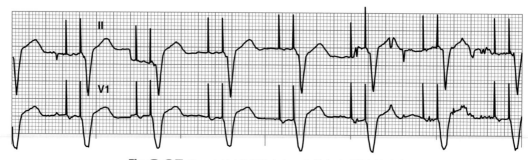

Fig. 8.25 (From Aehlert B: *ECG study cards,* St. Louis, 2004, Mosby.)

23. **Fig. 8.25**

Atrial paced activity? _____ Ventricular paced activity? _____

Pacemaker malfunction? _____ Interpretation: _____

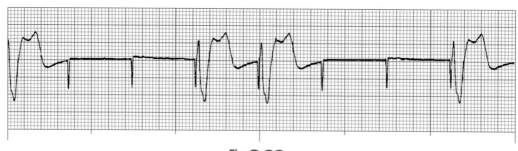

Fig. 8.26

24. **Fig. 8.26**

Atrial paced activity? _____ Ventricular paced activity? _____

Pacemaker malfunction? _____ Interpretation: _____

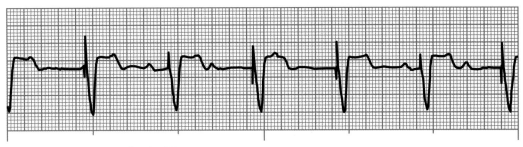

Fig. 8.27 (From Aehlert B: *ECG study cards,* St. Louis, 2004, Mosby.)

25. **Fig. 8.27**. This rhythm strip is from a 90-year-old woman with shortness of breath.

    Atrial paced activity? _____ Ventricular paced activity? _____

    Pacemaker malfunction? _____ Interpretation: _____

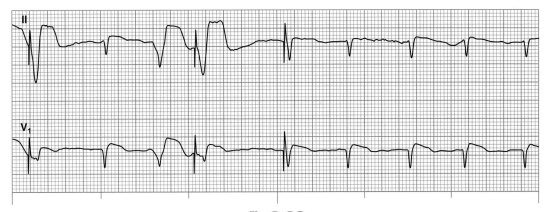

Fig. 8.28

26. **Fig. 8.28**

    Atrial paced activity? _____ Ventricular paced activity? _____

    Pacemaker malfunction? _____ Interpretation: _____

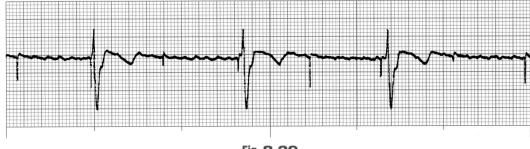

Fig. 8.29

27. **Fig. 8.29**

    Atrial paced activity? _____ Ventricular paced activity? _____

    Pacemaker malfunction? _____ Interpretation: _____

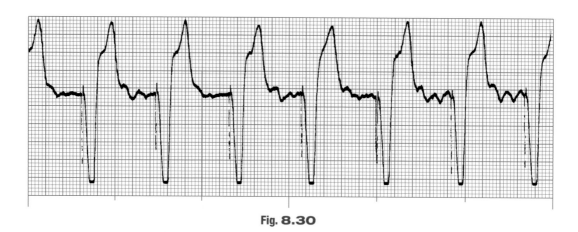

Fig. 8.30

28. **Fig. 8.30**

Atrial paced activity? _____ Ventricular paced activity? _____

Pacemaker malfunction? _____ Interpretation: _____

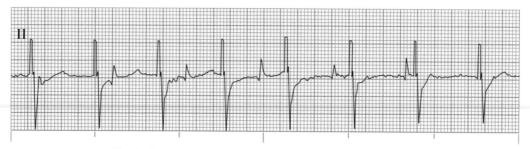

Fig. 8.31 (Modified from Aehlert B: *ECG study cards,* St. Louis, 2004, Mosby.)

29. **Fig. 8.31**. This rhythm strip is from an 80-year-old woman complaining of weakness.

Atrial paced activity? _____ Ventricular paced activity? _____

Pacemaker malfunction? _____ Interpretation: _____

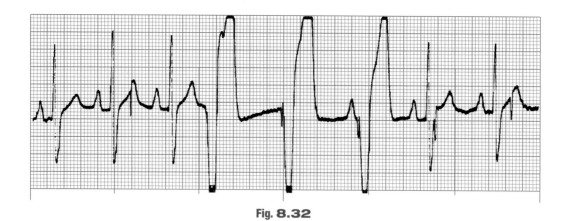

Fig. 8.32

30. **Fig. 8.32**

Atrial paced activity? _____ Ventricular paced activity? _____

Pacemaker malfunction? _____ Interpretation: _____

STOP & REVIEW / ANSWERS

1. H
2. L
3. F
4. N
5. C
6. A
7. E
8. J
9. O
10. B
11. K
12. G
13. M
14. D
15. I

Practice Rhythm Strip Answers

Note: Because of the distortion of ECGs that can occur during printing, a range of acceptable measurements is provided in the rhythm strip answers throughout this textbook.

16. Fig. 8.18

Atrial paced activity?   Yes
Ventricular paced activity?   No
Pacemaker malfunction?   No
Interpretation: Atrial paced rhythm with 100% capture at 79 pulses/min

17. Fig. 8.19

Atrial paced activity?   Yes
Ventricular paced activity?   Yes
Pacemaker malfunction?   No
Interpretation: Dual-chamber pacemaker rhythm with 100% capture at 79 pulses/min

18. Fig. 8.20

Atrial paced activity?   No
Ventricular paced activity?   Yes
Pacemaker malfunction?   Yes—failure to capture; 7 of 9 paced impulses captured
Interpretation: Ventricular paced rhythm at 65 pulses/min with failure to capture

19. Fig. 8.21

Atrial paced activity?   Yes
Ventricular paced activity?   Yes
Pacemaker malfunction?   No
Interpretation: Dual-chamber pacemaker rhythm with 100% capture at 88 pulses/min

20. Fig. 8.22

Atrial paced activity?   Yes
Ventricular paced activity?   Yes
Pacemaker malfunction?   Yes—failure to capture; 4 of 6 paced impulses captured
Interpretation: Dual-chamber pacemaker rhythm at 60 pulses/min with failure to capture

21. Fig. 8.23

Atrial paced activity?   No
Ventricular paced activity?   Yes
Pacemaker malfunction?   No
Interpretation: Ventricular paced rhythm with 100% capture at 68 pulses/min

22. Fig. 8.24

Atrial paced activity?   No
Ventricular paced activity?   Yes
Pacemaker malfunction?   No
Interpretation: Ventricular paced rhythm with 100% capture at 80 pulses/min

23. Fig. 8.25

Atrial paced activity?   Yes
Ventricular paced activity?   Yes
Pacemaker malfunction?   No
Interpretation: Dual-chamber pacemaker rhythm with 100% capture at 71 pulses/min

24. Fig. 8.26

Atrial paced activity?   No
Ventricular paced activity?   Yes
Pacemaker malfunction?   Yes—failure to capture; 3 of 7 paced impulses captured (the first complex is not counted because the pacer spike before the complex is not visible)
Interpretation: Ventricular paced rhythm at 79 pulses/min with failure to capture

25. Fig. 8.27

Atrial paced activity?   No
Ventricular paced activity?   Yes
Pacemaker malfunction?   No
Interpretation: Ventricular-paced rhythm with 100% capture at 60 pulses/min; underlying rhythm appears to be a third-degree AV block

26. Fig. 8.28

Atrial paced activity?   No
Ventricular paced activity?   Yes
Pacemaker malfunction?   No
Interpretation: Ventricular demand pacemaker at 60 pulses/min; underlying rhythm appears to be atrial fibrillation

27. Fig. 8.29

Atrial paced activity?   No
Ventricular paced activity?   Yes
Pacemaker malfunction?   Yes—failure to capture; 3 of 8 paced impulses captured
Interpretation: Ventricular demand pacemaker rhythm at 72 pulses/min with failure to capture

28. Fig. 8.30

Atrial paced activity?   No

Ventricular paced activity?   Yes

Pacemaker malfunction?   No

Interpretation: Ventricular paced rhythm with 100% capture at 74 pulses/min; underlying rhythm appears to be atrial flutter

29. Fig. 8.31

Atrial paced activity?   No

Ventricular paced activity?   Yes

Pacemaker malfunction?   No

Interpretation: Ventricular paced rhythm with 100% capture at 83 pulses/min

30. Fig. 8.32

Atrial paced activity?   No

Ventricular paced activity?   Yes

Pacemaker malfunction?   Yes—failure to sense (undersensing)

Interpretation: Sinus rhythm at 88 beats/min with a ventricular pacemaker and pacemaker malfunction (undersensing); note the pacer spikes in the T waves of the second and eighth beats from the left

REFERENCES

Bernstein, A. D., Daubert, J. C., Fletcher, R. D., Hayes, D. L., Lüderitz, B., Reynolds, D. W., & Sutton, R. (2002). The revised NASPE/BPEG generic code for antibradycardia, adaptive-rate, and multisite pacing. North American Society of Pacing and Electrophysiology/British Pacing and Electrophysiology Group. *Pacing Clin Electrophysiol, 25*(2), 260–264.

Introduction to the 12-Lead ECG

9

LEARNING OBJECTIVES

After reading this chapter, you should be able to:

1. Give examples of indications for using a 12-lead electrocardiogram (ECG).
2. Explain the term *electrical axis* and its significance.
3. Discuss the determination of electrical axis using leads I and aVF.
4. Recognize the changes on the ECG that may reflect evidence of myocardial ischemia, injury, or infarction.
5. Describe the appearance of right and left bundle branch block as seen in lead V_1.
6. Discuss the ECG changes that are characteristic of right atrial, left atrial, right ventricular, and left ventricular enlargement.
7. Identify the ECG changes characteristically produced by hyperkalemia, hypokalemia, hypercalcemia, and hypocalcemia.
8. Describe a systematic method for analyzing a 12-lead ECG.

KEY TERMS

bundle branch block (BBB): A disruption in impulse conduction from the bundle of His through the right or left bundle branch to the Purkinje fibers; a BBB may be intermittent or permanent

electrical axis: Net direction, or angle in degrees, in which the main vector of depolarization is pointed

vector: Quantity having direction and magnitude, usually depicted by a straight arrow whose length represents magnitude and whose head represents direction

INTRODUCTION

[Objective 1]

A standard 12-lead electrocardiogram (ECG) provides views of the heart in both the frontal and horizontal planes and views the surfaces of the left ventricle from 12 different angles. Multiple views of the heart can provide useful information including the following:

- Identification of ST-segment and T-wave changes associated with myocardial ischemia, injury, and infarction
- Identification of ECG changes associated with certain medications and electrolyte imbalances
- Recognition of bundle branch blocks (BBBs)

Indications for using a 12-lead ECG are shown in Box 9.1.

Box 9.1	Indications for Obtaining a 12-Lead ECG
<ul><li>Abdominal or epigastric pain</li><li>Assisting in dysrhythmia interpretation</li><li>Chest pain or discomfort</li><li>Diabetic ketoacidosis</li><li>Dizziness</li><li>Dyspnea</li><li>Electrical injuries</li><li>Known or suspected electrolyte imbalances</li></ul>	<ul><li>Known or suspected medication overdoses</li><li>Right or left ventricular failure</li><li>Status before and after electrical therapy (e.g., defibrillation, cardioversion, pacing)</li><li>Stroke</li><li>Syncope or near syncope</li><li>Unstable patient, unknown etiology</li></ul>

LAYOUT OF THE 12-LEAD ELECTROCARDIOGRAM

Most 12-lead monitors record all 12 leads simultaneously but display them in a conventional three-row by four-column format. The standard limb leads are recorded in the first column, the augmented limb leads in the second column, and the chest leads in the third and fourth columns (Table 9.1).

The 12-lead ECG provides a 2.5-second view of each lead because it is assumed that 2.5 seconds is long enough to capture at least one representative complex. Although most 12-lead ECG machines obtain the signals for all leads at the same time, other machines obtain the signals sequentially (i.e., all limb leads, then the augmented limb leads followed by leads V_1 through V_3 and finally leads V_4 through V_6). The 12-lead computer's interpretive program provides measurements of intervals and duration in milliseconds (msec). Seconds can be easily converted to milliseconds by moving the decimal point three places to the right. An example of a 12-lead ECG is shown in Fig. 9.1.

VECTORS

[Objective 2]

Leads have a negative (−) and positive (+) electrode pole that senses the magnitude and direction of the electrical force caused by the spread of waves of depolarization and repolarization throughout the myocardium. A **vector** (arrow) is a symbol representing this force. A vector points in the direction of depolarization. Leads that face the tip or point of a vector record a positive deflection on ECG paper. A *mean vector* identifies the average of depolarization waves in one portion of the heart. The *mean P vector* represents the average magnitude and direction of both right and left atrial

TABLE 9.1	Layout of a Four-Column 12-Lead ECG		
Limb Leads		**Chest Leads**	
Standard Leads	**Augmented Leads**	**V_1 to V_3**	**V_4 to V_6**
Column I	Column II	Column III	Column IV
I: Lateral	aVR: None	V_1: Septum	V_4: Anterior
II: Inferior	aVL: Lateral	V_2: Septum	V_5: Lateral
III: Inferior	aVF: Inferior	V_3: Anterior	V_6: Lateral

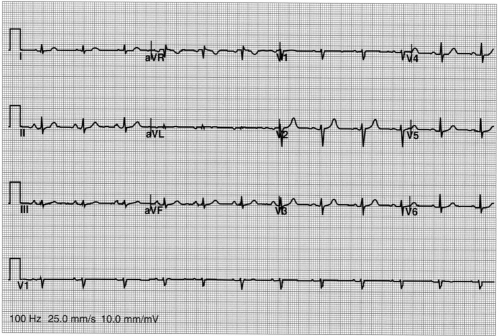

Female   Caucasian

Room:

Loc:

Vent. rate   77 bpm

PR interval   156 ms

QRS duration   80 ms

QT/QTc   356/402 ms

P-R-T axes   73 56 60

Normal sinus rhythm

Normal ECG

100 Hz 25.0 mm/s 10.0 mm/mV

Fig. 9.1 An example of a 12-lead electrocardiogram (ECG). Note the four-column format used on the majority of the page. A continuous recording of lead V_1 is shown at the bottom of the page. (From Phalen T, Aehlert BJ: *The 12-lead ECG in acute coronary syndromes,* ed 3, St. Louis, 2012, Mosby.)

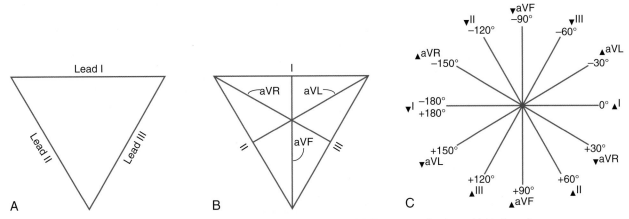

Fig. 9.2 A, Einthoven's equilateral triangle formed by leads I, II, and III. B, The augmented leads are added to the equilateral triangle. C, The hexaxial reference system derived from B. (From Chou T, Ramaiah LS: *Electrocardiography in clinical practice: adult and pediatric,* ed 4, Philadelphia, 1996, Saunders.)

depolarization. The *mean QRS vector* represents the average magnitude and direction of both right and left ventricular depolarization. The average direction of a mean vector is called the *mean axis* and is only identified in the frontal plane. An imaginary line joining the positive and negative electrodes of a lead is called the *axis* of the lead. **Electrical axis** refers to the net direction, or angle in degrees, in which the main vector of depolarization is pointed. When *axis* is used by itself, it refers to the QRS axis.

Axis

[Objectives 2, 3]

During normal ventricular depolarization, the left side of the interventricular septum is stimulated first. The electrical impulse then crosses the septum to stimulate the right side. The left and right ventricles are then depolarized simultaneously. Because the left ventricle is considerably larger than the right, right ventricular depolarization forces are overshadowed on the ECG. As a result, the mean QRS vector points down (i.e., inferior) and to the left.

The axes of leads I, II, and III form an equilateral triangle with the heart at the center (i.e., Einthoven's triangle) (Fig. 9.2, *A*). Einthoven's law states that the sum of the electrical currents recorded in leads I and III equals the sum of the electrical current recorded in lead II. This can be expressed as lead I + lead III = lead II.

If the augmented limb leads are added to the equilateral triangle and the axes of the six leads move in a way in which they bisect each other, the result is the *hexaxial reference system* (Fig. 9.2, *B*). The hexaxial reference system represents all of the frontal plane (limb) leads with the heart in the center and is the means used to express the location of the frontal plane axis. This system forms a 360-degree circle surrounding the heart. The positive end of lead I is designated at 0 degrees. The six frontal plane leads divide the circle into segments, each representing 30 degrees. All degrees

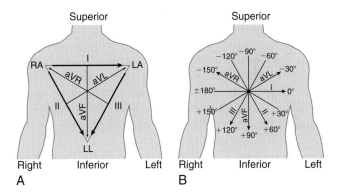

Fig. 9.3 Axis of electrical activation. A, Vectors for the limb leads in the frontal plane. B, Hexaxial reference for determining the frontal plane axis. Note that the vectors for leads I, II, and III are in the same direction as in *A,* but now, similar to the augmented limb leads, these standard limb lead vectors have been moved so that they emanate from the center of the figure. (From Goldman L, Ausiello DA, Arend W, et al: *Cecil medicine,* ed 23, Philadelphia, 2007, Saunders.)

in the upper hemisphere are labeled as negative degrees, and all degrees in the lower hemisphere are labeled as positive degrees (Fig. 9.2, *C*).

In the hexaxial reference system, the axes of some leads are perpendicular to each other. Lead I is perpendicular to lead aVF. Lead II is perpendicular to lead aVL, and lead III is perpendicular to lead aVR. If the electrical force moves toward a positive electrode, a positive (i.e., upright) deflection will be recorded. If the electrical force moves away from a positive electrode, a negative (i.e., downward) deflection will be recorded. If the electrical force is parallel to a given lead, the largest deflection in that lead will be recorded. If the electrical force is perpendicular to a lead axis, the resulting ECG complex will be isoelectric, equiphasic, or both in that lead. Notice that leads III and aVL are positioned on opposite (i.e., reciprocal) sides of the hexaxial reference system (Fig. 9.3). Axis determination can provide clues in the differential diagnosis of wide QRS tachycardia and localization of accessory pathways.

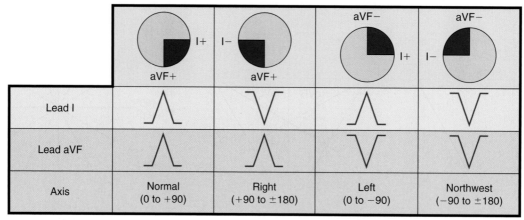

Lead I	∧	∨	⌐∨⌐	∨
Lead aVF	∧	∧	∨	∨
Axis	Normal (0 to +90)	Right (+90 to ±180)	Left (0 to −90)	Northwest (−90 to ±180)

Fig. 9.4 Determination of QRS axis quadrant by noting predominant QRS polarity in leads I and aVF. Normal axis: If the QRS is primarily positive in both I and aVF, the axis falls within the normal quadrant from 0 to 90 degrees. Right axis deviation: If the QRS complex is primarily negative in I and positive in aVF, right axis deviation is present. Left axis deviation: If the QRS complex is predominantly positive in I and negative in aVF, left axis deviation is present. Indeterminate axis: If the QRS is primarily negative in both I and aVF, a markedly abnormal "indeterminate" or "northwest" axis is present. (From Urden LD, Stacy KM, Lough ME: *Critical care nursing,* ed 8, St. Louis, 2018, Mosby.)

To determine electrical axis, look at the 12-lead ECG in Fig. 9.1. Because the hexaxial reference system is derived from the limb leads, we will be focusing on the leads shown in the two columns on the left side of the figure (leads I, II, III, aVR, aVL, and aVF). Look for the most equiphasic or iso-electric QRS complexes in these leads. Lead aVL shows QRS complexes that most closely reflect our criteria. The patient's QRS axis is perpendicular to the positive electrode in lead aVL. Look at the hexaxial reference system diagram (see Fig. 9.3) to determine which ECG lead is perpendicular to lead aVL. Lead II is perpendicular to lead aVL. Now we know that the patient's QRS axis is moving along the same vector as lead II. Note that the values associated with lead II in the hexaxial reference system diagram are −120 degrees and +60 degrees. To determine if the QRS axis is moving in a positive or negative direction, look at lead II in Fig. 9.1 and determine if the QRS complex is primarily positive or negative in this lead. You will see that the QRS is primarily positive in lead II; therefore, this patient's QRS axis is approximately +60 degrees. At the top of Fig. 9.1, you will see the computer's calculation of the patient's P-QRS-T axes. The computer calculated the patient's QRS axis at +56 degrees. Our estimate of +60 degrees was very close!

In adults, the normal QRS axis is considered to be between −30 and +90 degrees in the frontal plane. Current flow to the right of normal is called *right axis deviation* (between +90 and ±180 degrees). Current flow in the direction opposite of normal is called *indeterminate,* "no man's land," *northwest,* or *extreme right axis deviation* (between −90 and ±180 degrees). Current flow to the left of normal is called *left axis deviation* (between −30 and −90 degrees).

Shortcuts exist to determine axis deviation. Leads I and aVF divide the heart into four quadrants. These two leads can be used to quickly estimate electrical axis. In leads I and aVF, the QRS complex is normally positive. If the QRS complex in either or both of these leads is negative, axis deviation is present (Fig. 9.4).

Right axis deviation may be a normal variant, particularly in the young and in thin individuals. Other causes of right axis deviation include mechanical shifts associated with inspiration or emphysema, right ventricular hypertrophy, chronic obstructive pulmonary disease, Wolff-Parkinson-White syndrome, and pulmonary embolism.

Left axis deviation may be a normal variant, particularly in older and obese individuals. Other causes of left axis deviation include mechanical shifts associated with expiration; a high diaphragm caused by pregnancy, ascites, or abdominal tumors; hyperkalemia; emphysema; left atrial hypertrophy; and dextrocardia.

ACUTE CORONARY SYNDROMES

[Objective 4]

You will recall from Chapter 1 that acute coronary syndromes (ACSs) are conditions that are caused by an abrupt reduction in coronary artery blood flow. Partial or intermittent blockage of a coronary artery may result in no clinical signs and symptoms (silent ischemia), unstable angina (UA), non–ST-elevation MI (NSTEMI), or, possibly, sudden death. Complete blockage of a coronary artery may result in ST-elevation MI (STEMI) or sudden death. UA and NSTEMI are often grouped together as *non–ST-elevation acute coronary syndromes* (NSTE-ACS) because ECG changes associated with these conditions usually include ST-segment depression and T-wave inversion in the leads that face the affected area. Cardiac biomarkers (e.g., troponins) are elevated when an infarction is present. Biomarkers are not elevated in patients with UA because there is no tissue death.

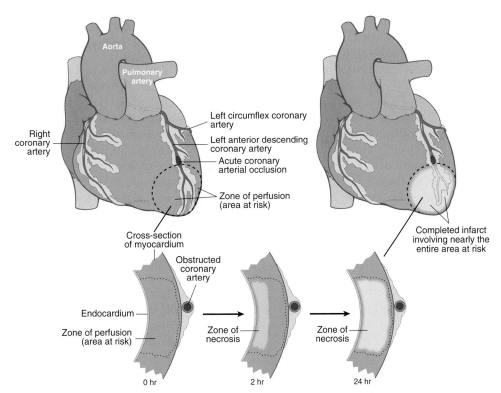

Fig. 9.5 Progression of a myocardial infarction. (From Kumar V, Abbas AK, Aster JC: *Robbins basic pathology,* ed 9, Philadelphia, 2013, Saunders.)

The diagnosis of an ACS is made on the basis of the patient's clinical presentation, history, ECG findings, and cardiac biomarker results. If ST segments are elevated in two contiguous leads and elevated cardiac biomarkers are present, the diagnosis is STEMI. If ST-segment elevation (STE) is not present but biomarker levels are elevated, the diagnosis is NSTEMI. If the ST segments are not elevated and cardiac biomarkers are not elevated, the diagnosis is UA (Thygesen et al, 2012).

In caring for any patient with an ACS, time is muscle. The region of the heart supplied by the blocked artery is called the *area at risk* (Fig. 9.5). The longer the area at risk is deprived of oxygen and nutrients, the greater the likelihood of permanent damage. Therefore, if myocardium is to be saved, the blockage must be removed before irreversible tissue death occurs. If blood flow is quickly restored, the area at risk can potentially be salvaged. Of the patients who are experiencing ACSs, those who are experiencing a STEMI are most likely to benefit from reperfusion therapy. The benefits of reperfusion therapy are often time dependent. The primary choices for reperfusion therapy are fibrinolysis and percutaneous coronary intervention (PCI). Fibrinolytics are medications that are administered to break up blood clots. A PCI is a procedure in which a catheter is used to open a coronary artery that has been blocked or narrowed by coronary artery disease.

The area supplied by a blocked coronary artery goes through a sequence of events that have been identified as zones of ischemia, injury, and infarction. Each zone is associated

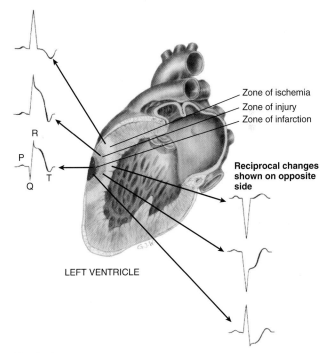

Fig. 9.6 Zones of ischemia, injury, and infarction showing indicative electrocardiogram changes and reciprocal changes corresponding to each zone. (Modified from Urden LD, Stacy KM, Lough ME: *Critical care nursing,* ed 8, St. Louis, 2018, Mosby.)

with characteristic ECG changes that affect the shape of the QRS complex, the ST segment, and the T wave (Fig. 9.6).

Because most infarctions occur in the left ventricle and a standard 12-lead ECG views the surfaces of the left ventricle from multiple angles, obtaining and reviewing a 12-lead

ECG is an important component of the initial care provided to a patient presenting with ischemic chest discomfort. The first 12-lead ECG should be obtained within 10 minutes of patient contact in all patients with symptoms of suspected ACS. Obtain a repeat 12-lead ECG with each set of vital signs, when the patient's symptoms change, and as often as necessary. After the 12-lead ECG has been obtained, carefully review it for signs of ischemia, injury, and infarction. Look closely at each lead for STE or ST-segment depression. If present, compare the ST segment deviation to the isoelectric line using the TP segment for this comparison and document the degree of displacement in millimeters. Examine the T waves for any changes in orientation, shape, and size. Next, look at each lead for the presence of a Q wave. If a Q wave is present, measure its duration.

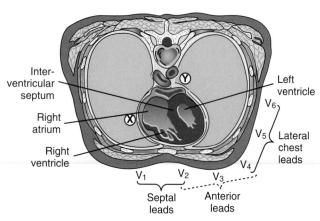

Fig. 9.7 The areas of the heart as seen by the chest leads. Leads V_1, V_2, and V_3 are contiguous. Leads V_3, V_4, and V_5 are contiguous as well as V_4, V_5, and V_6. Note that neither the right ventricular wall *(X)* nor the inferobasal (posterior) surface of the left ventricle *(Y)* is well visualized by any of the usual six chest leads. (From Grauer K: *A practical guide to ECG interpretation,* ed 2, St. Louis, 1998, Mosby.)

Anatomic Location of a Myocardial Infarction

The left ventricle has been divided into regions where a myocardial infarction (MI) may occur: septal, anterior, lateral, inferior, and inferobasal (i.e., posterior). You will recall that ECG changes are considered significant if they are viewed in two or more anatomically contiguous leads (Fig. 9.7). Color has been added to Table 9.2 so you can quickly recognize contiguous lead groups.

In the standard 12-lead ECG, leads II, III, and aVF view the inferior wall of the left ventricle, which is supplied by the right coronary artery (RCA) in most people. If an ECG shows STE in these leads, it is reasonable to suppose that these ECG changes are caused by partial or complete blockage of the RCA (Phalen & Aehlert, 2012a). When indicative changes appear in the leads viewing the septal, anterior, and/or lateral walls of the left ventricle (i.e., V_1 to V_6, I, and aVL), it is reasonable to suspect that the left coronary artery is partially or completely blocked (Phalen & Aehlert, 2012a).

To evaluate the relative extent or size of an infarction, determine how many leads show indicative changes. An ECG showing changes in only a few leads suggests a smaller infarction than one that produces changes in many leads. In general, the more proximal the blockage in the vessel, the larger the infarction and the greater the number of leads showing indicative changes (Phalen & Aehlert, 2012a). Table 9.3 summarizes the pattern in which coronary arteries most commonly supply the myocardium.

CLINICAL CORRELATION

It is important to remember that some areas of the heart are not shown on a standard 12-lead ECG. It is also essential to recall that some infarctions do not show changes on the 12-lead ECG. Therefore, if infarct changes are seen on the 12-lead ECG, the greater the number of leads showing indicative changes, the larger the infarction. But if the patient presents with signs and symptoms suggestive of an ACS and the 12-lead ECG does not show indicative changes, an MI cannot be ruled out based solely on the ECG findings.

TABLE **9.2**	Localizing ECG Changes		
I: Lateral	aVR: None	V_1: Septum	V_4: Anterior
II: Inferior	aVL: Lateral	V_2: Septum	V_5: Lateral
III: Inferior	aVF: Inferior	V_3: Anterior	V_6: Lateral

TABLE **9.3**	Localizing a Myocardial Infarction	
MI Location	**ECG Leads**	**Probable Culprit Coronary Artery**
Anterior wall	Indicative changes: V_3, V_4 Reciprocal changes: III, aVF	LAD
Ventricular septum	Indicative changes: V_1, V_2	LAD
Lateral wall	Indicative changes: I, aVL, V_5, V_6 Reciprocal changes: II, III, aVF (if high lateral MI)	Cx, LAD, or RCA
Inferior wall	Indicative changes: II, III, aVF Reciprocal changes: I, aVL	RCA (most common) or Cx
Inferobasal (posterior) wall	Indicative changes: V_7, V_8, V_9 Reciprocal changes: V_1, V_2, V_3	RCA or Cx
Right ventricle	Indicative changes: V_1R-V_6R Reciprocal changes: I, aVL	RCA

Cx, Circumflex artery; *ECG,* electrocardiogram; *LAD,* left anterior descending artery; *MI,* myocardial infarction; *RCA,* right coronary artery; *STEMI,* ST-elevation myocardial infarction.

It is important to emphasize that the approach discussed here with regard to localization of an infarction (i.e., determining which and how many coronary arteries are affected) works reasonably well for STEMI. However, ST-segment depression and T-wave changes that suggest the presence of myocardial ischemia, as in NSTE-ACS, are less reliable in localizing the culprit vessel because these ECG changes reflect subendocardial rather than transmural ischemia (Halim et al, 2010). Furthermore, recognition of STEMI is often difficult in the presence of right BBBs (RBBBs) and left BBBs (LBBBs), left ventricular hypertrophy, pericarditis, and paced ventricular rhythms because these conditions can cause STE, mimicking STEMI. Factors including the anatomic position and size of the heart, the patient's unique pattern of coronary artery distribution, the location of the occlusion along the length of the coronary artery, the presence of collateral circulation, previous infarctions, and related drug- and electrolyte-related ECG changes may also affect the perceived location of an infarction versus its actual location.

ANTERIOR INFARCTION

[Objective 4]

The left main coronary artery supplies the left anterior descending (LAD) artery and the circumflex (Cx) artery (Fig. 9.8). Blockage of the proximal portion of the LAD artery (i.e., the "widow maker") often leads to cardiogenic shock and death if reperfusion does not occur promptly.

An anterior wall myocardial infarction (AWMI) occurs when the blood supply to the LAD artery is disrupted (Fig. 9.9). Evidence of an AWMI can be seen in leads V_3 and V_4, which face the anterior wall of the left ventricle. Septal involvement is evidenced by changes in leads V_1 and V_2 (Fig. 9.10). If an infarction involves the anterior wall and septum, ECG changes will be visible in V_1, V_2, V_3, and V_4, and the descriptive name *anteroseptal* MI is used (Fig. 9.11).

Because the LAD artery supplies a large portion of the left ventricle, a blockage in this area can lead to more widespread myocardial damage and complications (e.g., heart failure, cardiogenic shock) than infarctions involving other areas of

the heart. Increased sympathetic nervous system activity is common with anterior MIs with resulting sinus tachycardia, hypertension, or both. A blockage in the septal area may result in BBBs, second-degree atrioventricular (AV) block type II, and third-degree AV block. BBBs are discussed later in this chapter.

R-Wave Progression

The wave of ventricular depolarization in the major portions of the ventricles is normally from right to left and in

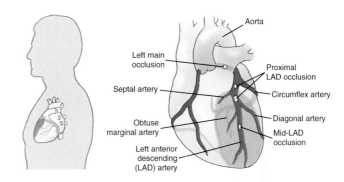

I Lateral	aVR	V₁ Septum	V₄ Anterior
II Inferior	aVL Lateral	V₂ Septum	V₅ Lateral
III Inferior	aVF Inferior	V₃ Anterior	V₆ Lateral

Fig. 9.9 Anterior infarction. Occlusion of the midportion of the left anterior descending (LAD) artery results in an anterior infarction. Proximal occlusion of the LAD may become an anteroseptal infarction if the septal branch is involved or an anterolateral infarction if the marginal branch is involved. If the occlusion occurs proximal to both the septal and diagonal branches, an extensive anterior infarction will result. (From Phalen T, Aehlert BJ: *The 12-lead ECG in acute coronary syndromes,* ed 3, St. Louis, 2012, Mosby.)

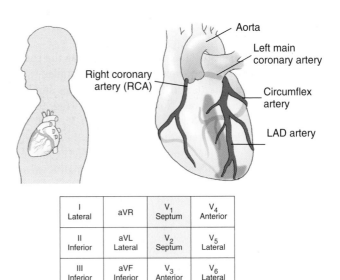

I Lateral	aVR	V₁ Septum	V₄ Anterior
II Inferior	aVL Lateral	V₂ Septum	V₅ Lateral
III Inferior	aVF Inferior	V₃ Anterior	V₆ Lateral

Fig. 9.10 Septal infarction. *LAD,* Left anterior descending. (From Phalen T, Aehlert BJ: *The 12-lead ECG in acute coronary syndromes,* ed 3, St. Louis, 2012, Mosby.)

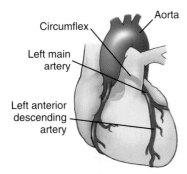

Fig. 9.8 The left main coronary artery supplies the left anterior descending artery and the circumflex artery. (From Phalen T, Aehlert BJ: *The 12-lead ECG in acute coronary syndromes,* ed 3, St. Louis, 2012, Mosby.)

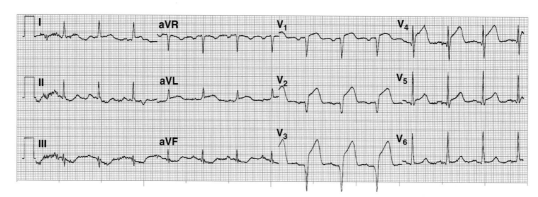

Fig. 9.11 Anteroseptal infarction. Note the ST-segment elevation in leads V_1 through V_4. (From Phalen T, Aehlert BJ: *The 12-lead ECG in acute coronary syndromes,* ed 3, St. Louis, 2012, Mosby.)

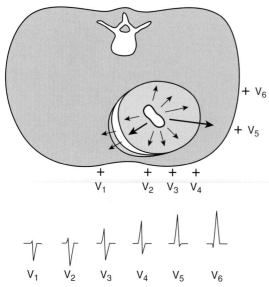

Fig. 9.12 Ventricular activation and R-wave progression as viewed in the chest leads. In normal R-wave progression, the QRS complex is negative in V_1, positive in V_6, and switches from negative to positive in the V_3 to V_4 transition zone. (From Conover MB: *Understanding electrocardiography,* ed 8, St. Louis, 2003, Mosby.)

an anterior to posterior direction. When viewing the chest leads in a normal heart, the R wave becomes taller (i.e., increases in amplitude), and the S wave becomes smaller as the electrode is moved from right to left (Fig. 9.12). This pattern is called *R-wave progression*. In V_1 and V_2, the QRS deflection is predominantly negative (i.e., moving away from the positive chest electrode), reflecting depolarization of the septum and right ventricle (small R wave) and the left ventricle (large S wave). As the chest electrode is placed farther left, the wave of depolarization is moving toward the positive electrode. The *transition zone* is the area at which the amplitude of the R wave begins to exceed the amplitude of the S wave (Ganz, 2012). This usually occurs in the area of leads V_3 and V_4. The phrase *early transition* is used when the transition is seen in V_2. *Late transition* describes a delay in transition until leads V_4 and

V_5. Electrode placement in the correct intercostal space is critical in evaluating R-wave progression.

Poor R-wave progression is a phrase used to describe R waves that decrease in size from V_1 to V_4 (Fig. 9.13). This may be a nonspecific indicator of an anterior wall infarction, but it may be a normal variant in young people, particularly in young women. Other causes of poor R-wave progression include left BBB, right or left ventricular hypertrophy, and severe chronic obstructive pulmonary disease (particularly emphysema).

LATERAL INFARCTION

[Objective 4]

Leads I, aVL, V_5, and V_6 view the lateral wall of the left ventricle. Because the lateral wall of the left ventricle may be supplied by the Cx artery, the LAD artery, or a branch of the RCA, a lateral infarction may be associated with an anterior, inferior, or posterior infarction (Fig. 9.14). An isolated lateral infarction is most commonly associated with a Cx artery occlusion (Brown, 2013). An example of an infarction involving the lateral wall is shown in Fig. 9.15.

INFERIOR INFARCTION

[Objective 4]

Leads II, III, and aVF view the inferior surface of the left ventricle. In most individuals, the inferior wall of the left ventricle is supplied by the posterior descending branch of the RCA (Fig. 9.16). Increased parasympathetic nervous system activity is common with inferior MIs, resulting in bradydysrhythmias. Conduction delays (e.g., first-degree AV block, second-degree AV block type I) are common and are usually transient. An example of an infarction involving the inferior wall is shown in Fig. 9.17.

INFEROBASAL INFARCTION

[Objective 4]

Inferobasal (i.e., posterior) infarctions usually occur in conjunction with an inferior or lateral infarction. The inferobasal

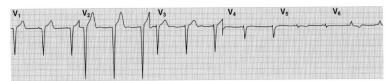

Fig. 9.13 Poor R-wave progression in V_1 through V_4, QRS greater than 0.12 second, and left bundle branch block. (From Khan M: *Rapid ECG interpretation,* Philadelphia, 1997, Saunders.)

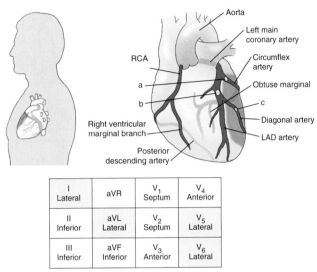

I Lateral	aVR	V_1 Septum	V_4 Anterior
II Inferior	aVL Lateral	V_2 Septum	V_5 Lateral
III Inferior	aVF Inferior	V_3 Anterior	V_6 Lateral

Fig. 9.14 Lateral wall infarction. Coronary artery anatomy shows blockage of the circumflex (Cx) artery (*a*), blockage of the proximal left anterior descending artery (*b*), and blockage of the diagonal artery (*c*). *LAD,* Left anterior descending; *RCA,* right coronary artery. (From Phalen T, Aehlert BJ: *The 12-lead ECG in acute coronary syndromes,* ed 3, St. Louis, 2012, Mosby.)

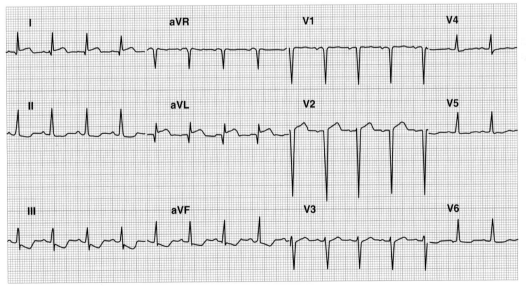

Fig. 9.15 Lateral infarction. Lead I shows a small Q wave with ST-segment elevation (STE). A larger Q wave with STE can be seen in lead aVL. This patient had an anterior non–ST-segment elevation infarction 4 days earlier with STE and T-wave inversion in leads V_2 through V_6. A coronary arteriogram at that time showed a blocked left anterior descending artery distal to its first large septal perforator. The STE evolved and the T waves in all of the chest leads had become upright the day before this tracing was recorded. The patient then had another episode of chest pain associated with the appearance of signs of acute lateral infarction as shown in this tracing. A repeat coronary arteriogram showed new blockage of the obtuse marginal branch of the circumflex (Cx) artery. (From Surawicz B, Knilans TK: *Chou's electrocardiography in clinical practice: adult and pediatric,* ed 5, Philadelphia, 2001, Saunders.)

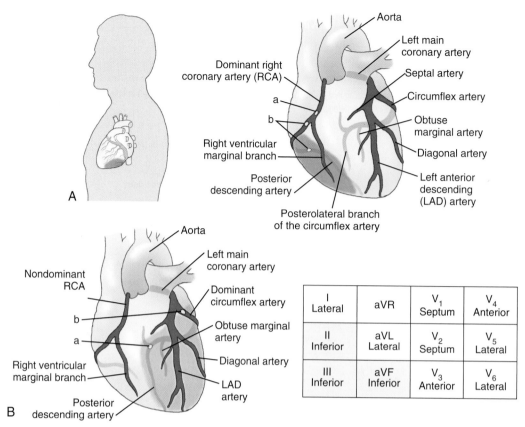

Fig. 9.16 A, Inferior wall infarction. Coronary anatomy shows a dominant right coronary artery (RCA). A blockage at point *a* results in an inferior infarction and right ventricular infarction. A blockage at point *b* involves only the inferior wall, sparing the right ventricle. B, Inferior wall infarction. Coronary anatomy shows a dominant circumflex (Cx) artery. A blockage at point *a* results in an inferior infarction. A blockage at point *b* may result in a lateral and inferobasal infarction. *LAD,* Left anterior descending. (From Phalen T, Aehlert BJ: *The 12-lead ECG in acute coronary syndromes,* ed 3, St. Louis, 2012, Mosby.)

The table within the figure:

I Lateral	aVR	V$_1$ Septum	V$_4$ Anterior
II Inferior	aVL Lateral	V$_2$ Septum	V$_5$ Lateral
III Inferior	aVF Inferior	V$_3$ Anterior	V$_6$ Lateral

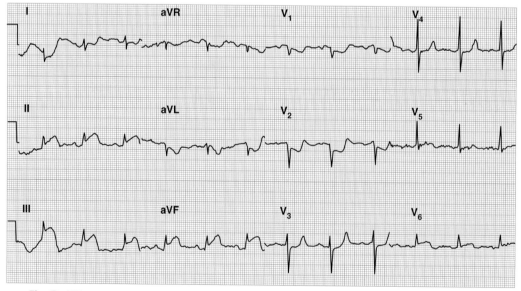

Fig. 9.17 Inferior infarction. Note the ST-segment elevation in leads II, III, and aVF and the reciprocal ST-segment depression in leads I and aVL. (From Goldberger AL: *Clinical electrocardiography: a simplified approach,* ed 7, St. Louis, 2006, Mosby.)

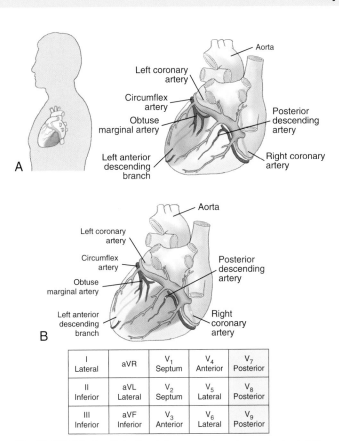

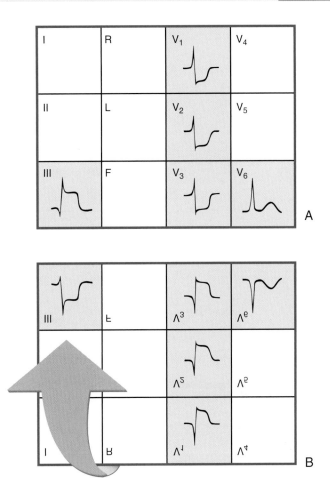

I Lateral	aVR	V$_1$ Septum	V$_4$ Anterior	V$_7$ Posterior
II Inferior	aVL Lateral	V$_2$ Septum	V$_5$ Lateral	V$_8$ Posterior
III Inferior	aVF Inferior	V$_3$ Anterior	V$_6$ Lateral	V$_9$ Posterior

Fig. 9.18 Inferobasal infarction. A, Coronary anatomy shows a dominant right coronary artery (RCA). Occlusion of the RCA commonly results in an inferior and inferobasal infarction. B, Coronary anatomy shows a dominant circumflex artery. Occlusion of a marginal branch is the cause of most isolated inferobasal infarctions. (From Phalen T, Aehlert BJ: *The 12-lead ECG in acute coronary syndromes,* ed 3, St. Louis, 2012, Mosby.)

Fig. 9.19 Application of the mirror test. This test is most helpful in assessing a patient with an acute inferior infarction, in whom you suspect an acute inferobasal infarction. A, Schematic 12-lead ECG with indicative changes of inferior infarction in lead III. Note the tall R wave in lead V$_1$ and the ST-segment depression in leads V$_1$, V$_2$, and V$_3$. B, The tracing in A is now flipped over. Looking through the paper (as it is held up to the light), you now see Q waves and ST-segment elevation in leads V$_1$, V$_2$, and V$_3$. This is a positive mirror test and suggests that the lead changes observed in A may reflect associated acute inferobasal infarction. (From Grauer K: *A practical guide to ECG interpretation,* ed 2, St. Louis, 1998, Mosby.)

wall of the left ventricle is supplied by the Cx artery in most patients; however, in some patients, it is supplied by the RCA (Fig. 9.18). Because no leads of a standard 12-lead ECG directly view the posterior wall of the left ventricle, additional chest leads (V$_7$ to V$_9$) may be used to view the heart's posterior surface. Indicative changes of a posterior wall infarction include STE in these leads. If placement of posterior chest leads is not feasible, the mirror test may be helpful in the recognition of ECG changes suggesting an inferobasal MI (Fig. 9.19).

Complications of a posterior wall MI may include left ventricular dysfunction. If the posterior wall is supplied by the RCA, complications may include dysrhythmias involving the sinoatrial (SA) node, AV node, and bundle of His. An example of an inferobasal MI is shown in Fig. 9.20.

RIGHT VENTRICULAR INFARCTION

[Objective 4]

A right ventricular infarction (RVI) is usually a consequence of RCA occlusion (Fig. 9.21). However, the Cx artery supplies a significant proportion of the right ventricle in about 10% of patients (Hutchinson & Rudakewich, 2009).

Although RVI may occur by itself, it has been estimated that about one third of patients with inferior MI experience an RVI (O'Gara et al, 2013). Right-sided chest leads should be used to evaluate for evidence of RVI in all patients with inferior STEMI, with V$_4$R having the highest sensitivity (Kurz et al, 2014). Because the STE associated with RVI is present for a much shorter period than that of the STE associated with an inferior infarction, it is important to record leads V$_3$R and V$_4$R as soon as possible after the patient's onset of ischemic symptoms (Wagner et al, 2009). An example of an infarction involving the right ventricle is shown in Fig. 9.22. Because patients experiencing an RVI are often preload sensitive, they can develop hypotension of varying degrees in response to medications that reduce preload such as nitrates and diuretics. Other complications associated with RVI include bradycardias, AV blocks, and ventricular dysrhythmias.

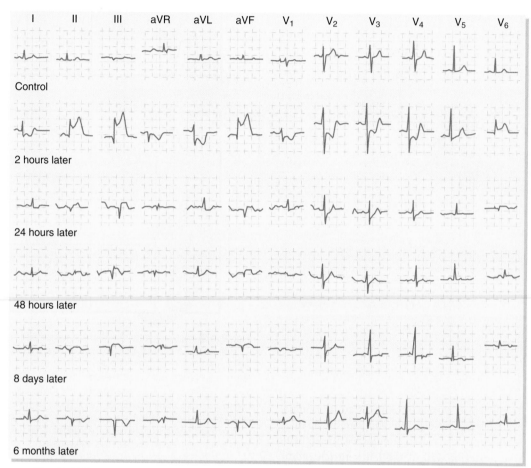

Fig. 9.20 Evolutionary changes in a posteroinferior myocardial infarction (MI). Control tracing is normal. The tracing recorded 2 hours after onset of chest pain demonstrated development of early Q waves; marked ST-segment elevation; and hyperacute T waves in leads II, III, and aVF. In addition, a larger R wave, ST-segment depression, and negative T waves have developed in leads V_1 and V_2. These are early changes indicating acute posteroinferior MI. The 24-hour tracing demonstrates evolutionary changes. In leads II, III, and aVF, the Q wave is larger, the ST segments have almost returned to baseline, and the T wave has begun to invert. In leads V_1 to V_2, the duration of the R wave now exceeds 0.04 second, the ST segment is depressed, and the T wave is upright. (In this example, electrocardiogram [ECG] changes of true posterior involvement extend past lead V_2; ordinarily, only leads V_1 and V_2 may be involved.) Only minor further changes occur through the 8-day tracing. Finally, 6 months later, the ECG illustrates large Q waves, isoelectric ST segments, and inverted T waves in leads II, III, and aVF and large R waves, isoelectric ST segments, and upright T waves in leads V_1 and V_2, indicative of an old posteroinferior MI. (From Andreoli TE, Benjamin I, Griggs RC, et al: *Andreoli and Carpenter's Cecil essentials of medicine,* ed 9, Philadelphia, 2016, Saunders.)

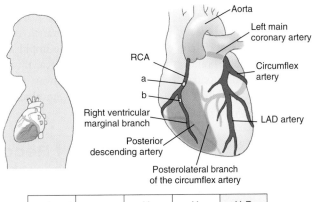

I Lateral	aVR	V$_1$ Septum	V$_4$ Anterior	V$_4$R Rt vent
II Inferior	aVL Lateral	V$_2$ Septum	V$_5$ Lateral	V$_5$R Rt vent
III Inferior	aVF Inferior	V$_3$ Anterior	V$_6$ Lateral	V$_6$R Rt vent

Fig. 9.21 Right ventricular infarction (RVI). At *a*, blockage of the right coronary artery proximal to the right ventricular marginal branch results in an inferior infarction and RVI. At *b*, blockage of the right ventricular marginal branch results in an isolated RVI. *LAD*, Left anterior descending; *RCA*, right coronary artery. (From Phalen T, Aehlert BJ: *The 12-lead ECG in acute coronary syndromes,* ed 3, St. Louis, 2012, Mosby.)

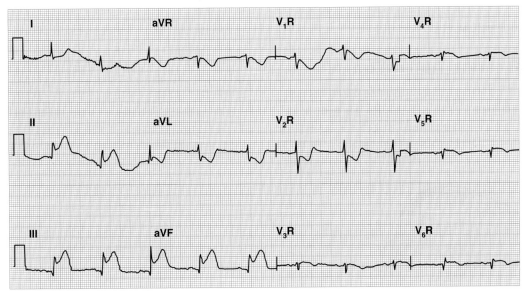

Fig. 9.22 Inferior infarction, right ventricular infarction. (From Goldberger AL: *Clinical electrocardiography: a simplified approach,* ed 7, St. Louis, 2006, Mosby.)

INTRAVENTRICULAR CONDUCTION DELAYS

Structures of the Intraventricular Conduction System

After passing through the AV node, the electrical impulse enters the bundle of His, which is normally the only electrical connection between the atria and the ventricles. The bundle of His conducts the electrical impulse to the right and left bundle branches (Fig. 9.23). A **bundle branch block (BBB)** is a disruption in impulse conduction from the bundle of His through either the right or left bundle branch to the Purkinje fibers. A BBB may be intermittent or permanent, complete or incomplete.

The right bundle branch travels down the right side of the interventricular septum to conduct the electrical impulse to the right ventricle. Structurally, the right bundle branch is long, thin, and more fragile than the left. Because of its structure, a relatively small lesion in the right bundle branch can result in delays or interruptions in electrical impulse transmission.

The left bundle branch begins as a single structure that is short and thick and then divides into two subdivisions that are called the *anterior fascicle* and the *posterior fascicle*. The anterior fascicle spreads the electrical impulse to the anterior portions of the left ventricle. This fascicle is thin and vulnerable to disruptions in electrical impulse transmission. The posterior fascicle relays the impulse to the posterior portions of the left ventricle. It is short, thick, and rarely disrupted because of its structure and dual blood supply from both the LAD artery and the RCA. In some people, a third fascicle, called the *medial fascicle* or *septal fascicle*, emerges from the left bundle itself or its posteroinferior division (Latcu & Nadir, 2010).

Bundle Branch Activation

The wave of normal ventricular depolarization moves from the endocardium to the epicardium. The left side of the interventricular septum, which is stimulated by the left posterior fascicle, is stimulated first. The electrical impulse (i.e., wave of depolarization) then traverses the septum to stimulate the right side. The left and right ventricles are then depolarized at the same time (Fig. 9.24).

A delay or block can occur in any part of the intraventricular conduction system. If a delay or block occurs in one of the bundle branches, the ventricles will not be depolarized at the same time. The electrical impulse travels first down the unblocked branch and stimulates that ventricle. Because of the block, the impulse must then travel from cell to cell through the myocardium, rather than through the normal conduction pathway, to stimulate the other ventricle. The ventricle with the blocked bundle branch is the last to be depolarized.

How Do I Recognize It?

Essentially, two conditions must exist to suspect BBB. First, the QRS complex must have an abnormal duration (i.e., 0.12 second or more in duration if a complete BBB), and second, the QRS complex must arise as the result of supraventricular activity (this excludes paced beats and beats that originate from the ventricles) (Phalen & Aehlert, 2012b). If these two conditions are met, delayed ventricular conduction is assumed to be present, and BBB is the most common (but not the only) cause of this abnormal conduction.

When one of the bundles becomes blocked, the impulse that is normally conducted by that bundle branch is interrupted, and it does not depolarize the intended ventricle. Meanwhile, the other bundle branch is conducting its impulse and depolarizing its respective ventricle. For the second ventricle to depolarize, the electrical impulses must trudge through myocardial cells, which are not specialized for electrical conduction. Thus, the impulses from one ventricle must be transmitted, cell by cell, to the other ventricle. Because the impulses are not traveling down the normal conduction pathway, ventricular depolarization takes longer to occur. This delay is evidenced in the form of a wide QRS complex.

Variation in QRS duration from lead to lead is often seen and may produce confusion about whether the complex is or is not wide. As a rule, use the widest QRS complex to determine width. Try to pinpoint the exact beginning and end of

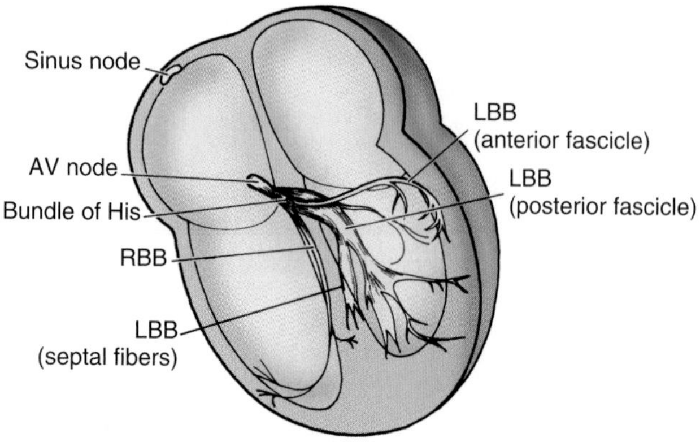

Fig. 9.23 Cardiac conduction system. *AV,* Atrioventricular; *LBB,* left bundle branch; *RBB,* right bundle branch. (From Conover MB: *Understanding electrocardiography,* ed 7, St. Louis, 1995, Mosby.)

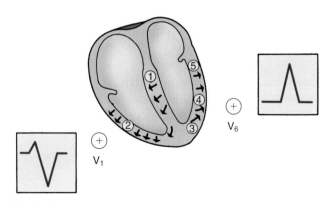

Fig. 9.24 Sequence of normal ventricular depolarization and resulting QRS complex, as seen in leads V₁ and V₆. (From Urden LD, Stacy KM, Lough ME: *Critical care nursing,* ed 8, St. Louis, 2018, Mosby.)

the QRS complex. This can be difficult to do and is sometimes impossible. Therefore, *when measuring for BBB, select the widest QRS complex with a discernible beginning and end.*

The criteria for BBB recognition may be identified in any lead of the ECG. However, in differentiating RBBB from LBBB, pay particular attention to the QRS morphology (i.e., shape) in specific leads. Lead V_1 is probably the single best lead to use in differentiating between RBBB and LBBB.

 Lead In_____

ECG Criteria for Bundle Branch Block

To be considered a BBB, the following ECG criteria must be met:
- QRS duration of 0.12 second or more in adults (if a *complete* RBBB or LBBB); if a BBB pattern is discernible and the QRS duration is between 0.11 and 0.119 second in adults, it is called an *incomplete* right or left BBB (Surawicz et al, 2009). (If the QRS is wide but there is no BBB pattern, the term *wide QRS* or *intraventricular conduction delay* is used to describe the QRS.)
- Visible QRS complexes are produced by supraventricular activity (i.e., the QRS complex is not a paced beat, and it does not originate in the ventricles).

DIFFERENTIATING RIGHT BUNDLE BRANCH BLOCK FROM LEFT BUNDLE BRANCH BLOCK

[Objective 5]

When BBB is suspected, an examination of V_1 can reveal whether the block affects the right or the left bundle branch. Following are descriptions of how each type of block affects the direction of electrical current and produces its own distinct QRS morphology (Phalen & Aehlert, 2012b).

Right Bundle Branch Block

With RBBB, the electrical impulse travels through the AV node and down the left bundle branch into the interventricular septum. The septum is activated by the left posterior fascicle and is depolarized in a left-to-right direction (Fig. 9.25).

Thus, septal depolarization moves in a left-to-right direction, which is toward V_1, and produces an initial small R wave. As the left bundle continues to conduct impulses, the entire left ventricle is depolarized from right to left. This produces movement away from V_1 and results in a negative deflection (i.e., an S wave). Now the impulses that depolarized the left ventricle conduct through the myocardial cells and depolarize the right ventricle. This depolarization creates a movement of electrical activity in the direction of V_1, and so a second positive deflection is recorded (R′). The rSR′ pattern is characteristic of RBBB. The rSR′ pattern is sometimes referred to as an "M" or "rabbit ear" pattern.

Left Bundle Branch Block

With LBBB, the septum is depolarized by the right bundle branch, as is the right ventricle. The septum is part of the left ventricle and is normally depolarized by the left bundle branch. Because the left bundle branch is blocked, depolarization of the septum by the right bundle branch occurs in an abnormal direction (i.e., from right to left); thus, the wave of myocardial depolarization begins with the net movement of current going away from V_1 and is recorded as an initial negative deflection (Fig. 9.26). The right ventricle is depolarized next. Because the wave of depolarization moves briefly toward the positive electrode in lead V_1, a small upright notch in the QRS complex is seen on the ECG. As the remainder of the left ventricle is depolarized, the QRS complex is inscribed in lead V_1 as a deep, negative deflection (i.e., an S wave), which is a reflection of the left ventricle's large muscle mass. Sometimes depolarization of the left ventricle overshadows that of the right ventricle on the ECG. When this occurs, a QS deflection is inscribed in lead V_1, and the small upright notch that is usually seen with right ventricular depolarization is absent.

Unfortunately not every BBB presents with a clear pattern as previously described, which makes the differentiation between RBBB and LBBB less clear. Variant patterns of BBB as seen in lead V_1 appear in Fig. 9.27.

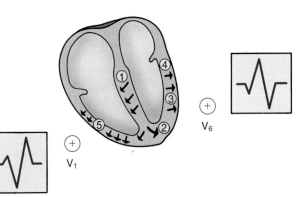

Fig. 9.25 Sequence of ventricular depolarization for a right bundle branch block and resulting QRS complex, as seen in leads V_1 and V_6. (From Urden LD, Stacy KM, Lough ME: *Critical care nursing*, ed 8, St. Louis, 2018, Mosby.)

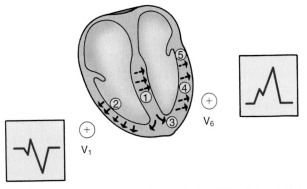

Fig. 9.26 Sequence of ventricular depolarization for a left bundle branch block and resulting QRS complex, as seen in leads V_1 and V_6. (From Urden LD, Stacy KM, Lough ME: *Critical care nursing*, ed 8, St. Louis, 2018, Mosby.)

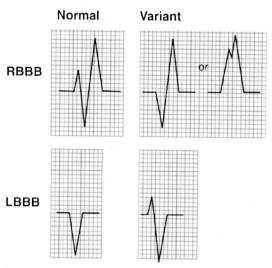

Fig. 9.27 Variant patterns of bundle branch block as seen in lead V₁. *LBBB,* Left bundle branch block; *RBBB,* right bundle branch block. (From Phalen T, Aehlert BJ: *The 12-lead ECG in acute coronary syndromes,* ed 3, St. Louis, 2012, Mosby.)

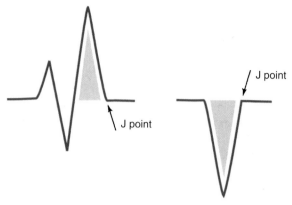

Fig. 9.28 Determining the direction of the terminal force. In lead V₁, move from the J point into the QRS complex and determine whether the terminal portion (last 0.04 second) of the QRS complex is a positive (upright) or negative (downward) deflection. (From Phalen T, Aehlert BJ: *The 12-lead ECG in acute coronary syndromes,* ed 3, St. Louis, 2012, Mosby.)

An Easier Way

Remember that in the setting of BBB, the ventricles are not depolarized in their normal simultaneous manner. Instead, they are depolarized sequentially. The last ventricle to be depolarized is, of course, the ventricle with the blocked bundle branch. Therefore, if it is possible to determine which ventricle was depolarized last, it becomes possible to determine which bundle branch was blocked. For example, if the right ventricle was depolarized last, it is because the impulse traveled down the left bundle branch, depolarized the left ventricle first, and then marched through and depolarized the right ventricle. It stands to reason that if one ventricle is depolarized late, its depolarization makes up the later portion of the QRS complex.

The final portion of the QRS complex is referred to as the *terminal force.* Examination of the terminal force of the QRS complex reveals the ventricle that was depolarized last and therefore the bundle that was blocked. To identify the terminal force, first locate the J point. From the J point, move backward into the QRS and determine if the last electrical activity produced an upward or downward deflection. An example of the terminal force in both RBBB and LBBB is illustrated in Fig. 9.28. If the right bundle branch is blocked, then the right ventricle will be depolarized last, and the current will be moving from the left ventricle to the right. This will create a positive deflection of the terminal force of the QRS complex in V₁. If the left bundle branch is blocked, the left ventricle will be depolarized last, and the current will flow from right to left. This will produce a negative deflection of the terminal force of the QRS complex seen in V₁. Therefore, to differentiate RBBB from LBBB, look at V₁ and determine whether the terminal force of the QRS complex is a positive or negative deflection. If it is directed upward, an RBBB is present (i.e., the current is moving toward the

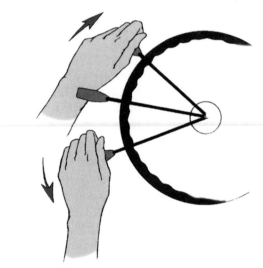

Fig. 9.29 Differentiating between right and left bundle branch blocks. The "turn signal" theory is that right is up and left is down. (From Phalen T, Aehlert BJ: *The 12-lead ECG in acute coronary syndromes,* ed 3, St. Louis, 2012, Mosby.)

right ventricle and toward V₁). An LBBB is present when the terminal force of the QRS complex is directed downward (i.e., the current is moving away from V₁ and toward the left ventricle). This rule is especially helpful when rSR′ and QS variants are present.

A simple way to remember this rule has been suggested by Mike Taigman and Syd Canan and is demonstrated in Fig. 9.29. They recognized the similarity between this rule and the turn signal on a car. To indicate a right turn, you lift up the arm of the turn signal. Likewise, when an RBBB is present, the terminal force of the QRS complex points up. Conversely, left turns and LBBB move downward.

EXCEPTIONS

Two notable exceptions must be mentioned to complete the discussion of BBB. The first involves the criteria used to recognize BBB, and the second relates to differentiating LBBB from RBBB.

The criteria used to recognize BBB are valid but lack some sensitivity and specificity. The sensitivity can be limited by junctional rhythms because there may be no discernible P waves when the AV junction is the pacemaker site. The AV junction is a supraventricular pacemaker, but this presents as an exception to the two-part rule of BBB recognition. Specificity is limited by Wolff-Parkinson-White (WPW) syndrome and other conditions that produce wide QRS complexes resulting from atrial activity. If the characteristic delta wave and shortened PR interval are recognized, WPW syndrome should be suspected.

As for differentiating LBBB from RBBB, a third category exists: nonspecific intraventricular conduction delay (NSIVCD). These blocks do not display the typical V_1 morphologies generally produced by BBB. Their origin may not be the result of a complete BBB but are often the result of several factors, of which incomplete BBB may be one. Atypical patterns of BBB can be attributed to NSIVCD.

What Causes It?

Right BBB can occur in individuals with no underlying heart disease, but it occurs more commonly in the presence of organic heart disease, with coronary artery disease being the most common cause. Acute RBBB may occur secondary to an RVI. LBBB may be acute or chronic. Acute LBBB may occur secondary to an anteroseptal (more common) or inferior MI, acute heart failure, and acute pericarditis or myocarditis, among other causes.

Other causes of BBBs include aortic valve disease; congenital, hypertensive, and rheumatic heart disease; and trauma (e.g., cardiac surgery). Sometimes the ECG will show occasional QRS complexes that have a RBBB or LBBB morphology interspersed with normal QRS complexes. When the intermittent BBB is related to the patient's heart rate, it is referred to as a *rate-related BBB* (i.e., the R-R intervals of the QRS complexes that show BBB are shorter when compared with the R-R intervals of the normal QRS complexes) (Litwin, 2010). Nonischemic diseases are also capable of producing a BBB.

What Do I Do About It?

Because the LAD artery supplies much of the bundle branches, patients experiencing septal and anteroseptal infarctions are most likely to develop BBB. Of course, an infarcting patient presenting with BBB may have had it as a preexisting condition. Unless a previous ECG is available for comparison or the BBB develops during the infarction, it can be difficult to determine which came first, the infarction or the BBB. BBB in the setting of infarction also identifies patients with a higher likelihood of developing third-degree AV block. Another significant aspect of BBB is its ability to mimic the infarct pattern on the ECG. For the patient who is experiencing chest discomfort, the presence of LBBB can complicate the diagnosis of an acute MI because LBBB can produce STE and wide Q waves that look remarkably similar to infarction. Close ECG monitoring and frequent patient reassessment are essential.

 CLINICAL CORRELATION

When BBB is present, STE is often seen in leads with negatively deflected QRS complexes. RBBB rarely produces STE because most of the leads remain positively deflected. Occasionally, when the inferior leads (II, III, and aVF) happen to be negatively deflected, an RBBB may produce STE in those leads and may occasionally mimic an inferior wall infarction. Although this combination is possible, LBBB is by far the more common cause of STE.

The presence of a BBB in an asymptomatic patient requires no specific treatment. RBBB generally requires no specific treatment; however, when RBBB occurs in the setting of an acute MI, close ECG monitoring for the development of symptomatic AV conduction system disturbances is essential.

Because of its association with organic heart disease, patients with LBBB should be evaluated for cardiomyopathies, coronary disease, hypertension, valvular heart disease, and other conditions associated with LBBB. Insertion of a permanent pacemaker is generally required for patients with LBBB who develop second-degree AV block type II or third-degree AV block.

CHAMBER ENLARGEMENT

[Objective 6]

Cardiomyopathy is a general term that is used to describe different types of heart diseases involving the heart muscle and resulting in abnormal enlargement. *Cardiac enlargement* refers to either dilation of a heart chamber or hypertrophy of the heart muscle (Goldberger et al, 2013). With dilation, stretching of a chamber of the heart muscle occurs, resulting in enlargement of that chamber. Dilation may be acute or chronic. *Cardiac hypertrophy* refers to thickening of the heart muscle, with resultant enlargement of a heart chamber. Hypertrophy is commonly accompanied by dilation. In evaluating the ECG for indications of chamber enlargement, it is particularly important to check the calibration marker to ensure that it is 10 mm (1 mV) tall.

Cardiomyopathies can be classified into three physiologic categories: (1) dilated cardiomyopathy, (2) hypertrophic cardiomyopathy, and (3) restrictive cardiomyopathy (Fig. 9.30). Of these categories, dilated cardiomyopathy is the most common, and restrictive cardiomyopathy is the least common (Kumar et al, 2013).

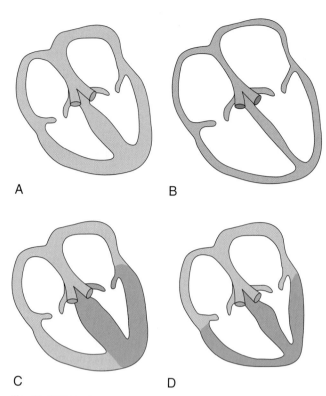

Fig. 9.30 The three types of cardiomyopathy. A, Normal heart. B, Dilated cardiomyopathy demonstrating enlargement of all four chambers. C, Hypertrophic cardiomyopathy showing a thickened left ventricle. D, Restrictive cardiomyopathy characterized by a small left ventricular volume. (From Copstead-Kirkhorn LE, Banasik JL: *Pathophysiology,* ed 5, St. Louis, 2013, Saunders.)

Dilated cardiomyopathy (DCM) is characterized by enlargement of all heart chambers (Otto, 2013) with progressive dilation of both the right and left ventricles that results in impaired contractile (systolic) function, usually with concurrent hypertrophy (Kumar et al, 2013). Patients with DCM usually present with signs and symptoms of heart failure, but atypical presentations do occur.

Hypertrophic cardiomyopathy (HCM) is characterized by significant myocardial hypertrophy without ventricular dilation that results in a markedly reduced stroke volume because of impaired diastolic filling. Most cases of HCM have a genetic origin. Patients with HCM may be asymptomatic or present with atrial and ventricular dysrhythmias, syncope after exercise, palpitations, or symptoms of heart failure and angina or with sudden death with no previous diagnosis (Otto, 2013). When sudden cardiac death occurs in athletes younger than 35 years of age, HCM is the underlying cause in nearly one third of cases (Kumar et al, 2013).

Restrictive cardiomyopathy is characterized by increased ventricular wall stiffness that impedes ventricular filling, reduced diastolic volume of either or both ventricles, and normal or nearly normal systolic function. Although the ventricles are typically of normal size or are only slightly enlarged, dilation of both atria is common because of poor ventricular filling and pressure overload (Kumar et al, 2013). Restrictive cardiomyopathy may be caused by conditions

such as amyloidosis, myocardial fibrosis, or an unknown cause. Patients often present with signs and symptoms that are consistent with progressive left- and right-sided heart failure.

Atrial Abnormalities

The first half of the P wave is recorded when the electrical impulse that originated in the SA node stimulates the right atrium and reaches the AV node. The downslope of the P wave reflects stimulation of the left atrium. The appearance of abnormal P waves on the ECG may be caused by delayed intraatrial conduction, elevated atrial pressure, atrial dilation, and atrial muscular hypertrophy, among other causes. In the past, terms used to describe atrial abnormalities have included *P-mitrale, P-pulmonale, left atrial enlargement, right atrial enlargement, atrial hypertrophy,* and *atrial overload,* among others. Today, experts recommend that the terms *left atrial abnormality* and *right atrial abnormality* be used because a combination of several factors that may not be distinguishable can result in abnormal P waves (Hancock et al, 2009).

You will recall that the normal P wave is the result of atrial depolarization with the initial portion of the P wave representing depolarization of the right atrium and the middle and end portions representing left atrial depolarization. Because these events normally occur nearly at the same time, they fuse into a single, smooth rounded waveform.

Right atrial abnormality (RAA) produces changes in the initial part of the P wave. The P wave is tall (more than 2.5 mm in height), peaked, and usually of normal duration (Hancock et al, 2009) (Fig. 9.31). The abnormal P waves characteristic of RAA are usually best seen in leads II, III, aVF, and sometimes V_1 (Goldberger et al, 2013). Lead V_1 may reveal a biphasic P wave. Examples of conditions that may cause right atrial abnormality include chronic obstructive pulmonary disease with or without pulmonary hypertension, congenital heart disease, and right ventricular failure.

With left atrial abnormality (LAA), the middle and end of the P wave is prolonged because depolarization of the left atrium begins and ends later than right atrial depolarization (Surawicz & Knilans, 2008). Notched P waves are usually visible and correspond with the delay in left atrial activation because the right and left atrial peaks that are normally nearly simultaneous and fused into a single peak become more widely separated (Hancock et al, 2009) (see Fig. 9.31). Notched P waves are generally most easily seen in the limb leads. The P wave may be biphasic in lead V_1 with a small initial positive deflection and a prominent, wide negative deflection (Goldberger et al, 2013). A P wave amplitude of more than 2.5 mm has been observed in about 5% to 10% of patients with LAA resulting from left-sided valvular disease or hypertensive heart disease (Surawicz & Knilans, 2008). Examples of conditions in which LAA may occur include coronary artery disease, cardiomyopathies, hypertensive

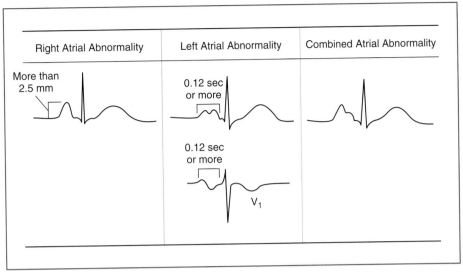

Fig. 9.31 Criteria for atrial abnormalities.

heart disease, and valvular heart disease. When the ECG reflects features of both right atrial and left atrial abnormality, the term *combined atrial abnormality* is used.

Ventricular Abnormalities

With right ventricular hypertrophy (RVH), current travels between hypertrophied cells and moves through the enlarged right ventricle, producing higher-than-normal voltages on the body surface (Mirvis & Goldberger, 2015) (Fig. 9.32). Because the right ventricle is normally considerably smaller than the left, it must become extremely enlarged before changes are visible on the ECG. Characteristic ECG changes associated with RVH include tall R waves in leads V_1 through V_3 and deeper than normal S waves in leads I, aVL, V_5, and V_6. (Litwin, 2010) (Fig. 9.33). Right axis deviation is usually present, and evidence of right atrial abnormality may be seen. Causes of RVH include pulmonary hypertension and chronic pulmonary diseases, valvular heart disease, and congenital heart disease.

Left ventricular hypertrophy (LVH) is recognized on the ECG by increased QRS amplitude and changes in the ST segment and T wave (see Fig. 9.32). Typically, R waves in leads I, aVL, V_5, and V_6 are taller than normal, and S waves in leads V_1 through V_2 are deeper than normal (Mirvis & Goldberger, 2015). The QRS duration is often increased in LVH and may be attributed to the longer time required to activate the thickened wall of the left ventricle (Hancock et al, 2009) and the slower-than-normal conduction within the working myocardium (Mirvis & Goldberger, 2015). Causes of LVH include systemic hypertension, hypertrophic cardiomyopathy, aortic stenosis, and aortic insufficiency. LVH may be accompanied by left axis deviation.

Although several formulas exist to assist in its recognition, the Cornell voltage criterion is often used to check

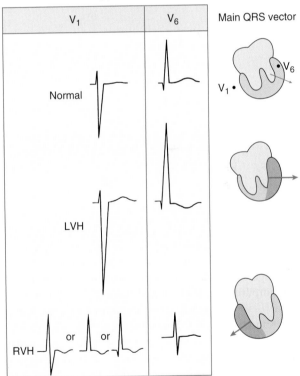

Fig. 9.32 Left ventricular hypertrophy (LVH) increases the amplitude of electrical forces directed to the left and posteriorly. In addition, repolarization abnormalities can cause ST-segment depression and T-wave inversion in leads with a prominent R wave. Right ventricular hypertrophy (RVH) can shift the QRS vector to the right, usually with an R, RS, or qR complex in lead V_1, especially when caused by severe pressure overload. T-wave inversion may be present in the right chest leads. (From Goldberger AL: *Clinical electrocardiography: a simplified approach*, ed 8, Philadelphia, 2013, Saunders.)

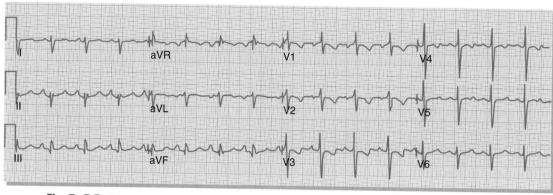

Fig. 9.33 Right ventricular hypertrophy with tall R wave in right chest leads, downsloping ST depression in the chest leads, right axis deviation, and evidence of right atrial enlargement. (From Andreoli TE, Benjamin I, Griggs RC, et al: *Andreoli and Carpenter's Cecil essentials of medicine,* ed 9, Philadelphia, 2016, Saunders.)

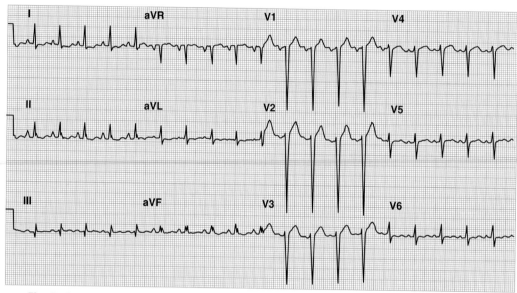

Fig. 9.34 Left ventricular hypertrophy. Note that the ST segment is elevated in leads V_1, V_2, and V_3. (From Phalen T, Aehlert BJ: *The 12-lead ECG in acute coronary syndromes,* ed 3, St. Louis, 2012, Mosby.)

for the presence of LVH. To use this formula, add the S wave amplitude in lead V_3 and the R wave amplitude in lead aVL. A total greater than 20 mm (2 mV) in women and 28 mm or more (2.8 mV) in men suggests that LVH is present (Ganz, 2012). A 12-lead ECG's interpretive algorithm checks for the presence of LVH using preprogrammed criteria, including formulas, to measure voltage. If the 12-lead machine determines that an ECG meets the criteria for LVH, a message is displayed such as "Meets voltage criteria for left ventricular hypertrophy" (Phalen & Aehlert, 2012a).

An example of LVH is shown in Fig. 9.34. Note that the ST segment in Fig. 9.34 is elevated in leads V_1, V_2, and V_3. Also note the ST-segment depression shown in leads V_5 and V_6. Recall that when the QRS complexes of left BBBs, ventricular rhythms, and ventricular paced rhythms are

negatively deflected (i.e., a QS configuration), the ST segments and T waves are in the opposite direction of the last portion of the QRS complex. Similarly, when the QRS complex of LVH is negatively deflected, these ECG findings are shared by LVH, making the identification of ECG changes associated with acute MI difficult. Careful correlation of the patient's ECG, his or her clinical presentation, and the results of other diagnostic studies is essential (Phalen & Aehlert, 2012a).

ELECTROLYTE DISTURBANCES

Because electrolyte imbalances may increase cardiac irritability and cause cardiac dysrhythmias, a patient's ECG can be evaluated for evidence of electrolyte disturbances. It is important to keep in mind that ECG changes associated with electrolyte imbalances can vary widely from patient to patient.

Sodium

Sodium is the most abundant electrolyte in the body and makes up 90% of the positively charged ions (i.e., cations) in the extracellular fluid (Huether, 2012). It is important in maintaining water balance, is necessary for the normal conduction of impulses in nerve and muscle fibers (in conjunction with potassium and calcium), and plays an important role in the voltage of action potentials (Speakman & Weldy, 2002). The diet is the primary source of sodium. In healthy individuals, excess sodium is excreted in the urine.

HYPERNATREMIA

Hypernatremia (sodium excess) may result from the retention of relatively more sodium than water, or it may be caused by a loss of relatively more water than sodium (Felver, 2013). Possible causes of hypernatremia because of the retention of relatively more sodium than water include excess aldosterone secretion, excess secretion of adrenocorticotropic hormone (ACTH), or hypertonic parenteral fluid administration, inadequate fluid intake, or ingestion of abnormal amounts of sodium. Possible causes of hypernatremia because of a loss of relatively more water than sodium include diabetes insipidus, severe watery diarrhea, and severe insensible water losses (e.g., heat stroke, prolonged high fever).

The patient may present with restlessness, irritability, thirst, dry and flushed skin, dry mucous membranes, decreased urine output, seizures, and coma. Hypernatremia does not cause any significant changes on the ECG.

HYPONATREMIA

Hyponatremia (sodium deficit) may result from an inadequate intake of sodium, from dilution of sodium by water excess, or when there is loss of sodium (Huether, 2012). Hyponatremia alters the action potential in neurons and muscle because of changes in the cell's ability to depolarize and repolarize (Huether, 2012). Possible causes of hyponatremia include inadequate sodium intake, prolonged diuretic therapy, excessive diaphoresis, excessive loss of sodium from trauma (e.g., burns), adrenal insufficiency, renal disease, severe gastrointestinal (GI) fluid losses from gastric suctioning or lavage, and prolonged vomiting or diarrhea. Some medications, such as morphine and barbiturates, may impair water excretion and contribute to hyponatremia (Speakman & Weldy, 2002).

The patient may present with irritability, fatigue, headache, nausea and vomiting, abdominal cramps, and muscle weakness. Hyponatremia does not cause any significant changes on the ECG.

Box 9.2	ECG Signs of Hyperkalemia

- Tall, peaked (tented), narrow, symmetric T waves
- QRS duration increases as potassium level increases
- P waves decrease in amplitude as potassium level increases
- PR interval duration increases as potassium level increases

Potassium

Potassium is the primary intracellular fluid cation. It is important for many cell functions, including cardiac and neuromuscular activity, resting membrane potential, growth, and regulation of the fluid volume and pH within the cell (Stanton & Koeppen, 2010).

HYPERKALEMIA

[Objective 7]

Hyperkalemia (potassium excess) may occur because of acute or chronic renal failure, excessive administration of intravenous (IV) potassium, metabolic acidosis, ingestion of excessive amounts of salt substitutes, medications (e.g., spironolactone, angiotensin-converting enzyme inhibitors, nonsteroidal antiinflammatory drugs), or widespread cell damage (e.g., crush injuries, burns). The patient may present with anxiety, restlessness, cardiac dysrhythmias, skeletal muscle weakness, abdominal muscle cramping, and diarrhea.

The effects of hyperkalemia depend on the tissue involved, with the atrial myocardium being the most sensitive, the ventricular myocardium less sensitive, and the SA node and bundle of His the least sensitive (El-Sherif et al, 2012). When the potassium level exceeds 5.5 mEq/L, tall, peaked T waves may be seen on the ECG (Box 9.2). However, 50% of patients with potassium levels higher than 6.5 mEq/L will not manifest any ECG changes (El-Sherif et al, 2012). As the potassium level rises, PR intervals lengthen and the QRS duration increases, reflecting slowed conduction. When the potassium level nears 10 mEq/L, intraventricular conduction delays and dysrhythmias such as ventricular tachycardia, ventricular fibrillation, and asystole may develop. Examples of the effects of hyperkalemia on the ECG are shown in Fig. 9.35.

HYPOKALEMIA

[Objective 7]

Hypokalemia (potassium deficit) is one of the most common electrolyte disorders (Stanton & Koeppen, 2010). It may occur because of prolonged diuretic therapy with thiazide diuretics or furosemide, an inadequate dietary intake of potassium, administration of potassium-deficient parenteral fluids, starvation, severe GI fluid losses from gastric suctioning or lavage, prolonged vomiting or diarrhea, or laxative use without replacement of potassium. It has been estimated that

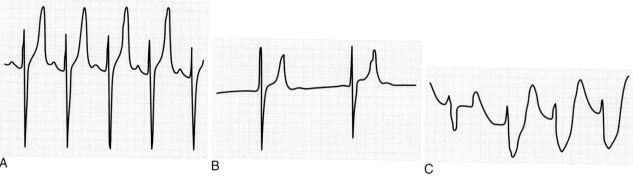

A   B   C

Fig. 9.35 The effects of progressive hyperkalemia on the electrocardiogram. All of the illustrations are from lead V₃. A, Serum potassium concentration (K⁺) was 6.8 mEq/L; note the peaked T waves together with sinus rhythm. B, Serum K⁺ was 8.9 mEq/L; note the peaked T waves and absent P waves. C, Serum K⁺ was greater than 8.9 mEq/L; note the classic sine wave with absent P waves, marked prolongation of the QRS complex, and peaked T waves. (From Goldman L, Schafer AI, *Goldman-Cecil medicine,* ed 25, Philadelphia, 2015, Saunders.)

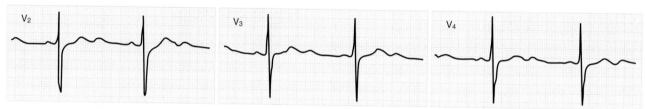

V₂   V₃   V₄

Fig. 9.36 The electrocardiographic manifestations of hypokalemia. The serum potassium concentration was 2.2 mEq/L. The ST segment is prolonged, primarily because of a U wave after the T wave, and the T wave is flattened. (From Goldman L, Schafer AI, *Goldman-Cecil medicine,* ed 25, Philadelphia, 2015, Saunders.)

Box **9.3**	**ECG Signs of Hypokalemia**

- ST-segment depression
- Decrease in T wave amplitude
- Prominent U waves; amplitude of U waves may exceed that of T waves in the same lead with marked hypokalemia
- P wave amplitude and duration are usually increased
- Slight prolongation of PR interval
- Increased QRS duration with severe hypokalemia

as many as 10% to 40% of patients taking thiazide diuretics and almost 50% of patients resuscitated from out-of-hospital ventricular fibrillation have low potassium levels (El-Sherif et al, 2012).

The patient may present with skeletal muscle weakness, fatigue, paresthesias, and cardiac dysrhythmias (e.g., sinus bradycardia, AV blocks). Electrophysiologic effects of hypokalemia include increased automaticity, decreased conduction velocity, shortening of the effective refractory period, and prolongation of the relative refractory period (El-Sherif et al, 2012). Possible ECG manifestations of hypokalemia are shown in Box 9.3 and Fig. 9.36.

Calcium

Calcium is important in bone formation, nerve and muscle function, and blood clotting.

HYPERCALCEMIA

[Objective 7]

Causes of hypercalcemia (calcium excess) include chronic and acute renal failure, excessive vitamin D or vitamin A intake, hyperthyroidism, hyperparathyroidism, adrenal insufficiency, cancer (e.g., breast, ovarian, multiple myeloma), excessive use of calcium-containing antacids, and an excessive intake of calcium supplements.

The patient may present with nausea, vomiting, acute mental status changes ranging from mild confusion to coma, skeletal muscle weakness, constipation, and cardiac dysrhythmias. ECG changes associated with hypercalcemia appear in Box 9.4.

Box **9.4**	**ECG Signs of Hypercalcemia**

- Shortening of the ST segment
- Decreased QT interval duration

HYPOCALCEMIA

[Objective 7]

Hypocalcemia (calcium deficit) may result from an inadequate intake of calcium or from increased excretion of calcium from the body (Speakman & Weldy, 2002). Possible causes include acute or chronic renal failure, dietary deficiency of calcium and vitamin D, pancreatic disease, malabsorption because of small bowel disease, and hypoparathyroidism.

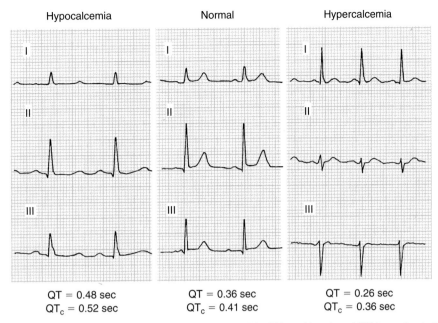

Fig. 9.37 With hypocalcemia, the ST segment is lengthened, and the QT interval is prolonged. With hypercalcemia, the ST segment is shortened, and the duration of the QT interval is decreased. (From Goldberger AL: *Clinical electrocardiography: a simplified approach,* ed 8, Philadelphia, 2013, Saunders.)

The patient may present with irritability and confusion, tingling of the nose, mouth, ears, fingers, or toes; nausea, vomiting, and diarrhea; cardiac dysrhythmias; hyperactive deep tendon reflexes; carpal spasms (Trousseau sign); facial muscle contraction (Chvostek sign); and pathologic fractures. ECG changes associated with hypocalcemia are shown in Box 9.5. Possible ECG manifestations of hypocalcemia and hypercalcemia are shown in Fig. 9.37.

Box 9.5	ECG Signs of Hypocalcemia

- Lengthening of the ST segment
- Increased QT interval duration

Magnesium

Magnesium is important for many biological processes, including enzyme reactions, neuromuscular function (including cardiac muscle contractility), and the production and use of adenosine triphosphate (Speakman & Weldy, 2002).

HYPERMAGNESEMIA

Causes of hypermagnesemia (magnesium excess) include renal failure, excessive use of parenteral magnesium, and excessive use of magnesium-containing antacids or laxatives.

The patient may present with drowsiness, flushing, hypotension, decreased rate and depth of breathing, and diminished deep tendon reflexes. Hypermagnesemia depresses AV and intraventricular conduction (El-Sherif et al, 2012). Hypermagnesemia does not produce significant ECG changes.

HYPOMAGNESEMIA

Hypomagnesemia (magnesium deficit) may occur because of prolonged or excessive diuretic therapy, excessive calcium or vitamin D intake, administration of IV fluids or total parenteral nutrition without magnesium replacement, hypercalcemia, malabsorption associated with disease of the small intestine, malnutrition, and alcoholism.

The patient may present with acute mental status changes, tachycardia, cardiac dysrhythmias, muscle tremors and muscle cramps, and hyperactive deep tendon reflexes. Although hypomagnesemia does not produce significant ECG changes, it has been implicated as a possible cause of torsades de pointes.

ANALYZING THE 12-LEAD ELECTROCARDIOGRAM

[Objective 8]

It is important to use a systematic method when analyzing a 12-lead ECG. Before beginning an in-depth review, take a moment to "take in" the entire 12-lead and get an overall impression of the tracing. Does the rate look as if it is normal, fast, or slow? Do the ST segments look markedly elevated or depressed? Is there evidence of premature beats, pauses, baseline wander, or artifact? If baseline wander or artifact is present to any significant degree, note it. If the presence of either of these conditions interferes with the assessment of any lead, use a modifier such as "possible" or "apparent" in your interpretation. After initially surveying the tracing, consider using the following approach when reviewing a 12-lead ECG:

1. Identify the rate and underlying rhythm. Identify any premature beats and pauses, if present.

2. Using leads I and aVF, determine the QRS axis.

3. Identify and examine waveforms and measure intervals. Before examining waveforms, quickly look at the calibration marker and determine if it is standard, half-standard, or twice the standard. Next, examine each lead, selecting one good representative waveform or complex in each lead. Inspect each waveform, noting any changes in orientation, shape, size, and duration.

4. Examine for evidence of ischemia, injury, and infarction. "**I See All Leads**" is a commonly used mnemonic to recall the lead groupings when localizing an infarction and predicting which coronary artery is occluded. **I** (inferior) = II, III, aVF; **S** (septal) = V_1, V_2; **A** (anterior) = V_3, V_4; **L** (lateral) = I, aVL, V_5, V_6. Look for the presence of ST-segment displacement (i.e., STE or ST-segment depression).

5. Look for evidence of chamber enlargement, look for effects of electrolyte imbalances, and ascertain if conditions that mimic MI are present (e.g., LVH, left BBB, ventricular rhythm, ventricular paced rhythm).

STOP & REVIEW

True/False

Indicate whether the statement is true or false.

_____ 1. In a patient presenting with an acute coronary syndrome, the presence of STE on the ECG suggests that myocardial injury is in progress.

_____ 2. Evidence of sodium disturbances is typically viewed on the ECG as marked increases in the amplitude of P waves and T waves.

_____ 3. An abnormal (i.e., pathologic) Q wave indicates the presence of dead myocardial tissue.

Multiple Choice

Identify the choice that best completes the statement or answers the question.

_____ 4. Although an RVI may occur by itself, it is more commonly associated with a(n) _____ wall MI.
   a. anterior
   b. lateral
   c. septal
   d. inferior

_____ 5. Lead I is perpendicular to lead
   a. II.
   b. III.
   c. aVF.
   d. aVL.

_____ 6. Which of the following are commonly seen ECG changes in hyperkalemia?
   a. Tall, peaked T waves
   b. Shortened PR intervals
   c. Elevated ST segments
   d. Peaked P waves

_____ 7. Patients experiencing _____ infarctions are most likely to develop BBB.
   a. inferior and lateral
   b. anterior and inferobasal
   c. septal and anteroseptal
   d. inferior and septal

_____ 8. When leads I and aVF are used to determine electrical axis, left axis deviation is present if
   a. the QRS is positive in lead I and positive in lead aVF.
   b. the QRS is positive in lead I and negative in lead aVF.
   c. the QRS is negative in lead I and negative in lead aVF.
   d. the QRS is negative in lead I and positive in lead aVF.

_____ 9. Which of the following statements is true regarding ventricular hypertrophy?
   a. Hypertrophy increases the QRS amplitude.
   b. Hypertrophy increases the duration of the QRS complex.
   c. Leads I, aVL, V_5, and V_6 are the best leads to use in looking for ECG evidence of hypertrophy.
   d. ECG evidence of right ventricular hypertrophy is usually more readily evident than left ventricular hypertrophy.

_____ 10. In a patient experiencing an acute coronary syndrome, T wave inversion suggests the presence of
   a. injury.
   b. ischemia.
   c. infarction.
   d. cardiogenic shock.

_____ 11. Normal electrical axis lies between _____ in the frontal plane.
   a. −30 and +90 degrees
   b. +90 and ±180 degrees
   c. −90 and ±180 degrees
   d. −30 and −90 degrees

_____ 12. In evaluating the ECG for indications of enlargement, an ECG machine's sensitivity must be calibrated so that a 1-mV electrical signal will produce a deflection measuring exactly _____ mm tall.
   a. 0.5
   b. 1
   c. 5
   d. 10

_____ 13. Which of the following ECG changes is one of the earliest to occur during a STEMI but may have resolved by the time the patient seeks medical assistance?
   a. Pathologic Q waves
   b. Hyperacute T waves
   c. Horizontal ST segments
   d. Lengthening of the QT interval

_____ 14. A 66-year-old man presents with persistent chest pain that has been present for 1 hour. His 12-lead ECG reveals STE in leads V_2, V_3, and V_4, and his cardiac biomarkers are elevated. You suspect
   a. stable angina.
   b. unstable angina.
   c. STEMI.
   d. NSTEMI.

_____ 15. Which of the following is probably the single best lead to use in differentiating between RBBB and LBBB?
   a. Lead II
   b. Lead V_1
   c. Lead V_4
   d. Lead aVR

Completion

Complete each statement.

16. A _____ BBB produces an rSR′ pattern in lead V_1.

17. A _____ BBB produces a QS pattern in lead V_1.

Matching

Match the terms below with their descriptions by placing the letter of each correct answer in the space provided.

a. Left anterior descending artery
b. STEMI
c. Cardiac enlargement
d. V_1, V_2
e. Positive
f. Dilated cardiomyopathy
g. I and aVF
h. Terminal force
i. Right atrial abnormality
j. QS
k. I, aVL, V_5, V_6
l. rSR′
m. Right coronary artery
n. Tall R waves in leads V_1 through V_3 and deeper than normal S waves in leads I, aVL, V_5, and V_6
o. LBBB
p. Non–ST-elevation acute coronary syndromes
q. Intraventricular conduction delay
r. Hypertrophic cardiomyopathy
s. Increased QRS amplitude and changes in the ST segment and T wave
t. Left atrial abnormality

____ **18.** This can produce ST-segment elevation and wide Q waves that look remarkably similar to infarction
____ **19.** Term that refers to either dilation of a heart chamber or hypertrophy of the heart muscle
____ **20.** Leads commonly used to determine axis deviation
____ **21.** NSTEMI and unstable angina
____ **22.** Cardiac biomarkers (e.g., troponins) are elevated when this is present
____ **23.** Leads that view the septum
____ **24.** QRS pattern that is characteristic of RBBB
____ **25.** Most common form of cardiomyopathy
____ **26.** Term used to describe a wide QRS that is not associated with a BBB pattern
____ **27.** The P wave is tall, peaked, and usually of normal duration
____ **28.** Vessel that is usually blocked with an inferior MI
____ **29.** Deflection of the terminal force of the QRS complex in V_1 in RBBB
____ **30.** Vessel that is usually blocked with an anterior MI
____ **31.** Characteristic ECG changes associated with right ventricular hypertrophy
____ **32.** Leads that view the lateral wall of the left ventricle
____ **33.** The final portion of the QRS complex
____ **34.** Characteristic ECG changes associated with left ventricular hypertrophy
____ **35.** QRS pattern that is characteristic of LBBB
____ **36.** Type of cardiomyopathy characterized by significant myocardial hypertrophy without ventricular dilation that results in a markedly reduced stroke volume because of impaired diastolic filling
____ **37.** Associated with prolongation of the middle and end of the P wave

12-Lead Electrocardiograms—Practice

38. Analyze this 12-lead ECG and record your findings below.

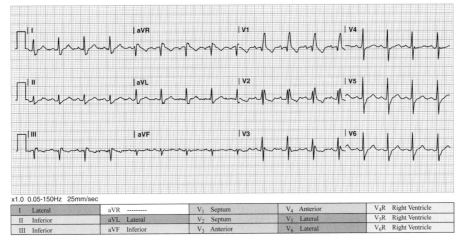

x1.0 0.05-150Hz 25mm/sec

I	Lateral	aVR	---------	V₁	Septum	V₄	Anterior	V₄R	Right Ventricle
II	Inferior	aVL	Lateral	V₂	Septum	V₅	Lateral	V₅R	Right Ventricle
III	Inferior	aVF	Inferior	V₃	Anterior	V₆	Lateral	V₆R	Right Ventricle

Fig. 9.38 (From Phalen T, Aehlert BJ: *The 12-lead ECG in acute coronary syndromes,* ed 3, St. Louis, 2012, Mosby.)

Rhythm and rate: _____ QRS axis: _____

PR interval: _____ QRS duration: _____ QT interval: _____

ST depression: _____ ST elevation: _____ Other findings: _____

Interpretation: _____

39. Analyze this 12-lead ECG and record your findings below.

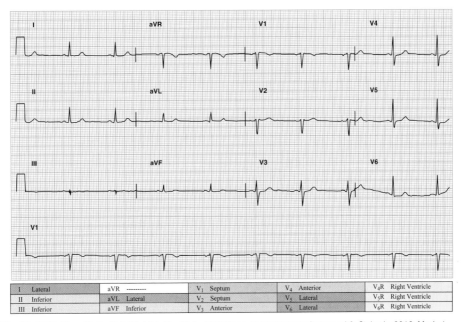

I	Lateral	aVR	---------	V₁	Septum	V₄	Anterior	V₄R	Right Ventricle
II	Inferior	aVL	Lateral	V₂	Septum	V₅	Lateral	V₅R	Right Ventricle
III	Inferior	aVF	Inferior	V₃	Anterior	V₆	Lateral	V₆R	Right Ventricle

Fig. 9.39 (From Phalen T, Aehlert BJ: *The 12-lead ECG in acute coronary syndromes,* ed 3, St. Louis, 2012, Mosby.)

Rhythm and rate: _____ QRS axis: _____

PR interval: _____ QRS duration: _____ QT interval: _____

ST depression: _____ ST elevation: _____ Other findings: _____

Interpretation: _____

40. Analyze this 12-lead ECG and record your findings below.

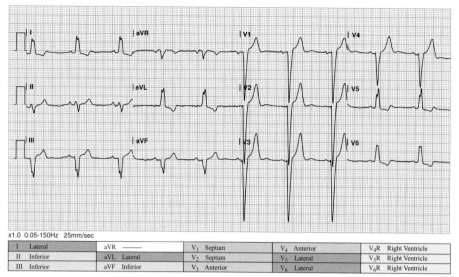

I	Lateral	aVR	---------	V₁	Septum	V₄	Anterior	V₄R	Right Ventricle
II	Inferior	aVL	Lateral	V₂	Septum	V₅	Lateral	V₅R	Right Ventricle
III	Inferior	aVF	Inferior	V₃	Anterior	V₆	Lateral	V₆R	Right Ventricle

Fig. 9.40 (From Phalen T, Aehlert BJ: *The 12-lead ECG in acute coronary syndromes,* ed 3, St. Louis, 2012, Mosby.)

Rhythm and rate: _____   QRS axis: _____

PR interval: _____   QRS duration: _____   QT interval: _____

ST depression: _____   ST elevation: _____   Other findings: _____

Interpretation: _____

41. Analyze this 12-lead ECG and record your findings below.

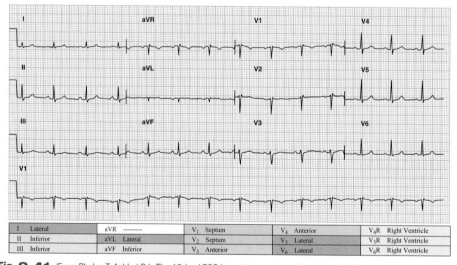

I	Lateral	aVR	---------	V₁	Septum	V₄	Anterior	V₄R	Right Ventricle
II	Inferior	aVL	Lateral	V₂	Septum	V₅	Lateral	V₅R	Right Ventricle
III	Inferior	aVF	Inferior	V₃	Anterior	V₆	Lateral	V₆R	Right Ventricle

Fig. 9.41 (From Phalen T, Aehlert BJ: *The 12-lead ECG in acute coronary syndromes,* ed 3, St. Louis, 2012, Mosby.)

Rhythm and rate: _____   QRS axis: _____

PR interval: _____   QRS duration: _____   QT interval: _____

ST depression: _____   ST elevation: _____   Other findings: _____

Interpretation: _____

42. Analyze this 12-lead ECG and record your findings below.

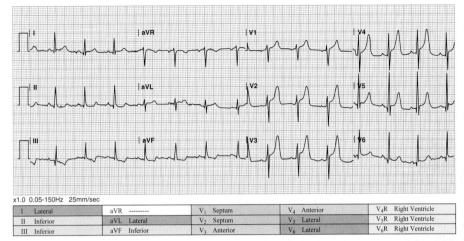

x1.0 0.05-150Hz 25mm/sec

I Lateral	aVR ---------	V₁ Septum	V₄ Anterior	V₄R Right Ventricle
II Inferior	aVL Lateral	V₂ Septum	V₅ Lateral	V₅R Right Ventricle
III Inferior	aVF Inferior	V₃ Anterior	V₆ Lateral	V₆R Right Ventricle

Fig. 9.42 (From Phalen T, Aehlert BJ: *The 12-lead ECG in acute coronary syndromes,* ed 3, St. Louis, 2012, Mosby.)

Rhythm and rate: _____ QRS axis: _____

PR interval: _____ QRS duration: _____ QT interval: _____

ST depression: _____ ST elevation: _____ Other findings: _____

Interpretation: _____

43. Analyze this 12-lead ECG and record your findings below.

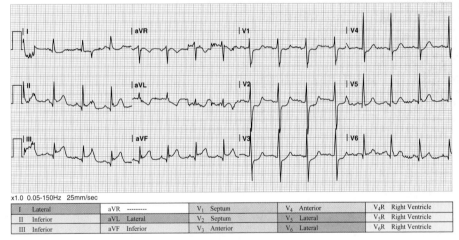

x1.0 0.05-150Hz 25mm/sec

I Lateral	aVR ---------	V₁ Septum	V₄ Anterior	V₄R Right Ventricle
II Inferior	aVL Lateral	V₂ Septum	V₅ Lateral	V₅R Right Ventricle
III Inferior	aVF Inferior	V₃ Anterior	V₆ Lateral	V₆R Right Ventricle

Fig. 9.43 (From Phalen T, Aehlert BJ: *The 12-lead ECG in acute coronary syndromes,* ed 3, St. Louis, 2012, Mosby.)

Rhythm and rate: _____ QRS axis: _____

PR interval: _____ QRS duration: _____ QT interval: _____

ST depression: _____ ST elevation: _____ Other findings: _____

Interpretation: _____

44. Analyze this 12-lead ECG and record your findings below.

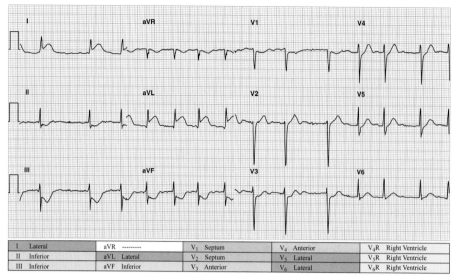

Fig. 9.44 (From Phalen T, Aehlert BJ: *The 12-lead ECG in acute coronary syndromes,* ed 3, St. Louis, 2012, Mosby.)

Rhythm and rate: _____ QRS axis: _____

PR interval: _____ QRS duration: _____ QT interval: _____

ST depression: _____ ST elevation: _____ Other findings: _____

Interpretation: _____

45. Analyze this 12-lead ECG and record your findings below.

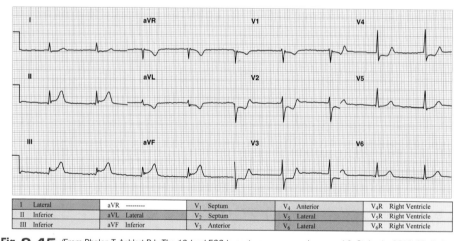

Fig. 9.45 (From Phalen T, Aehlert BJ: *The 12-lead ECG in acute coronary syndromes,* ed 3, St. Louis, 2012, Mosby.)

Rhythm and rate: _____ QRS axis: _____

PR interval: _____ QRS duration: _____ QT interval: _____

ST depression: _____ ST elevation: _____ Other findings: _____

Interpretation: _____

46. Analyze this 12-lead ECG and record your findings below.

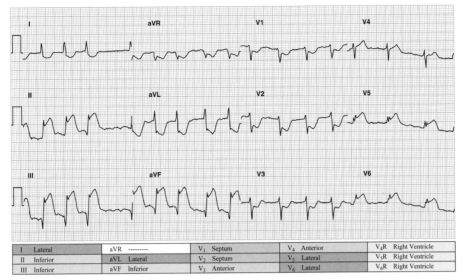

I	Lateral	aVR	---------	V₁	Septum	V₄	Anterior	V₄R	Right Ventricle
II	Inferior	aVL	Lateral	V₂	Septum	V₅	Lateral	V₅R	Right Ventricle
III	Inferior	aVF	Inferior	V₃	Anterior	V₆	Lateral	V₆R	Right Ventricle

Fig. 9.46 (From Phalen T, Aehlert BJ: *The 12-lead ECG in acute coronary syndromes,* ed 3, St. Louis, 2012, Mosby.)

Rhythm and rate: _____ QRS axis: _____

PR interval: _____ QRS duration: _____ QT interval: _____

ST depression: _____ ST elevation: _____ Other findings: _____

Interpretation: _____

47. Analyze this 12-lead ECG and record your findings below.

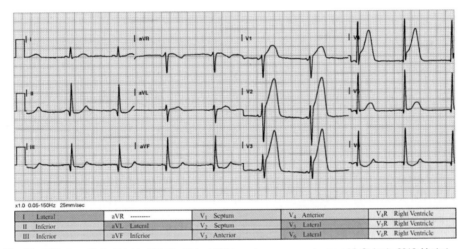

x1.0 0.05-150Hz 25mm/sec

I	Lateral	aVR	---------	V₁	Septum	V₄	Anterior	V₄R	Right Ventricle
II	Inferior	aVL	Lateral	V₂	Septum	V₅	Lateral	V₅R	Right Ventricle
III	Inferior	aVF	Inferior	V₃	Anterior	V₆	Lateral	V₆R	Right Ventricle

Fig. 9.47 (From Phalen T, Aehlert BJ: *The 12-lead ECG in acute coronary syndromes,* ed 3, St. Louis, 2012, Mosby.)

Rhythm and rate: _____ QRS axis: _____

PR interval: _____ QRS duration: _____ QT interval: _____

ST depression: _____ ST elevation: _____ Other findings: _____

Interpretation: _____

48. Analyze this 12-lead ECG and record your findings below.

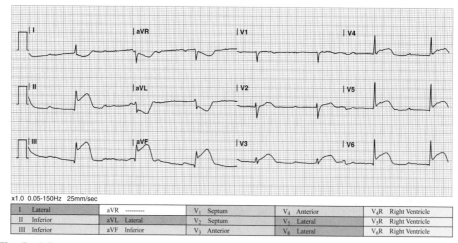

x1.0 0.05-150Hz 25mm/sec

I	Lateral	aVR	---------	V₁	Septum	V₄	Anterior	V₄R	Right Ventricle
II	Inferior	aVL	Lateral	V₂	Septum	V₅	Lateral	V₅R	Right Ventricle
III	Inferior	aVF	Inferior	V₃	Anterior	V₆	Lateral	V₆R	Right Ventricle

Fig. 9.48 (From Phalen T, Aehlert BJ: *The 12-lead ECG in acute coronary syndromes,* ed 3, St. Louis, 2012, Mosby.)

Rhythm and rate: _____ QRS axis: _____

PR interval: _____ QRS duration: _____ QT interval: _____

ST depression: _____ ST elevation: _____ Other findings: _____

Interpretation: _____

49. Analyze this 12-lead ECG and record your findings below.

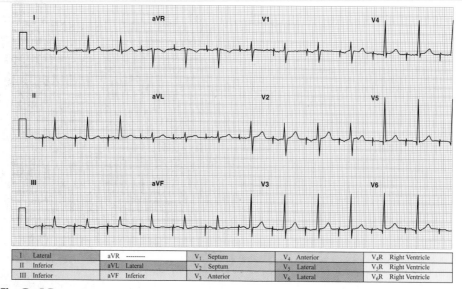

I	Lateral	aVR	---------	V₁	Septum	V₄	Anterior	V₄R	Right Ventricle
II	Inferior	aVL	Lateral	V₂	Septum	V₅	Lateral	V₅R	Right Ventricle
III	Inferior	aVF	Inferior	V₃	Anterior	V₆	Lateral	V₆R	Right Ventricle

Fig. 9.49 (From Phalen T, Aehlert BJ: *The 12-lead ECG in acute coronary syndromes,* ed 3, St. Louis, 2012, Mosby.)

Rhythm and rate: _____ QRS axis: _____

PR interval: _____ QRS duration: _____ QT interval: _____

ST depression: _____ ST elevation: _____ Other findings: _____

Interpretation: _____

50. Analyze this 12-lead ECG and record your findings below.

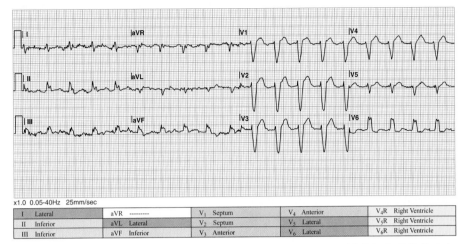

I	Lateral	aVR	---------	V₁	Septum	V₄	Anterior	V₄R	Right Ventricle
II	Inferior	aVL	Lateral	V₂	Septum	V₅	Lateral	V₅R	Right Ventricle
III	Inferior	aVF	Inferior	V₃	Anterior	V₆	Lateral	V₆R	Right Ventricle

Fig. 9.50 (From Phalen T, Aehlert BJ: *The 12-lead ECG in acute coronary syndromes,* ed 3, St. Louis, 2012, Mosby.)

Rhythm and rate: _____ QRS axis: _____

PR interval: _____ QRS duration: _____ QT interval: _____

ST depression: _____ ST elevation: _____ Other findings: _____

Interpretation: _____

1. T. In a patient presenting with an acute coronary syndrome, STE may develop, indicating myocardial injury in progress. STE may occur within the first hour or first few hours of infarction.
OBJ: Recognize the changes on the ECG that may reflect evidence of myocardial ischemia, injury, or infarction.

2. F. Sodium disturbances do not cause any significant changes on the ECG.
OBJ: Identify the ECG changes characteristically produced by hyperkalemia, hypokalemia, hypercalcemia, and hypocalcemia.

3. T. An abnormal (i.e., pathologic) Q wave is more than 0.04 second in duration or more than one third the height of the following R wave in that lead. MI is one possible cause of abnormal Q waves. In the early hours of infarction, an abnormal Q wave may not have developed to its full width or amplitude. Therefore, a single ECG tracing may not identify an abnormal Q wave. In a patient with a suspected MI, be sure to look at Q waves closely. Even if the initial ECG tracings do not show Q waves that are more than 0.04 second in duration or equal to or more than one third of the amplitude of the QRS complex, pathology must be considered if the Q waves become wider or deeper in each subsequent tracing.
OBJ: Recognize the changes on the ECG that may reflect evidence of myocardial ischemia, injury, or infarction.

4. D. The right ventricle is supplied by the right ventricular marginal branch of the RCA. An occlusion of the right ventricular marginal branch results in an isolated RVI. Occlusion of the RCA proximal to the right ventricular marginal branch results in an inferior and RVI. RVI should be suspected when ECG changes suggesting an inferior infarction are seen.
OBJ: Recognize the changes on the ECG that may reflect evidence of myocardial ischemia, injury, or infarction.

5. C. In the hexaxial reference system, the axes of some leads are perpendicular to each other. Lead I is perpendicular to lead aVF. Lead II is perpendicular to aVL, and lead III is perpendicular to aVR.
OBJ: Discuss the determination of electrical axis using leads I and aVF.

6. A. When the potassium level exceeds 5.5 mEq/L, tall, peaked T waves may be seen on the ECG; however, 50% of patients with potassium levels higher than 6.5 mEq/L will not manifest any ECG changes (El-Sherif et al, 2012).
OBJ: Identify the ECG changes characteristically produced by hyperkalemia, hypokalemia, hypercalcemia, and hypocalcemia.

7. C. The septum, which contains the bundle of His and bundle branches, is normally supplied by the left anterior descending coronary artery. ECG changes of infarction are seen in leads V_1 and V_2 if the site of infarction is limited to the septum. If the entire anterior wall is involved, ECG changes will be visible in V_1, V_2, V_3, and V_4. A blockage in this area may result in both RBBB and LBBB, second-degree AV block type II, and third-degree AV block.
OBJ: Recognize the changes on the ECG that may reflect evidence of myocardial ischemia, injury, or infarction.

8. B. Current flow to the left of normal is called *left axis deviation* (between −30 and −90 degrees). If the QRS complex is predominantly positive in I and negative in aVF, left axis deviation is present.
OBJ: Discuss the determination of electrical axis using leads I and aVF.

9. A. Ventricular muscle thickens (i.e., hypertrophies) when it sustains a persistent pressure overload. Dilatation occurs because of persistent volume overload. The two often go hand in hand. Hypertrophy increases the QRS amplitude and is often associated with ST-segment depression and asymmetric T-wave inversion. Because the right ventricle is normally considerably smaller than the left, it must become extremely enlarged before changes are visible on the ECG. Leads V_1, V_5, and V_6 are used when looking for ECG evidence of hypertrophy.
OBJ: Discuss the ECG changes that are characteristic of right atrial, left atrial, right ventricular, and left ventricular enlargement.

10. B. In a patient experiencing an acute coronary syndrome, T-wave inversion suggests the presence of myocardial ischemia.
OBJ: Recognize the changes on the ECG that may reflect evidence of myocardial ischemia, injury, or infarction.

11. A. In adults, the normal QRS axis is considered to be between −30 and +90 degrees in the frontal plane. Current flow to the right of normal is called *right axis deviation* (between +90 and ±180 degrees). Current flow in the direction opposite of normal is called *indeterminate*, "no man's land," *northwest*, or *extreme right axis deviation* (between −90 and ±180 degrees). Current flow to the left of normal is called *left axis deviation* (between −30 and −90 degrees).
OBJ: Explain the term *electrical axis* and its significance.

12. D. In evaluating the ECG for indications of chamber enlargement, it is particularly important to check the calibration marker to ensure that it is 10 mm (1 mV) tall.
OBJ: Discuss the ECG changes that are characteristic of right atrial, left atrial, right ventricular, and left ventricular enlargement.

13. B. Hyperacute (i.e., tall) T waves are sometimes called *tombstone T waves* and typically measure more than

50% of the preceding R wave. In addition to an increase in height, the T wave becomes more symmetric and may become pointed. These changes are often not recorded on the ECG because they have typically resolved by the time the patient seeks medical assistance.
OBJ: Recognize the changes on the ECG that may reflect evidence of myocardial ischemia, injury, or infarction.

14. C. The diagnosis of an acute coronary syndrome is made on the basis of the patient's clinical presentation, history, ECG findings, and cardiac biomarker results. If ST segments are elevated in two contiguous leads and elevated cardiac biomarkers are present, the diagnosis is STEMI. If ST elevation is not present but biomarker levels are elevated, the diagnosis is NSTEMI. If the ST segments are not elevated and cardiac biomarkers are not elevated, the diagnosis is unstable angina (Thygesen et al, 2012).
OBJ: Recognize the changes on the ECG that may reflect evidence of myocardial ischemia, injury, or infarction.

15. B. The criteria for BBB recognition may be identified in any lead of the ECG. However, when differentiating RBBB from LBBB, pay particular attention to the QRS morphology (i.e., shape) in specific leads. Lead V_1 is probably the single best lead to use in differentiating between RBBB and LBBB.
OBJ: Describe the appearance of RBBB and LBBB as seen in lead V_1.

16. An RBBB produces an RSR′ pattern in lead V_1.
OBJ: Describe the appearance of RBBB and LBBB as seen in lead V_1.

17. An LBBB produces a QS pattern in lead V_1.
OBJ: Describe the appearance of RBBB and LBBB as seen in lead V_1.

18. O
19. C
20. G
21. P
22. B
23. D
24. L
25. F
26. Q
27. I
28. M
29. E
30. A
31. N
32. K
33. H
34. S
35. J
36. R
37. T

Practice 12-Lead Electrocardiograms Answers

Note: Because of the distortion of ECGs that can occur during printing, a range of acceptable measurements is provided in the rhythm strip answers throughout this textbook.

38. **Fig. 9.38**
Rhythm and rate: Sinus tachycardia at 101 beats/min
QRS axis: Left
PR interval: 0.16 second
QRS duration: 0.13 second
QT interval: 0.35 second
ST depression/elevation: Depression in I, II, aVL, V_1 to V_2
Other findings: T waves inverted in V_1 to V_2
Interpretation: Sinus tachycardia at 101 beats/min with RBBB

39. **Fig. 9.39**
Rhythm and rate: Sinus bradycardia at 56 beats/min
QRS axis: Normal
PR interval: 0.12 second
QRS duration: 0.10 second
QT interval: 0.43 second
ST depression/elevation:
Other findings: T waves inverted in V_1
Interpretation: Sinus bradycardia at 56 beats/min, otherwise normal ECG

40. **Fig. 9.40**
Rhythm and rate: Sinus rhythm at 60 beats/min
QRS axis: Left
PR interval: 0.16 second
QRS duration: 0.14 second
QT interval: 0.42 second
ST depression/elevation: Elevation V_1 to V_4; depression in I, aVL, V_5, V_6
Other findings: T waves inverted in I, aVL, V_5, V_6
Interpretation: Sinus rhythm at 60 beats/min; possible STEMI/new onset LBBB; consider clinical presentation

41. **Fig. 9.41**
Rhythm and rate: Sinus rhythm at 84 beats/min
QRS axis: Normal
PR interval: 0.16 second
QRS duration: 0.08 second
QT interval: 0.34 second
ST depression/elevation:
Other findings:
Interpretation: Normal ECG

42. **Fig. 9.42**

Rhythm and rate: Sinus rhythm at 86 beats/min

QRS axis: Normal

PR interval: 0.14 second

QRS duration: 0.09 second

QT interval: 0.35 second

ST depression/elevation: Elevation noted in V_1 to V_4

Other findings: T waves inverted in III; tall, peaked in V_2 to V_4; baseline wander in V_6

Interpretation: Sinus rhythm at 86 beats/min. Anteroseptal infarction; STE noted in V_1 to V_4. Tall, peaked T waves in V_2 to V_4. Reciprocal changes noted in III, subtle changes in II and aVF.

43. **Fig. 9.43**

Rhythm and rate: Sinus rhythm at 92 beats/min

QRS axis: Normal

PR interval: 0.15 second

QRS duration: 0.11 second

QT interval: 0.36 second

ST depression/elevation: Elevation in II, III, aVF; depression in I, aVL, V_1 to V_4

Other findings: Pathologic Q waves in II, III, aVF; baseline wander in I, II, III

Interpretation: Sinus rhythm at 92 beats/min. Inferior STEMI; STE noted in II, III, and aVF. Obvious reciprocal change noted in aVL. ST depression in V_1 to V_4 suggests possible posterior involvement; consider obtaining posterior leads. Obtain V_4R to assess for RVI.

44. **Fig. 9.44**

Rhythm and rate: Atrial fibrillation at 81 beats/min

QRS axis: Left

PR interval: None

QRS duration: 0.09 second

QT interval: 0.39 second

ST depression/elevation: Elevation in I, aVL; depression in II, III, aVF

Other findings:

Interpretation: Atrial fibrillation at 81 beats/min. Lateral STEMI; reciprocal changes noted in II, III, and aVF.

45. **Fig. 9.45**

Rhythm and rate: Junctional rhythm at 55 beats/min

QRS axis: Normal

PR interval: None

QRS duration: 0.10 second

QT interval: 0.45 second

ST depression/elevation: Elevation in II, III, aVF; depression in I, aVL, V_1 to V_4

Other findings: T waves inverted in aVL, V_1

Interpretation: Junctional rhythm at 55 beats/min. Inferior STEMI; reciprocal changes noted in aVL. Obtain V_4R to assess for RVI.

46. **Fig. 9.46**

Rhythm and rate: Atrial fibrillation at 115 beats/min

QRS axis: Normal

PR interval:

QRS duration: 0.10 second

QT interval: 0.36 second

ST depression/elevation: Elevation in II, III, aVF, V_5, V_6; depression in I, aVL, V_1 to V_3

Other findings: T waves inverted in V_1, V_2

Interpretation: Atrial fibrillation at 115 beats/min. Inferolateral STEMI; reciprocal changes in I and aVL. Obtain V_4R to assess for RVI. ST-segment depression in V_1 to V_3 suggests possible posterior involvement; consider obtaining posterior leads.

47. **Fig. 9.47**

Rhythm and rate: Sinus bradycardia at 56 beats/min

QRS axis: Normal

PR interval: 0.11 second

QRS duration: 0.10 second

QT interval: 0.46 second

ST depression/elevation: Elevation in V_1 to V_4; depression in II, III, aVF

Other findings: Tall T waves in V_2 to V_4

Interpretation: Sinus bradycardia at 56 beats/min. Suspected anteroseptal STEMI; reciprocal changes noted in II, III, aVF. Short PR interval.

48. **Fig. 9.48**

Rhythm and rate: Supraventricular bradycardia at 42 beats/min

QRS axis: Normal

PR interval: None

QRS duration: 0.09 second

QT interval: 0.52 second

ST depression/elevation: Elevation in II, III, aVF, V_5 to V_6; depression in I, aVL

Other findings: Tall T waves in II, III, aVF

Interpretation: Supraventricular bradycardia at 42 beats/min. Inferolateral STEMI; reciprocal changes in I and aVL. Prolonged QT interval. Obtain V_4R to assess for RVI.

49. **Fig. 9.49**

Rhythm and rate: Electronic atrial pacemaker at 80 beats/min

QRS axis: Normal

PR interval: 0.26 second

QRS duration: 0.09 second

QT interval: 0.36 second

ST depression/elevation:

Other findings:

Interpretation: Atrial paced rhythm at 80 beats/min; no ECG evidence of STEMI

50. Fig. 9.50

Rhythm and rate: Sinus tachycardia at 113 beats/min with first-degree AV block and LBBB

QRS axis: Normal

PR interval: 0.33 second

QRS duration: 0.15 second

QT interval: 0.33 second

ST depression/elevation: Elevation in V_1 to V_3

Other findings: Artifact in limb leads

Interpretation: Sinus tachycardia at 113 beats/min with first-degree AV block. Possible anteroseptal STEMI; however, wide QRS and LBBB pattern are also present. Consider clinical presentation and obtain serial ECGs.

REFERENCES

Brown, D. F. (2013). Acute coronary syndrome. In J. G. Adams (Ed.), *Emergency medicine* (2nd ed.) (pp. 452–468). Philadelphia: Saunders.

El-Sherif, N., Turitto, G., & Robotis, D. (2012). Arrhythmias and electrolyte disorders. In S. Saksena & A. J. Camm (Eds.), *Electrophysiological disorders of the heart* (2nd ed.) (pp. 865–874). Philadelphia: Saunders.

Felver, L. (2013). Fluid and electrolyte homeostasis and imbalances. In L.-E. C. Copstead & J. L. Banasik (Eds.), *Pathophysiology* (5th ed.) (pp. 519–538). St. Louis: Saunders.

Ganz, L. (2012). Electrocardiography. In L. Goldman & A. I. Schafer (Eds.), *Goldman's Cecil medicine* (24th ed.) (pp. 272–278). Philadelphia: Saunders.

Goldberger, A. L., Goldberger, Z. D., & Shvilkin, A. (2013). Atrial and ventricular enlargement. In *Clinical electrocardiography: a simplified approach* (6th ed.) (pp. 45–74). Philadelphia: Saunders.

Halim, S. A., Newby, K., & Ohman, E. M. (2010). Diagnosis of acute myocardial ischemia and infarction. In M. H. Crawford, J. P. DiMarco, & W. J. Paulus (Eds.), *Cardiology* (3rd ed.) (pp. 345–360). Philadelphia: Elsevier.

Hancock, E. W., Deal, B. J., Mirvis, D. M., Okin, P., Kligfield, P., & Gettes, L. S. (2009). AHA/ACCF/HRS recommendations for the standardization and interpretation of the electrocardiogram: Part V: electrocardiogram changes associated with cardiac chamber hypertrophy. *J Am Coll Cardiol*, 53(11), 992–1002.

Huether, S. E. (2012). Fluids and electrolytes, acids and bases. In S. E. Huether & K. L. McCance (Eds.), *Understanding pathophysiology* (5th ed.) (pp. 98–118). St. Louis: Mosby.

Hutchinson, S. J., & Rudakewich, G. (2009). Right ventricular infarction. In *Complications of myocardial infarction: clinical diagnostic imaging atlas* (pp. 91–110). Philadelphia: Saunders.

Kumar, V., Abbas, A. K., & Aster, J. C. (2013). Heart. In *Robbins basic pathology* (9th ed.) (pp. 365–406). Philadelphia: Saunders.

Kurz, M. C., Mattu, A., & Brady, W. J. (2014). Acute coronary syndrome. In *Rosen's emergency medicine* (8th ed.) (pp. 997–1033). Philadelphia: Saunders.

Latcu, D.-G., & Nadir, S. (2010). Atrioventricular and intraventricular conduction disorders. In M. H. Crawford, J. P. DiMarco, & W. J. Paulus (Eds.), *Cardiology* (3rd ed.) (pp. 725–739). Philadelphia: Elsevier.

Litwin, S. E. (2010). Diagnostic tests and procedures in the patient with cardiovascular disease. In T. E. Andreoli, I. J. Benjamin, R. C. Griggs, & E. J. Wing (Eds.), *Andreoli and Carpenter's Cecil essentials of medicine* (8th ed.) (pp. 46–57). Philadelphia: Saunders.

Mirvis, D. M., & Goldberger, A. L. (2015). Electrocardiography. In D. L. Mann, D. P. Zipes, P. Libby, R. O. Bonow, & E. Braunwald (Eds.), *Braunwald's heart disease: a textbook of cardiovascular medicine* (10th ed.) (pp. 114–154). Philadelphia: Saunders.

O'Gara, P. T., Kushner, F. G., Ascheim, D. D., Casey, D. E., Jr., Chung, M. K., de Lemos, J. A., … & Zhao, D. X. (2013). 2013 ACCF/AHA guideline for the management of ST-elevation myocardial infarction. *J Am Coll Cardiol*, 61(4), e78–e140.

Otto, C. M. (2013). Cardiomyopathies, hypertensive and pulmonary heart disease. In *Textbook of clinical echocardiography* (5th ed.) (pp. 221–253). Philadelphia: Saunders.

Phalen, T., & Aehlert, B. (2012a). Myocardial infarction: recognition and localization. In *The 12-lead ECG in acute coronary syndromes* (3rd ed.) (pp. 75–130). Maryland Heights, Missouri: Mosby.

Phalen, T., & Aehlert, B. (2012b). Acute coronary syndrome imposters. In *The 12-lead ECG in acute coronary syndromes* (3rd ed.) (pp. 143–158). Maryland Heights, Missouri: Mosby.

Speakman, E., & Weldy, N. J. (2002). Electrolyte imbalance. In *Body fluids & electrolytes* (8th ed.) (pp. 113–190). St. Louis: Mosby.

Stanton, B. A., & Koeppen, B. M. (2010). Potassium, calcium, and phosphate homeostasis. In B. M. Koeppen & B. A. Stanton (Eds.), *Berne & Levy physiology* (6th ed.) (pp. 619–635). Philadelphia: Mosby.

Surawicz, B., & Knilans, T. K. (2008). Atrial abnormalities. In *Chou's electrocardiography in clinical practice* (6th ed.) (pp. 29–44). Philadelphia: Saunders.

Surawicz, B., Childers, R., Deal, B. J., & Gettes, L. S. (2009). AHA/ACCF/HRS Recommendations for the standardization and interpretation of the electrocardiogram: Part III: intraventricular conduction disturbances: a scientific statement from the American Heart Association Electrocardiography and Arrhythmias Committee. *J Am Coll Cardiol*, 53(11), 976–981.

Thygesen, K., Alpert, J. S., Jaffe, A. S., Simoons, M. L., Chaitman, B. R., & White, H. D. (2012). Third universal definition of myocardial infarction. *Circulation*, 126(16), 2020–2035.

Wagner, G. S., Macfarlane, P., Wellens, H., Josephson, M., Gorgels, A., Mirvis, D. M., … & Gettes, L. S. (2009). AHA/ACCF/HRS recommendations for the standardization and interpretation of the electrocardiogram: Part VI: Acute ischemia/infarction; a scientific statement from the American Heart Association Electrocardiography and Arrhythmias Committee. *J Am Coll Cardiol*, 53(11), 1003–1011.

Multiple Choice

Identify the choice that best completes the statement or answers the question.

____ 1. A branch of the _____ supplies the right atrium and right ventricle with blood.
  a. circumflex (Cx) artery
  b. right coronary artery (RCA)
  c. left main coronary artery
  d. left anterior descending (LAD) artery

____ 2. Stimulation of parasympathetic nerve fibers typically results in which of the following actions?
  a. Constriction of coronary blood vessels
  b. Increased strength of cardiac muscle contraction
  c. Increased rate of discharge of the sinoatrial (SA) node
  d. Slowed conduction through the atrioventricular (AV) node

____ 3. The contribution of blood that is added to the ventricles and results from atrial contraction is called
  a. afterload.
  b. atrial kick.
  c. cardiac output.
  d. peripheral resistance.

____ 4. Which of the following are semilunar valves?
  a. Aortic and pulmonic
  b. Aortic and tricuspid
  c. Pulmonic and mitral
  d. Tricuspid and mitral

____ 5. The left main coronary artery divides into the
  a. marginal and Cx branches.
  b. marginal and LAD branches.
  c. anterior and posterior descending branches.
  d. LAD and Cx branches.

____ 6. _____ cells are specialized cells of the electrical conduction system responsible for the spontaneous generation and conduction of electrical impulses.
  a. Working
  b. Pacemaker
  c. Mechanical
  d. Contractile

____ 7. The absolute refractory period
  a. begins with the onset of the P wave and terminates with the end of the QRS complex.
  b. begins with the onset of the QRS complex and terminates at approximately the apex of the T wave.
  c. begins with the onset of the QRS complex and terminates with the end of the T wave.
  d. begins with the onset of the P wave and terminates with the beginning of the QRS complex.

____ 8. Which of the following statements is true regarding the QT interval?
  a. The QT interval represents atrial depolarization followed immediately by atrial systole.
  b. The QT interval corresponds to atrial depolarization and impulse delay in the AV node.
  c. The QT interval represents ventricular depolarization followed immediately by ventricular systole.
  d. The QT interval represents the time from initial depolarization of the ventricles to the end of ventricular repolarization.

____ **9.** How do you determine whether the atrial rhythm on an electrocardiogram (ECG) tracing is regular or irregular?
 a. Compare QT intervals
 b. Compare PR intervals
 c. Compare R to R intervals
 d. Compare P to P intervals

____ **10.** Which of the following ECG leads use two distinct electrodes, one of which is positive and the other negative?
 a. Leads I, II, and III
 b. Leads V_1, V_2, and V_3
 c. Leads V_4, V_5, and V_6
 d. Leads aVR, aVL, and aVF

____ **11.** In sinus arrhythmia, a gradual decreasing of the heart rate is usually associated with
 a. expiration.
 b. inspiration.
 c. excessive caffeine intake.
 d. early signs of heart failure.

____ **12.** An ECG rhythm strip shows a ventricular rate of 46 beats/min, a regular rhythm, a PR interval of 0.14 second, a QRS duration of 0.06 second, and one upright P wave before each QRS. This rhythm is
 a. sinus arrest.
 b. sinus rhythm.
 c. SA block.
 d. sinus bradycardia.

____ **13.** SA block is a disorder of impulse _____, and sinus arrest is a disorder of impulse _____.
 a. formation, conduction
 b. conduction, formation

____ **14.** Signs and symptoms experienced during a tachy-dysrhythmia are usually primarily related to
 a. vasoconstriction.
 b. atrial irritability.
 c. slowed conduction through the AV node.
 d. decreased ventricular filling time and stroke volume.

____ **15.** Which of the following correctly reflects examples of ectopic (latent) pacemakers?
 a. The SA node and AV junction
 b. The AV junction and ventricles
 c. The SA node and right bundle branch
 d. The AV junction and left bundle branch

____ **16.** A wandering atrial pacemaker rhythm with a ventricular rate of 60 to 100 beats/min may also be referred to as
 a. atrial flutter.
 b. atrial fibrillation (AFib).
 c. multiform atrial rhythm.
 d. multifocal atrial tachycardia.

____ **17.** The most common type of supraventricular tachycardia (SVT) is
 a. atrial flutter.
 b. atrial tachycardia.
 c. AV reentrant tachycardia (AVRT).
 d. AV nodal reentrant tachycardia (AVNRT).

____ **18.** Which of the following is true with regard to treatment of a symptomatic patient with AFib?
 a. With rate control, the patient remains in AFib, but the ventricular rate is reduced (controlled) to decrease acute symptoms.
 b. With rate control, measures are taken (either pharmacologic or electrical) to reestablish sinus rhythm.

____ **19.** If the onset or end of paroxysmal atrial tachycardia or paroxysmal supraventricular tachycardia (PSVT) is not observed on the ECG, the dysrhythmia is called
 a. sinus tachycardia.
 b. junctional tachycardia.
 c. SVT.
 d. multifocal atrial tachycardia.

____ **20.** Which of the following is the most common sustained dysrhythmia in adults?
 a. AFib
 b. Sinus bradycardia
 c. Junctional rhythm
 d. Ventricular tachycardia (VT)

____ **21.** Which of the following statements is true regarding the differences between premature atrial complexes (PACs) and premature junctional complexes (PJCs) in leads II, III, and aVF?
 a. A PAC has a narrow QRS complex, and a PJC has a wide QRS complex.
 b. A PAC has a negative P wave before the QRS complex, and a PJC has a positive P wave before each QRS complex.
 c. A P wave may or may not be present with a PAC, whereas a PJC typically has a positive P wave before the QRS complex.
 d. A PAC typically has a positive P wave before the QRS complex, whereas a P wave may or may not be present with a PJC.

____ **22.** A Wolff-Parkinson-White (WPW) pattern is associated with a
 a. long PR interval, delta wave, and wide QRS complex.
 b. short PR interval, delta wave, and wide QRS complex.
 c. long PR interval, flutter waves, and narrow QRS complex.
 d. short PR interval, flutter waves, and narrow QRS complex.

_____ **23.** Which of the following ECG characteristics distinguishes atrial flutter from other atrial dysrhythmias?
   a. The presence of fibrillatory waves
   b. The presence of delta waves before the QRS
   c. Clearly identifiable P waves of varying size and amplitude
   d. The saw-tooth or picket-fence appearance of waveforms before the QRS

_____ **24.** When a junctional rhythm is viewed in lead II, where is the location of the P wave on the ECG if atrial and ventricular depolarization occur simultaneously?
   a. Before the QRS complex
   b. Within the QRS complex
   c. After the QRS complex

_____ **25.** The usual rate of nonparoxysmal junctional tachycardia is
   a. 50 to 80 beats/min.
   b. 80 to 120 beats/min.
   c. 101 to 140 beats/min.
   d. 150 to 300 beats/min.

_____ **26.** Junctional (or ventricular) complexes may come early (before the next expected sinus beat) or late (after the next expected sinus beat). If the complex is *early*, it is called a(n) _____. If the complex is *late*, it is called a(n) _____.
   a. escape beat; premature complex
   b. premature complex; escape beat

_____ **27.** Depending on the severity of the patient's signs and symptoms, management of slow rhythms may require therapeutic intervention including
   a. defibrillation.
   b. administration of atropine.
   c. synchronized cardioversion.
   d. vagal maneuvers and administration of adenosine.

_____ **28.** The term for three or more premature ventricular complexes (PVCs) occurring in a row at a rate of more than 100/min is
   a. ventricular trigeminy.
   b. ventricular fibrillation (VF).
   c. a run of VT.
   d. a run of ventricular escape beats.

_____ **29.** PVCs that look alike in the same lead and begin from the same anatomic site (i.e., focus) are called _____ PVCs.
   a. uniform
   b. isolated
   c. multiform
   d. interpolated

_____ **30.** Which of the following dysrhythmias has QRS complexes that vary in shape and amplitude from beat to beat and appear to twist from upright to negative or negative to upright and back, resembling a spindle?
   a. AFib
   b. Idioventricular rhythm
   c. Polymorphic VT (PMVT)
   d. Monomorphic VT

_____ **31.** When a delay or interruption in impulse conduction from the atria to the ventricles occurs as a result of a transient or permanent anatomic or functional impairment, the resulting dysrhythmia is called a(n)
   a. sinus arrest.
   b. SA block.
   c. bundle branch block (BBB).
   d. AV block.

_____ **32.** Whenever the criteria for BBB have been met and lead V_1 displays an rSR′ pattern, you should suspect a
   a. left bundle branch block (LBBB).
   b. right bundle branch block (RBBB).

_____ **33.** The PR interval of a first-degree AV block
   a. is constant and less than 0.12 second in duration.
   b. is constant and more than 0.20 second in duration.
   c. is generally progressive until a P wave appears without a QRS complex.
   d. gradually decreases in duration until a P wave appears without a QRS complex.

_____ **34.** Which of the following is an example of a complete AV block?
   a. First-degree AV block
   b. Second-degree AV block type I
   c. Second-degree AV block type II
   d. Third-degree AV block

_____ **35.** Which of the following statements is correct regarding 2:1 AV block?
   a. The atrial rhythm is irregular.
   b. The PR interval remains constant.
   c. The ventricular rate is twice the atrial rate.
   d. The level of the block is located within the SA node.

_____ **36.** The terms *advanced* or *high-grade* second-degree AV block may be used to describe one or more consecutive P waves that are not conducted.
   a. True
   b. False

_____ **37.** Which lead is probably the best to use when differentiating between RBBB and LBBB?
   a. V_1
   b. V_4
   c. II
   d. aVR

____ **38.** The term *capture*, as it pertains to pacing, refers to
  a. a vertical line on the ECG that indicates the pacemaker has discharged.
  b. the extent to which an artificial pacemaker recognizes intrinsic cardiac electrical activity.
  c. a pacemaker response in which the output pulse is suppressed when an intrinsic event is sensed.
  d. the successful conduction of an artificial pacemaker's impulse through the myocardium, resulting in depolarization.

____ **39.** The 12-lead ECG only provides a _____-second view of each lead.
  a. 1
  b. 2.5
  c. 4
  d. 6

Completion

Complete each statement.

42. The right atrium receives deoxygenated blood from the _____ _____ _____ (which carries blood from the head and upper extremities), the _____ _____ _____ (which carries blood from the lower body), and the _____ _____ (which receives blood from the intracardiac circulation).

43. A beat originating from the AV junction that appears later than the next expected sinus beat is called a(n) _____ _____ _____.

44. A rapid, wide-QRS rhythm associated with pulselessness, shock, or heart failure should be presumed to be _____ _____.

45. PACs associated with a wide QRS complex are called _____ _____ PACs, indicating that conduction through the ventricles is abnormal.

46. _____ is the period of relaxation during which a heart chamber is filling.

47. The thick, muscular middle layer of the heart wall that contains the atrial and ventricular muscle fibers necessary for contraction is the _____.

48. Delivery of an electrical current timed for delivery during the QRS complex is called _____ _____.

49. Sometimes when a PAC occurs very prematurely and close to the T wave of the preceding beat, only a P wave may be seen with no QRS after it (appearing as a pause). This type of PAC is termed a(n) _____ PAC.

____ **40.** Although a right ventricular infarction may occur by itself, it is more commonly associated with a(n) _____ wall myocardial infarction (MI).
  a. septal
  b. lateral
  c. inferior
  d. anterior

____ **41.** *Poor R-wave progression* is a phrase used to describe R waves that decrease in size from V_1 to V_4. This is often seen in an _____ infarction.
  a. inferobasal
  b. anteroseptal
  c. anterolateral
  d. inferoposterior

50. If the AV junction paces the heart, the electrical impulse must travel in a(n) _____ direction to activate the atria.

51. A demand pacemaker is also known as a(n) _____ pacemaker.

52. The axes of leads I, II, and III form an equilateral triangle with the heart at the center (Einthoven's triangle). If the augmented limb leads are added to this configuration and the axes of the six leads moved in a way in which they bisect each other, the result is the _____ _____ _____.

53. Indicate the heart surface viewed by each of the following.
  Leads II, III, aVF: _____
  Leads V_1, V_2: _____
  Leads V_3, V_4: _____
  Leads I, aVL, V_5, V_6: _____

Short Answer

54. Beginning with the right atrium, describe (by numbering) blood flow through the normal heart and lungs to the systemic circulation.
  _____ Right atrium   _____ Left ventricle
  _____ Mitral valve   _____ Pulmonary arteries
  _____ Aorta   _____ Tricuspid valve
  _____ Right ventricle   _____ Pulmonary veins
  _____ Pulmonic valve   _____ Aortic valve
  _____ Left atrium   _____ Systemic circulation

55. List five steps used in ECG rhythm analysis.
  1. _____
  2. _____
  3. _____
  4. _____
  5. _____

56. Explain the benefits of a dual-chamber pacemaker.

_____
_____
_____

57. List three uses for ECG monitoring.
  1. _____
  2. _____
  3. _____

58. Describe the appearance of a pathologic Q wave.

_____
_____
_____

59. What is the most important difference between sinus rhythm and sinus tachycardia?

_____
_____
_____

60. List three causes of artifact on an ECG tracing.
  1. _____
  2. _____
  3. _____

61. How do coarse and fine VF differ?

_____
_____
_____

62. List four reasons why the AV junction may assume responsibility for pacing the heart.
  1. _____
  2. _____
  3. _____
  4. _____

63. Explain why patients who experience AFib are at increased risk of having a stroke.

_____
_____
_____

64. On the ECG, what do the ST segment and T wave represent?

_____
_____
_____

65. Fill in the blank areas in the table below.

ECG Finding	AVNRT	Atrial Flutter	Atrial Fibrillation
Rhythm			
Rate (beats/min)			
P waves (lead II)			
PR interval			
QRS duration			

66. Explain the difference between electrical capture and mechanical capture.

_____
_____
_____

67. List four primary characteristics of cardiac cells.
  1. _____
  2. _____
  3. _____
  4. _____

68. Explain what is meant by the phrase "anatomically contiguous leads."

_____
_____
_____

69. Indicate the ECG criteria for the following dysrhythmias.

	Second-Degree AV Block Type II	2:1 AV Block
Ventricular rhythm		
PR interval		
QRS width		

70. Fill in the blank areas in the table below.

ECG Finding	Idioventricular Rhythm	Accelerated Idioventricular Rhythm	Monomorphic Ventricular Tachycardia
Rhythm			
Rate (beats/min)			
P waves (lead II)			
PR interval			
QRS duration			

Posttest Rhythm Strips

Use the five steps of rhythm interpretation to interpret each of the following rhythm strips. All rhythms were recorded in lead II unless otherwise noted.

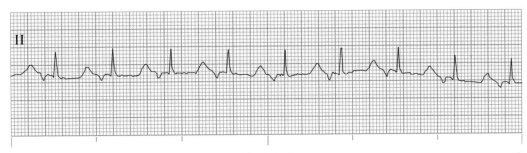

Fig. 10.1

71. **Fig. 10.1** This rhythm strip is from a 62-year-old woman with renal failure.

Rhythm: _____ Rate: _____ P waves: _____

PR interval: _____ QRS duration: _____ QT interval: _____

Interpretation: _____

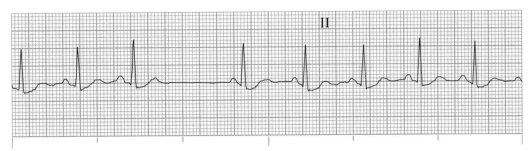

Fig. 10.2 (Modified from Aehlert B: *ECG study cards,* St. Louis, 2004, Mosby.)

72. **Fig. 10.2**

Rhythm: _____ Rate: _____ P waves: _____

PR interval: _____ QRS duration: _____ QT interval: _____

Interpretation: _____

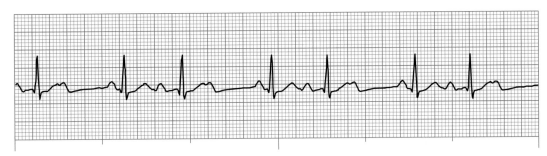

Fig. 10.3 (From Aehlert B: *ECG study cards,* St. Louis, 2004, Mosby.)

73. **Fig. 10.3**

Rhythm: _____ Rate: _____ P waves: _____

PR interval: _____ QRS duration: _____ QT interval: _____

Interpretation: _____

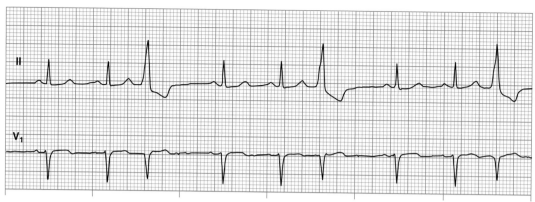

Fig. 10.4

74. **Fig. 10.4**

    Rhythm: _____ Rate: _____ P waves: _____

    PR interval: _____ QRS duration: _____ QT interval: _____

    Interpretation: _____

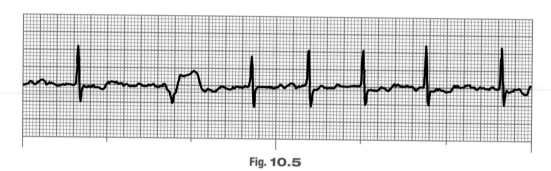

Fig. 10.5

75. **Fig. 10.5** This rhythm strip is from a 59-year-old man complaining of poor circulation in his legs.

    Rhythm: _____ Rate: _____ P waves: _____

    PR interval: _____ QRS duration: _____ QT interval: _____

    Interpretation: _____

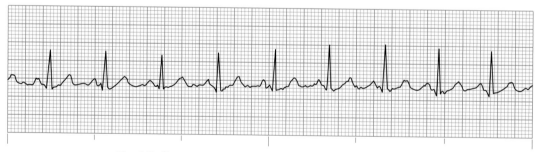

Fig. 10.6 (Modified from Aehlert B: *ECG study cards*, St. Louis, 2004, Mosby.)

76. **Fig. 10.6** This rhythm strip is from a 32-year-old woman complaining of dizziness and shortness of breath.

    Rhythm: _____ Rate: _____ P waves: _____

    PR interval: _____ QRS duration: _____ QT interval: _____

    Interpretation: _____

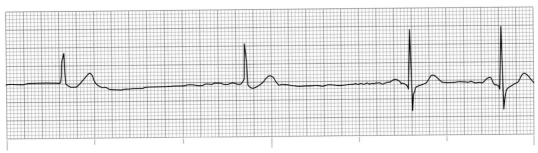

Fig. 10.7 (From Aehlert B: *ECG study cards,* St. Louis, 2004, Mosby.)

77. Fig. 10.7

Rhythm: _____ Rate: _____ P waves: _____

PR interval: _____ QRS duration: _____ QT interval: _____

Interpretation: _____

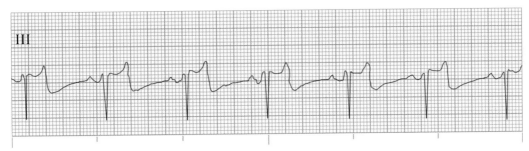

Fig. 10.8 (Modified from Aehlert B: *ECG study cards,* St. Louis, 2004, Mosby.)

78. Fig. 10.8 This rhythm strip is from a 76-year-old man who experienced a syncopal episode while playing golf.

Rhythm: _____ Rate: _____ P waves: _____

PR interval: _____ QRS duration: _____ QT interval: _____

Interpretation: _____

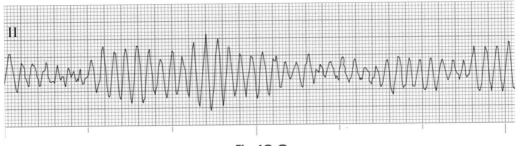

Fig. 10.9

79. Fig. 10.9 This rhythm strip is from a 54-year-old man complaining of chest pain.

Rhythm: _____ Rate: _____ P waves: _____

PR interval: _____ QRS duration: _____ QT interval: _____

Interpretation: _____

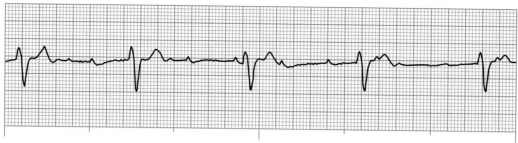

Fig. 10.10 (From Aehlert B: *ECG study cards,* St. Louis, 2004, Mosby.)

80. **Fig. 10.10**

Rhythm: _____ Rate: _____ P waves: _____

PR interval: _____ QRS duration: _____ QT interval: _____

Interpretation: _____

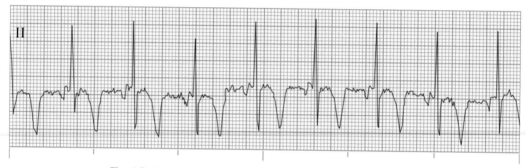

Fig. 10.11 (Modified from Aehlert B: *ECG study cards,* St. Louis, 2004, Mosby.)

81. **Fig. 10.11** This rhythm strip is from a 70-year-old woman with chronic obstructive pulmonary disease.

Rhythm: _____ Rate: _____ P waves: _____

PR interval: _____ QRS duration: _____ QT interval: _____

Interpretation: _____

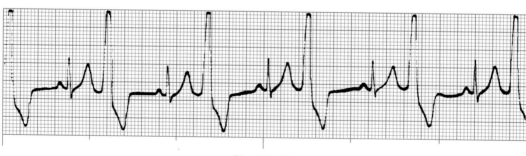

Fig. 10.12

82. **Fig. 10.12** This rhythm strip is from a 77-year-old man with chest pain. His chest hit the steering wheel during a motor vehicle crash.

Rhythm: _____ Rate: _____ P waves: _____

PR interval: _____ QRS duration: _____ QT interval: _____

Interpretation: _____

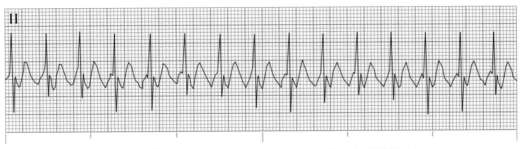

Fig. 10.13 (Modified from Aehlert B: *ECG study cards,* St. Louis, 2004, Mosby.)

83. **Fig. 10.13**

   Rhythm: _____ Rate: _____ P waves: _____

   PR interval: _____ QRS duration: _____ QT interval: _____

   Interpretation: _____

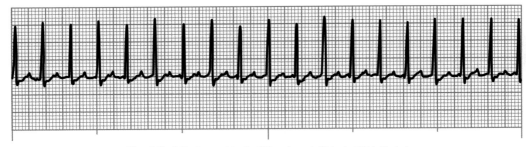

Fig. 10.14 (From Aehlert B: *ECG study cards,* St. Louis, 2004, Mosby.)

84. **Fig. 10.14** This rhythm strip is from a 20-year-old woman who collapsed on the sidewalk of her residence. A family member states that she has a history of SVT and takes atenolol.

   Rhythm: _____ Rate: _____ P waves: _____

   PR interval: _____ QRS duration: _____ QT interval: _____

   Interpretation: _____

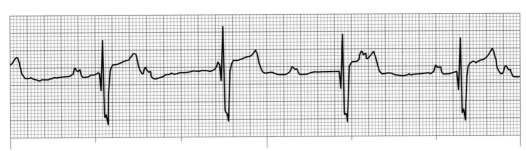

Fig. 10.15 (From Aehlert B: *ECG study cards,* St. Louis, 2004, Mosby.)

85. **Fig. 10.15** This rhythm strip is from a 42-year-old man with chest pain.

   Rhythm: _____ Rate: _____ P waves: _____

   PR interval: _____ QRS duration: _____ QT interval: _____

   Interpretation: _____

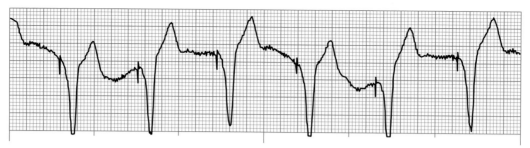

Fig. 10.16 (From Aehlert B: *ECG study cards,* St. Louis, 2004, Mosby.)

86. **Fig. 10.16** This rhythm strip is from a 76-year-old woman who is complaining of back pain. Her medical history includes an MI 2 years ago.

   Atrial paced activity? _____ Ventricular paced activity? _____

   Pacemaker malfunction? _____ Identification _____

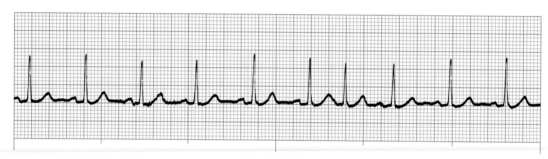

Fig. 10.17

87. **Fig. 10.17**

   Rhythm: _____ Rate: _____ P waves: _____

   PR interval: _____ QRS duration: _____ QT interval: _____

   Interpretation: _____

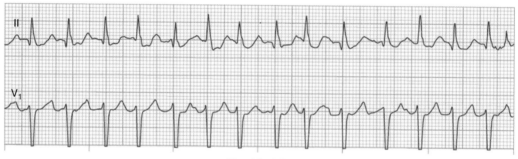

Fig. 10.18

88. **Fig. 10.18**

   Rhythm: _____ Rate: _____ P waves: _____

   PR interval: _____ QRS duration: _____ QT interval: _____

   Interpretation: _____

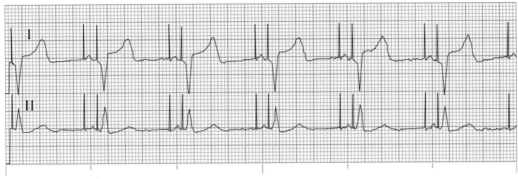

Fig. 10.19

89. **Fig. 10.19**

Atrial paced activity? _____ Ventricular paced activity? _____

Pacemaker malfunction? _____ Identification _____

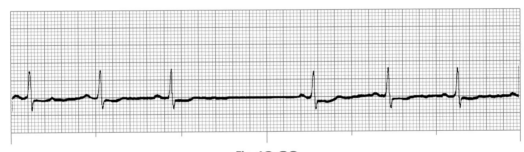

Fig. 10.20

90. **Fig. 10.20**

Rhythm: _____ Rate: _____ P waves: _____

PR interval: _____ QRS duration: _____ QT interval: _____

Interpretation: _____

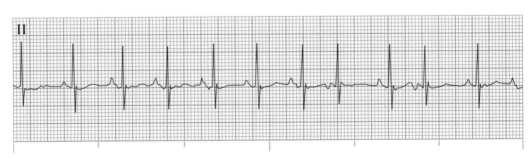

Fig. 10.21 (Modified from Aehlert B: *ECG study cards,* St. Louis, 2004, Mosby.)

91. **Fig. 10.21**

Rhythm: _____ Rate: _____ P waves: _____

PR interval: _____ QRS duration: _____ QT interval: _____

Interpretation: _____

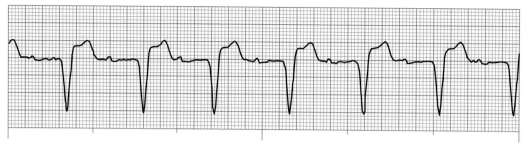

Fig. 10.22 (From Aehlert B: *ECG study cards,* St. Louis, 2004, Mosby.)

92. Fig. 10.22

Rhythm: _____ Rate: _____ P waves: _____

PR interval: _____ QRS duration: _____ QT interval: _____

Interpretation: _____

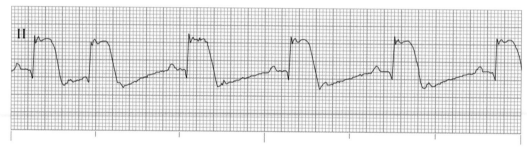

Fig. 10.23 (Modified from Aehlert B: *ECG study cards,* St. Louis, 2004, Mosby.)

93. Fig. 10.23

Rhythm: _____ Rate: _____ P waves: _____

PR interval: _____ QRS duration: _____ QT interval: _____

Interpretation: _____

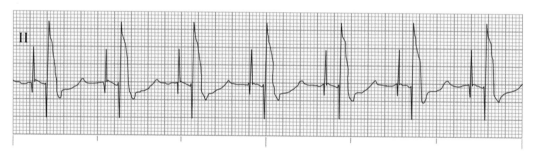

Fig. 10.24 (Modified from Aehlert B: *ECG study cards,* St. Louis, 2004, Mosby.)

94. Fig. 10.24 This rhythm strip is from a 79-year-old man who experienced a syncopal episode. He has a history of seizures.

Atrial paced activity? _____ Ventricular paced activity? _____

Pacemaker malfunction? _____ Identification: _____

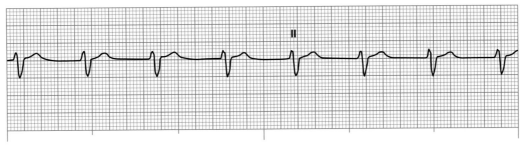

Fig. 10.25 (From Aehlert B: *ECG study cards,* St. Louis, 2004, Mosby.)

95. **Fig. 10.25** This rhythm strip is from an 81-year-old woman complaining of chest pain.

Rhythm: _____ Rate: _____ P waves: _____

PR interval: _____ QRS duration: _____ QT interval: _____

Interpretation: _____

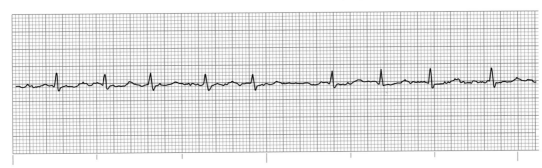

Fig. 10.26

96. **Fig. 10.26** This rhythm strip is from a 74-year-old woman complaining of difficulty breathing.

Rhythm: _____ Rate: _____ P waves: _____

PR interval: _____ QRS duration: _____ QT interval: _____

Interpretation: _____

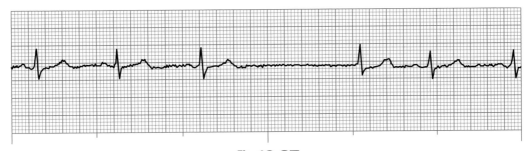

Fig. 10.27

97. **Fig. 10.27** This rhythm strip is from a 63-year-old woman complaining of dizziness.

Rhythm: _____ Rate: _____ P waves: _____

PR interval: _____ QRS duration: _____ QT interval: _____

Interpretation: _____

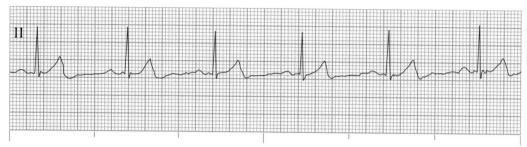

Fig. 10.28 (Modified from Aehlert B: *ECG study cards,* St. Louis, 2004, Mosby.)

98. Fig. 10.28 This rhythm strip is from a 53-year-old man complaining of chest pressure and shortness of breath. He has a history of a spinal cord injury and coronary artery disease.

Rhythm: _____ Rate: _____ P waves: _____

PR interval: _____ QRS duration: _____ QT interval: _____

Interpretation: _____

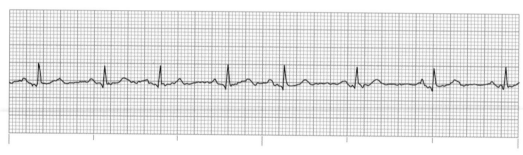

Fig. 10.29

99. Fig. 10.29 This rhythm strip is from an 82-year-old woman who had a ground-level fall.

Rhythm: _____ Rate: _____ P waves: _____

PR interval: _____ QRS duration: _____ QT interval: _____

Interpretation: _____

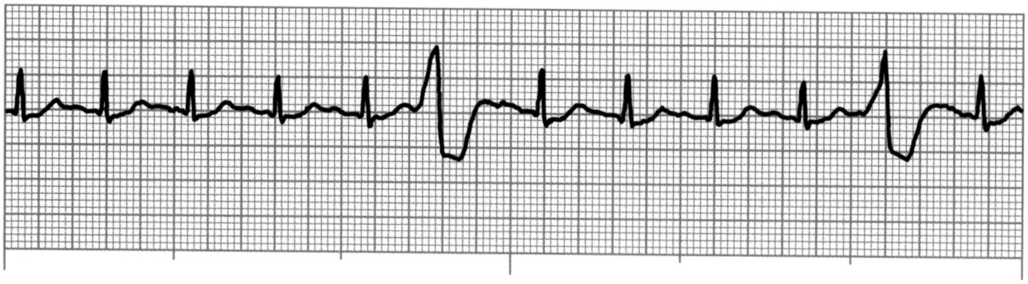

Fig. 10.30 (From Aehlert B: *ECG study cards,* St. Louis, 2004, Mosby.)

100. Fig. 10.30 This rhythm strip is from a 70-year-old man who is complaining of a sharp pain across his shoulders.

Rhythm: _____ Rate: _____ P waves: _____

PR interval: _____ QRS duration: _____ QT interval: _____

Interpretation: _____

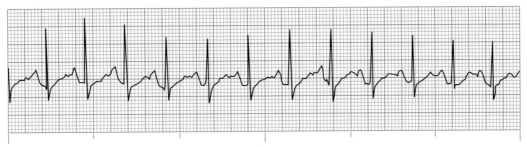

Fig. 10.31 (From Aehlert B: *ECG study cards,* St. Louis, 2004, Mosby.)

101. Fig. 10.31 This rhythm strip is from a 17-year-old man who experienced a syncopal episode while playing baseball in 110°F heat for 4 hours. His core temperature is 101.8°F.

Rhythm: _____ Rate: _____ P waves: _____

PR interval: _____ QRS duration: _____ QT interval: _____

Interpretation: _____

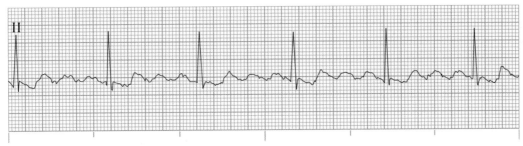

Fig. 10.32 (Modified from Aehlert B: *ECG study cards,* St. Louis, 2004, Mosby.)

102. Fig. 10.32 This rhythm strip is from a 71-year-old man who is complaining of abdominal pain.

Rhythm: _____ Rate: _____ P waves: _____

PR interval: _____ QRS duration: _____ QT interval: _____

Interpretation: _____

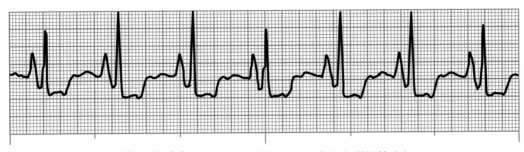

Fig. 10.33 (From Aehlert B: *ECG study cards,* St. Louis, 2004, Mosby.)

103. Fig. 10.33

Rhythm: _____ Rate: _____ P waves: _____

PR interval: _____ QRS duration: _____ QT interval: _____

Interpretation: _____

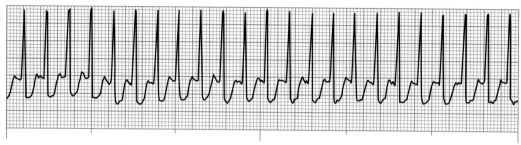

Fig. 10.34 (From Aehlert B: *ECG study cards,* St. Louis, 2004, Mosby.)

104. Fig. 10.34

Rhythm: _____ Rate: _____ P waves: _____

PR interval: _____ QRS duration: _____ QT interval: _____

Interpretation: _____

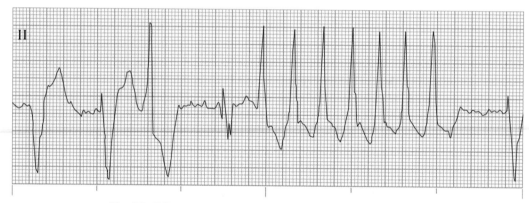

Fig. 10.35 (Modified from Aehlert B: *ECG study cards,* St. Louis, 2004, Mosby.)

105. Fig. 10.35

Atrial paced activity? _____ Ventricular paced activity? _____

Pacemaker malfunction? _____ Identification: _____

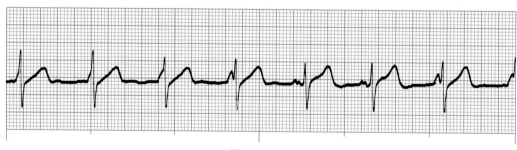

Fig. 10.36

106. Fig. 10.36

Rhythm: _____ Rate: _____ P waves: _____

PR interval: _____ QRS duration: _____ QT interval: _____

Interpretation: _____

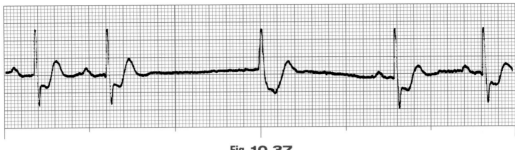

Fig. 10.37

107. Fig. 10.37

Rhythm: _____ Rate: _____ P waves: _____

PR interval: _____ QRS duration: _____ QT interval: _____

Interpretation: _____

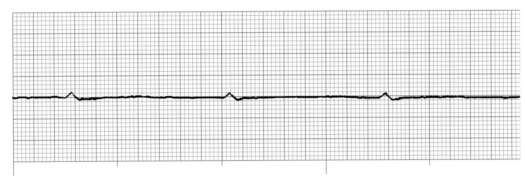

Fig. 10.38 (From Aehlert B: *ECG study cards,* St. Louis, 2004, Mosby.)

108. Fig. 10.38

Rhythm: _____ Rate: _____ P waves: _____

PR interval: _____ QRS duration: _____ QT interval: _____

Interpretation: _____

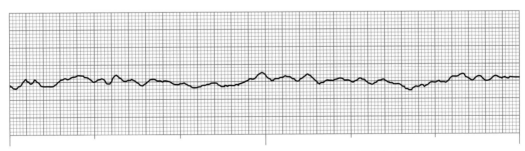

Fig. 10.39 (From Aehlert B: *ECG study cards,* St. Louis, 2004, Mosby.)

109. Fig. 10.39 This rhythm strip is from an 18-year-old man with a gunshot wound to his chest.

Rhythm: _____ Rate: _____ P waves: _____

PR interval: _____ QRS duration: _____ QT interval: _____

Interpretation: _____

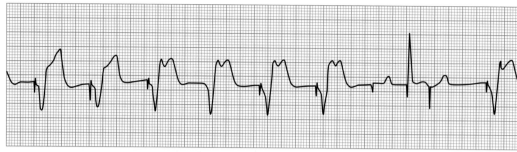

Fig. 10.40 (From Sole ML, Klein DG, Moseley MJ: *Introduction to critical care nursing,* ed 5, Philadelphia, 2008, Saunders.)

110. Fig. 10.40

Atrial paced activity? _____ Ventricular paced activity? _____

Pacemaker malfunction? _____ Identification: _____

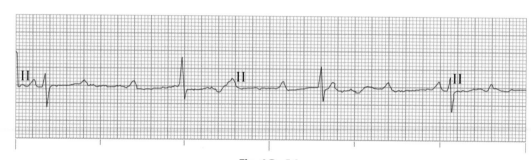

Fig. 10.41

111. Fig. 10.41

Rhythm: _____ Rate: _____ P waves: _____

PR interval: _____ QRS duration: _____ QT interval: _____

Interpretation: _____

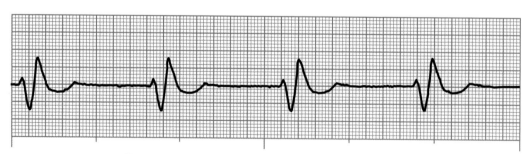

Fig. 10.42 (From Aehlert B: *ECG study cards,* St. Louis, 2004, Mosby.)

112. Fig. 10.42

Rhythm: _____ Rate: _____ P waves: _____

PR interval: _____ QRS duration: _____ QT interval: _____

Interpretation: _____

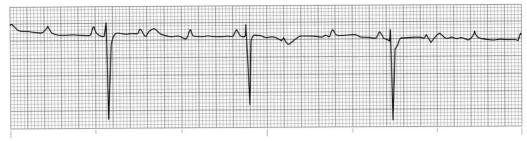

Fig. 10.43 (From Phillips RE, Feeney MK: *The cardiac rhythms: a systematic approach to interpretation,* ed 3, Philadelphia, 1990, Saunders.)

113. Fig. 10.43

Rhythm: _____ Rate: _____ P waves: _____

PR interval: _____ QRS duration: _____ QT interval: _____

Interpretation: _____

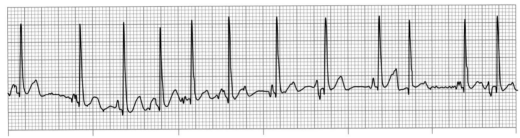

Fig. 10.44 (From Braunwald E, Libby P, Zipes DP, et al: *Heart disease: a textbook of cardiovascular medicine,* ed 6, St. Louis, 2001, Mosby.)

114. Fig. 10.44

Rhythm: _____ Rate: _____ P waves: _____

PR interval: _____ QRS duration: _____ QT interval: _____

Interpretation: _____

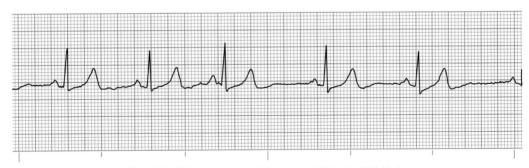

Fig. 10.45 (From Aehlert B: *ECG study cards,* St. Louis, 2004, Mosby.)

115. Fig. 10.45 This rhythm strip is from an 88-year-old woman complaining of dizziness.

Rhythm: _____ Rate: _____ P waves: _____

PR interval: _____ QRS duration: _____ QT interval: _____

Interpretation: _____

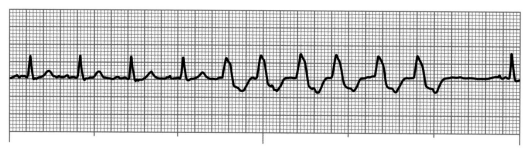

Fig. 10.46 (From Aehlert B: *ECG study cards,* St. Louis, 2004, Mosby.)

116. Fig. 10.46 This rhythm strip is from a 70-year-old man who sustained second-degree burns over 20% of his body. He has a history of diabetes, coronary artery disease, and hypertension.

Rhythm: _____ Rate: _____ P waves: _____

PR interval: _____ QRS duration: _____ QT interval: _____

Interpretation: _____

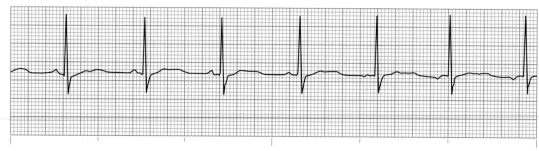

Fig. 10.47

117. Fig. 10.47

Rhythm: _____ Rate: _____ P waves: _____

PR interval: _____ QRS duration: _____ QT interval: _____

Interpretation: _____

Lead II (continuous)

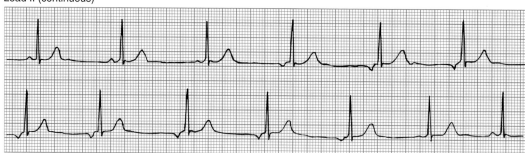

Fig. 10.48 (From Goldberger AL: *Clinical electrocardiography: a simplified approach,* ed 7, St. Louis, 2006, Mosby.)

118. Fig. 10.48

Rhythm: _____ Rate: _____ P waves: _____

PR interval: _____ QRS duration: _____ QT interval: _____

Interpretation: _____

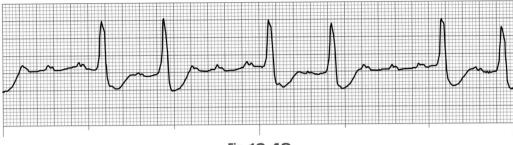

Fig. 10.49

119. Fig. 10.49

Rhythm: _____ Rate: _____ P waves: _____

PR interval: _____ QRS duration: _____ QT interval: _____

Interpretation: _____

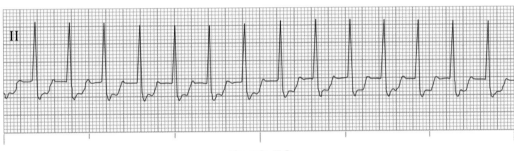

Fig. 10.50

120. Fig. 10.50

Rhythm: _____ Rate: _____ P waves: _____

PR interval: _____ QRS duration: _____ QT interval: _____

Interpretation: _____

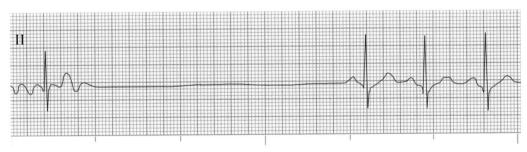

Fig. 10.51 (Modified from Aehlert B: *ECG study cards,* St. Louis, 2004, Mosby.)

121. Fig. 10.51

Rhythm: _____ Rate: _____ P waves: _____

PR interval: _____ QRS duration: _____ QT interval: _____

Interpretation: _____

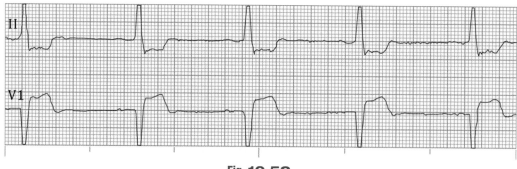

Fig. 10.52

122. Fig. 10.52

Rhythm: _____ Rate: _____ P waves: _____

PR interval: _____ QRS duration: _____ QT interval: _____

Interpretation: _____

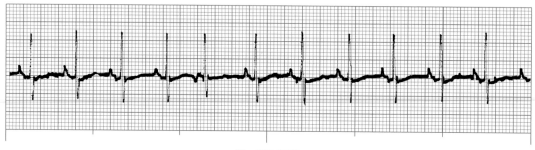

Fig. 10.53

123. Fig. 10.53

Rhythm: _____ Rate: _____ P waves: _____

PR interval: _____ QRS duration: _____ QT interval: _____

Interpretation: _____

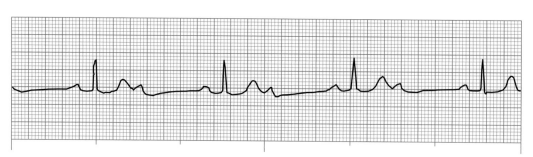

Fig. 10.54 (From Aehlert B: *ECG study cards,* St. Louis, 2004, Mosby.)

124. Fig. 10.54

Rhythm: _____ Rate: _____ P waves: _____

PR interval: _____ QRS duration: _____ QT interval: _____

Interpretation: _____

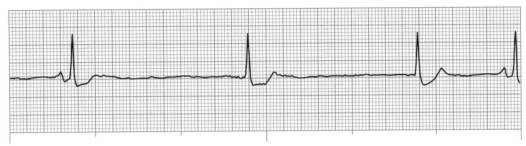

Fig. 10.55 (From Aehlert B: *ECG study cards,* St. Louis, 2004, Mosby.)

125. Fig. 10.55

Rhythm: _____ Rate: _____ P waves: _____

PR interval: _____ QRS duration: _____ QT interval: _____

Interpretation: _____

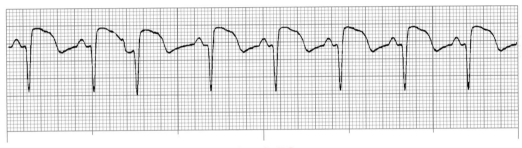

Fig. 10.56

126. Fig. 10.56

Rhythm: _____ Rate: _____ P waves: _____

PR interval: _____ QRS duration: _____ QT interval: _____

Interpretation: _____

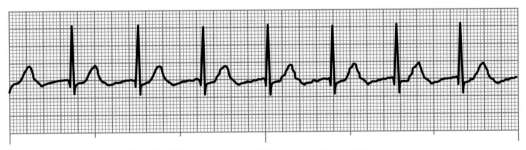

Fig. 10.57 (From Aehlert B: *ECG study cards,* St. Louis, 2004, Mosby.)

127. Fig. 10.57

Rhythm: _____ Rate: _____ P waves: _____

PR interval: _____ QRS duration: _____ QT interval: _____

Interpretation: _____

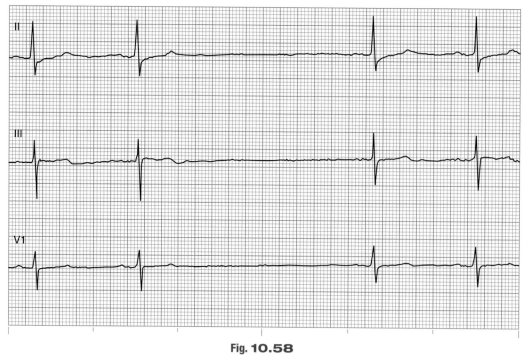

Fig. 10.58

128. **Fig. 10.58** These rhythm strips are from a 67-year-old woman complaining of dizziness and chest pain. She has a history of a three-vessel coronary artery bypass graft and hypertension.

Rhythm: _____ Rate: _____ P waves: _____

PR interval: _____ QRS duration: _____ QT interval: _____

Interpretation: _____

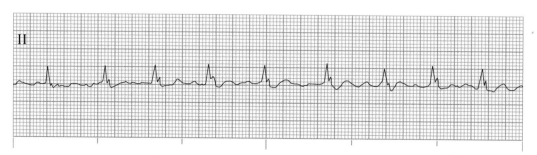

Fig. 10.59 (Modified from Aehlert B: *ECG study cards,* St. Louis, 2004, Mosby.)

129. **Fig. 10.59** This rhythm strip is from a 59-year-old man who was driving to work on the freeway when his internal defibrillator discharged. He was asymptomatic at the time this ECG was obtained a few minutes after the event.

Rhythm: _____ Rate: _____ P waves: _____

PR interval: _____ QRS duration: _____ QT interval: _____

Interpretation: _____

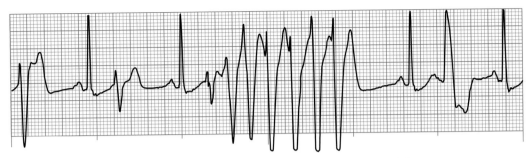

Fig. 10.60 (From Aehlert B: *ECG study cards,* St. Louis, 2004, Mosby.)

130. Fig. 10.60 This rhythm strip is from an 84-year-old man who is complaining of dizziness. He had a triple bypass 4 days ago.

Rhythm: _____ Rate: _____ P waves: _____

PR interval: _____ QRS duration: _____ QT interval: _____

Interpretation: _____

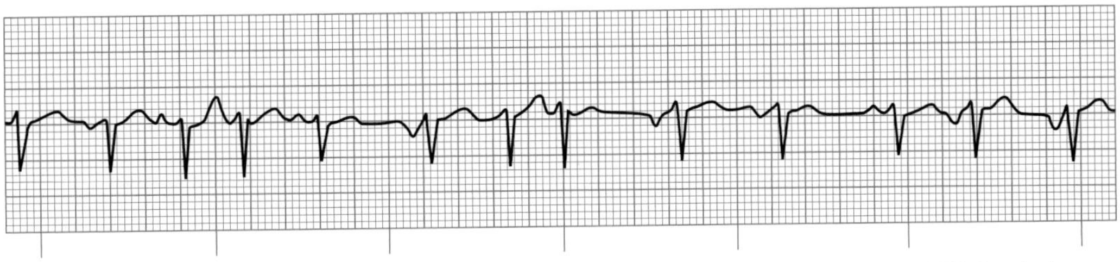

Fig. 10.61 (From Sole ML, Klein DG, Moseley MJ: *Introduction to critical care nursing,* ed 5, Philadelphia, 2008, Saunders.)

131. Fig. 10.61

Rhythm: _____ Rate: _____ P waves: _____

PR interval: _____ QRS duration: _____ QT interval: _____

Interpretation: _____

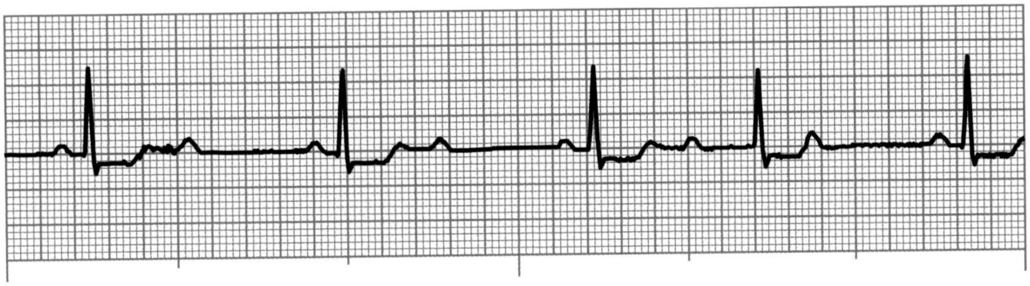

Fig. 10.62 (From Aehlert B: *ECG study cards,* St. Louis, 2004, Mosby.)

132. Fig. 10.62

Rhythm: _____ Rate: _____ P waves: _____

PR interval: _____ QRS duration: _____ QT interval: _____

Interpretation: _____

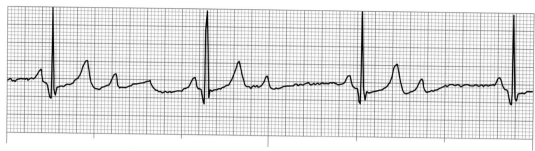

Fig. 10.63 (From Aehlert B: *ECG study cards,* St. Louis, 2004, Mosby.)

133. Fig. 10.63

Rhythm: _____ Rate: _____ P waves: _____

PR interval: _____ QRS duration: _____ QT interval: _____

Interpretation: _____

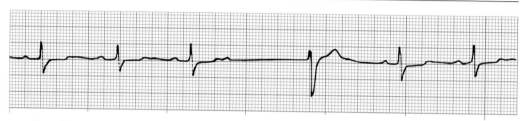

Fig. 10.64 (From Chou T, Ramaiah LS: *Electrocardiography in clinical practice: adult and pediatric,* ed 4, Philadelphia, 1996, Saunders.)

134. Fig. 10.64

Rhythm: _____ Rate: _____ P waves: _____

PR interval: _____ QRS duration: _____ QT interval: _____

Interpretation: _____

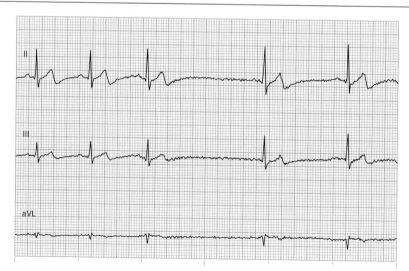

Fig. 10.65

135. Fig. 10.65

Rhythm: _____ Rate: _____ P waves: _____

PR interval: _____ QRS duration: _____ QT interval: _____

Interpretation: _____

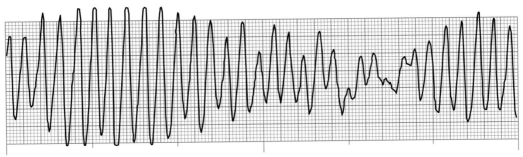

Fig. 10.66 (From Aehlert B: *ECG study cards,* St. Louis, 2004, Mosby.)

136. Fig. 10.66

Rhythm: _____ Rate: _____ P waves: _____

PR interval: _____ QRS duration: _____ QT interval: _____

Interpretation: _____

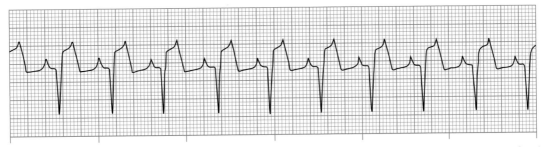

Fig. 10.67 (From Andreoli TE, Griggs R, Wing W, Fitz JG: *Andreoli and Carpenter's Cecil essentials of medicine,* ed 9, Philadelphia, 2016, Saunders.)

137. Fig. 10.67

Rhythm: _____ Rate: _____ P waves: _____

PR interval: _____ QRS duration: _____ QT interval: _____

Interpretation: _____

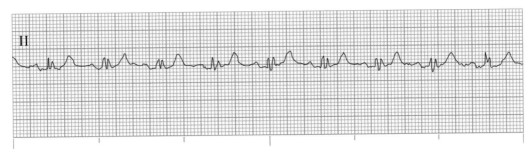

Fig. 10.68 (Modified from Aehlert B: *ECG study cards,* St. Louis, 2004, Mosby.)

138. Fig. 10.68 This rhythm strip is from a 61-year-old woman complaining of chest pain. She has a history of asthma and chronic obstructive pulmonary disease.

Rhythm: _____ Rate: _____ P waves: _____

PR interval: _____ QRS duration: _____ QT interval: _____

Interpretation: _____

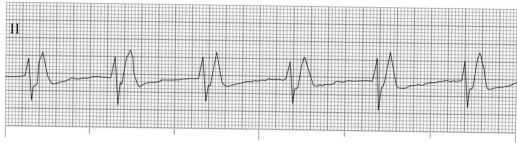

Fig. 10.69 (Modified from Aehlert B: *ECG study cards,* St. Louis, 2004, Mosby.)

139. Fig. 10.69 This rhythm strip is from a 52-year-old man found unresponsive, apneic, and pulseless.

Rhythm: _____ Rate: _____ P waves: _____

PR interval: _____ QRS duration: _____ QT interval: _____

Interpretation: _____

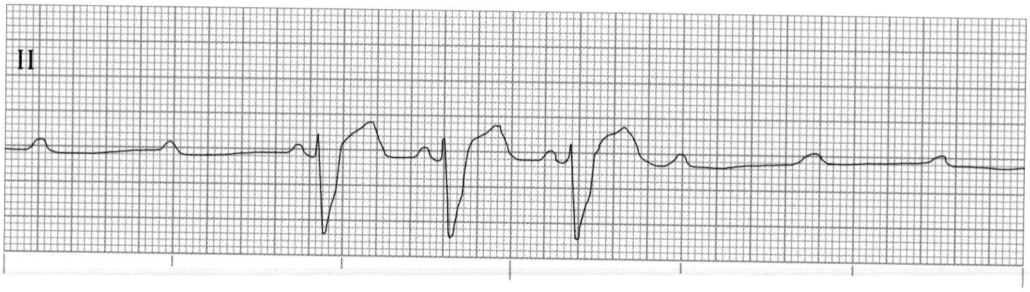

Fig. 10.70

140. Fig. 10.70

Rhythm: _____ Rate: _____ P waves: _____

PR interval: _____ QRS duration: _____ QT interval: _____

Interpretation: _____

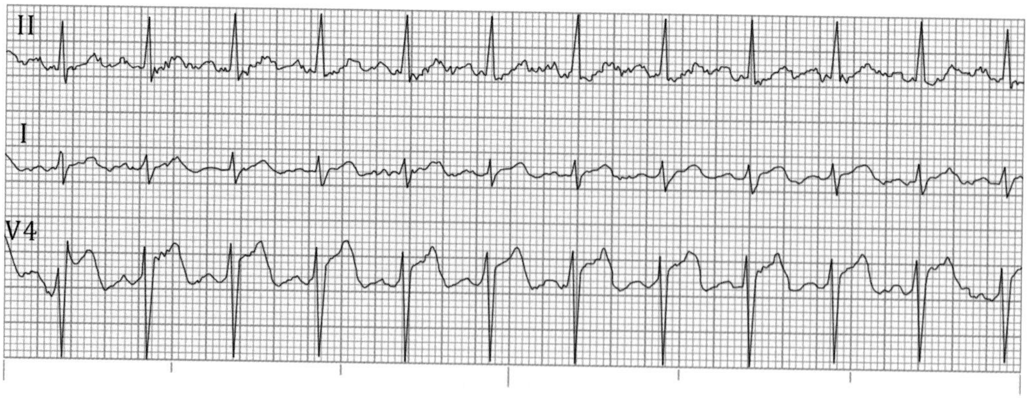

Fig. 10.71

141. Fig. 10.71

Rhythm: _____ Rate: _____ P waves: _____

PR interval: _____ QRS duration: _____ QT interval: _____

Interpretation: _____

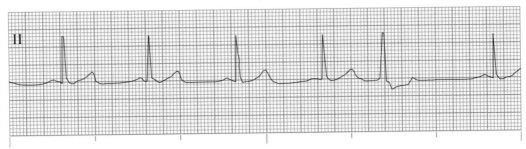

Fig. 10.72 (Modified from Aehlert B: *ECG study cards,* St. Louis, 2004, Mosby.)

142. Fig. 10.72

Rhythm: _____ Rate: _____ P waves: _____

PR interval: _____ QRS duration: _____ QT interval: _____

Interpretation: _____

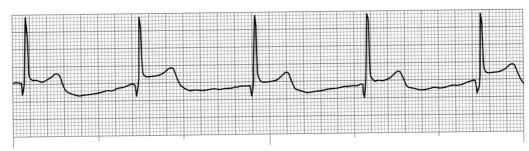

Fig. 10.73 (From Aehlert B: *ECG study cards,* St. Louis, 2004, Mosby.)

143. Fig. 10.73

Rhythm: _____ Rate: _____ P waves: _____

PR interval: _____ QRS duration: _____ QT interval: _____

Interpretation: _____

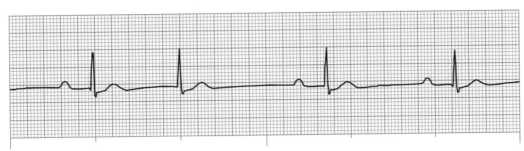

Fig. 10.74 (From Aehlert B: *ECG study cards,* St. Louis, 2004, Mosby.)

144. Fig. 10.74

Rhythm: _____ Rate: _____ P waves: _____

PR interval: _____ QRS duration: _____ QT interval: _____

Interpretation: _____

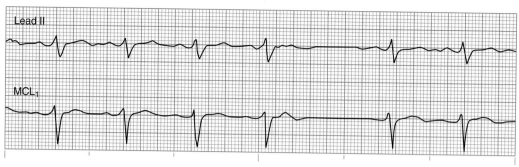

Fig. 10.75 (From Aehlert B: *ECG study cards*, St. Louis, 2004, Mosby.)

145. Fig. 10.75 These rhythm strips are from an 82-year-old man complaining of back pain.

Rhythm: _____   Rate: _____   P waves: _____

PR interval: _____   QRS duration: _____   QT interval: _____

Interpretation: _____

Posttest Answers

1. B. A branch of the <u>RCA</u> supplies the right atrium and right ventricle with blood.
OBJ: Name the primary branches and areas of the heart supplied by the right and left coronary arteries.

2. D. Parasympathetic (inhibitory) nerve fibers supply the SA node, atrial muscle, and AV bundle of the heart by the vagus nerves. Parasympathetic stimulation has the following actions:
- Slows the rate of discharge of the SA node
- Slows conduction through the AV node
- Decreases the strength of atrial contraction
- Can cause a small decrease in the force of ventricular contraction

OBJ: Compare and contrast the effects of sympathetic and parasympathetic stimulation of the heart.

3. B. The flow of blood from the superior and inferior venae cavae into the atria is normally continuous. About 70% of this blood flows directly through the atria and into the ventricles before the atria contract; this is called *passive filling*. When the atria contract, an additional 10% to 30% of the returning blood is added to filling of the ventricles. This additional contribution of blood resulting from atrial contraction is called *atrial kick*. Afterload is the pressure or resistance against which the ventricles must pump to eject blood. Cardiac output is the amount of blood pumped into the aorta each minute by the heart; it is defined as the stroke volume multiplied by the heart rate. Peripheral resistance is the resistance to the flow of blood determined by blood vessel diameter and the tone of the vascular musculature.
OBJ: Explain atrial kick.

4. A. The pulmonic and aortic valves are semilunar valves. The semilunar valves prevent backflow of blood from the aorta and pulmonary arteries into the ventricles. The tricuspid and mitral valves are AV valves, which separate the atria from the ventricles.
OBJ: Name and identify the location of the AV and semilunar valves.

5. D. The left main coronary artery supplies oxygenated blood to its two primary branches: the LAD artery, which is also called the *anterior interventricular artery*, and the Cx artery.
OBJ: Name the primary branches and areas of the heart supplied by the right and left coronary arteries.

6. B. In general, cardiac cells have either a mechanical (i.e., contractile) or an electrical (i.e., pacemaker) function. Pacemaker cells are specialized cells of the electrical conduction system. Pacemaker cells can also be called *conducting cells* or *automatic cells*. They are responsible for the spontaneous generation and conduction of electrical impulses.
OBJ: Describe the two basic types of cardiac cells in the heart, where they are found, and their function.

7. B. During the absolute refractory period, the cell will not respond to further stimulation within itself. This means that the myocardial working cells cannot contract and that the cells of the electrical conduction system cannot conduct an electrical impulse, no matter how strong the internal electrical stimulus. On the ECG, the absolute refractory period begins with the onset of the QRS complex and terminates at approximately the apex of the T wave.
OBJ: Define the absolute, effective, relative refractory, and supernormal periods and their location in the cardiac cycle.

8. D. The QT interval, measured from the beginning of the QRS complex to the end of the T wave, represents the time from initial depolarization of the ventricles to the end of ventricular repolarization.
OBJ: Define and describe the significance of each of the following as they relate to cardiac electrical activity: the P wave, QRS complex, T wave, U wave, PR segment, TP segment, ST segment, PR interval, QRS duration, and QT interval.

9. D. To evaluate the rhythmicity of the atrial rhythm, the interval between two consecutive P waves is measured and compared to succeeding P-P intervals.
OBJ: Describe a systematic approach to the analysis and interpretation of cardiac dysrhythmias.

10. A. A bipolar lead is an ECG lead that has a positive and negative electrode. Each lead records the difference in electrical potential (i.e., voltage) between two selected electrodes. Although all ECG leads are technically bipolar, leads I, II, and III use two distinct electrodes, one of which is connected to the positive input of the ECG machine and the other to the negative input.
OBJ: Describe correct anatomic placement of the standard limb leads, the augmented leads, and the chest leads.

11. A. In sinus arrhythmia, the heart rate increases gradually during inspiration (R-R intervals shorten) and decreases with expiration (R-R intervals lengthen).
OBJ: Describe the ECG characteristics, possible causes, signs and symptoms, and emergency management of sinus arrhythmia.

12. D. The rate of a sinus bradycardia is less than 60 beats/min. R-R and P-P intervals are regular; P waves are positive in lead II, and one precedes each QRS complex. The PR interval is within normal limits, and the QRS duration is 0.11 second or less unless it is abnormally conducted.
OBJ: Describe the ECG characteristics, possible causes, signs and symptoms, and emergency management of sinus bradycardia.

13. B. During SA block, also called *sinus exit block*, the pacemaker cells within the SA node initiate an impulse but it is blocked as it exits the SA node; thus, SA block is a disorder of impulse conduction. Sinus arrest, also called *sinus pause* or *SA arrest*, is a disorder of impulse formation. In sinus arrest, the pacemaker cells of the SA node fail to initiate an electrical impulse for one or more beats, resulting in absent PQRST complexes on the ECG.
OBJ: Describe the ECG characteristics, possible causes, signs and symptoms, and emergency management of SA block and sinus arrest.

14. D. Signs and symptoms experienced during a tachydysrhythmia are usually primarily related to decreased ventricular filling time and stroke volume. The heart's demand for oxygen increases as the heart rate increases. As the heart rate increases, there is less time for the ventricles to fill and less blood for the ventricles to pump out with each contraction, which can lead to decreased cardiac output. Because the coronary arteries fill when the ventricles are at rest, rapid heart rates decrease the time available for coronary artery filling. This decreases the heart's blood supply. Chest discomfort can result if the supplies of blood and oxygen to the heart are inadequate.
OBJ: Describe the ECG characteristics, possible causes, signs and symptoms, and emergency management of sinus tachycardia.

15. B. The terms *ectopic*, which means out of place, or *latent* are used to describe an impulse that originates from a source other than the SA node. Ectopic pacemaker sites include the cells of the AV junction and Purkinje fibers, although their intrinsic rates are slower than that of the SA node.
OBJ: Describe the location, the function, and, when appropriate, the intrinsic rate of the following structures: SA node, AV bundle, and Purkinje fibers.

16. C. *Multiform atrial rhythm* is an updated term for the rhythm formerly known as *wandering atrial pacemaker*. With this rhythm, the size, shape, and direction of the P waves vary, sometimes from beat to beat. The difference in the look of the P waves is a result of the gradual shifting of the dominant pacemaker between the SA node, the atria, and the AV junction. Wandering atrial pacemaker is associated with a normal or slow rate and irregular P-P, R-R, and PR intervals because of the different sites of impulse formation.
OBJ: Describe the ECG characteristics, possible causes, signs and symptoms, and initial emergency care for wandering atrial pacemaker (multiform atrial rhythm).

17. D. AVNRT is the most common type of SVT.
OBJ: Describe the ECG characteristics, possible causes, signs and symptoms, and initial emergency care for AVNRT.

18. D. Treatment decisions are based on the ventricular rate, the duration of the rhythm, the patient's general health, and how he or she is tolerating the rhythm. It is best to consult a cardiologist when considering specific therapies for AFib. The two primary treatment strategies used to control symptoms associated with AFib are rate control and rhythm control. With rate control, the patient remains in AFib, but the ventricular rate is controlled to decrease acute symptoms, reduce signs of ischemia, and reduce or prevent signs of heart failure from developing. With rhythm control, sinus rhythm is reestablished.
OBJ: Describe the ECG characteristics, possible causes, signs and symptoms, and initial emergency care for AFib.

19. C. The term *paroxysmal* is used to describe a rhythm that starts or ends suddenly. Atrial tachycardia that begins or ends suddenly is called PSVT, once called *paroxysmal atrial tachycardia* (PAT). PSVT may last for minutes, hours, or days. If the onset or end of PSVT is not observed on the ECG, the dysrhythmia is simply called *SVT*.
OBJ: Explain the terms *PAT* and *PSVT*.

20. A. AFib is the most common sustained dysrhythmia in adults, and it occurs because of altered automaticity in one or several rapidly firing sites in the atria or reentry involving one or more circuits in the atria.
OBJ: Describe the ECG characteristics, possible causes, signs and symptoms, and initial emergency care for AFib.

21. D. You can usually tell the difference between a PAC and a PJC by the P wave. A PAC typically has an upright P wave before the QRS complex in leads II, III, and aVF. A P wave may or may not be present with a PJC. If a P wave is present, it is inverted (retrograde) and may precede or follow the QRS. PJCs can be misdiagnosed when the P wave of a PAC is buried in the preceding T wave.
OBJ: Describe the ECG characteristics, possible causes, signs and symptoms, and initial emergency care for PJCs.

22. B. Characteristic ECG findings with a WPW pattern include a short PR interval, QRS widening, and a delta wave. A delta wave is an initial slurred deflection at the beginning of the QRS complex that results from the initial activation of the QRS by conduction over the accessory pathway.
OBJ: Describe the ECG characteristics, possible causes, signs and symptoms, and initial emergency care for AVNRT.

23. D. In atrial flutter, atrial waveforms are produced that resemble the teeth of a saw or the boards of a picket fence; these are called *flutter waves*, which are best observed in leads II, III, aVF, and V_1.
OBJ: Describe the ECG characteristics, possible causes, signs and symptoms, and initial emergency care for atrial flutter.

24. B. If the AV junction paces the heart, the electrical impulse must travel in a backward (retrograde) direction to activate the atria. If the atria depolarize before the ventricles, an inverted P wave will be seen *before* the QRS complex, and the PR interval will usually measure 0.12 second or less. The PR interval is shorter than usual because an impulse that begins in the AV junction does not have to travel as far to stimulate the ventricles. If the atria and ventricles depolarize at the same time, a P wave will not be visible because it will be hidden in the QRS complex. When the atria are depolarized after the ventricles, the P wave typically distorts the end of the QRS complex, and an inverted P wave will appear *after* the QRS.
OBJ: Describe the ECG characteristics, possible causes, signs and symptoms, and initial emergency care for a junctional escape rhythm.

25. C. Nonparoxysmal (i.e., gradual onset) junctional tachycardia usually starts as an accelerated junctional rhythm, but the heart rate gradually increases to more than 100 beats/min. The usual ventricular rate for nonparoxysmal junctional tachycardia is 101 to 140 beats/min. Paroxysmal junctional tachycardia, which is also known as focal or automatic junctional tachycardia, is an uncommon dysrhythmia that starts and ends suddenly and that is often precipitated by a PJC. The ventricular rate for paroxysmal junctional tachycardia is generally faster, at a rate of 140 beats/min or more.
OBJ: Describe the ECG characteristics, possible causes, signs and symptoms, and initial emergency care for junctional tachycardia.

26. B. Junctional (or ventricular) complexes may come early (before the next expected sinus beat) or late (after the next expected sinus beat). If the complex is *early*, it is called a <u>premature complex</u>—more specifically, a premature junctional (or ventricular) complex. If the complex is *late,* it is called a junctional (or ventricular) <u>escape beat</u>. To determine if a complex is early or late, you need to see at least two sinus beats in a row to establish the regularity of the underlying rhythm.
OBJ: Explain the difference between PJCs and junctional escape beats.

27. B. The term *symptomatic bradycardia* is used to describe a patient who experiences signs and symptoms of hemodynamic compromise related to a slow heart rate. Treatment of a symptomatic bradycardia should include assessing the patient's oxygen saturation level and determining if signs of increased work of breathing are present (e.g., retractions, tachypnea, paradoxic abdominal breathing). Give supplemental oxygen if oxygenation is inadequate. Assist breathing if ventilation is inadequate, establish intravenous access, and obtain a 12-lead ECG. Intravenous administration of atropine, the drug of choice for symptomatic bradycardia, may be necessary if the patient's symptoms warrant it. Reassess the patient's response and continue monitoring him or her.
OBJ: Describe the ECG characteristics, possible causes, signs and symptoms, and initial emergency care for a junctional escape rhythm.

28. C. Three or more sequential PVCs are termed a *run or burst*, and three or more PVCs that occur in a row at a rate of more than 100 beats/min are considered a run of VT.
OBJ: Explain the terms *bigeminy, trigeminy, quadrigeminy*, and *run* when used to describe premature complexes.

29. A. PVCs that look alike in the same lead and begin from the same anatomic site (i.e., focus) are called <u>uniform</u> PVCs.
OBJ: Describe the ECG characteristics, possible causes, signs and symptoms, and initial emergency care for PVCs.

30. C. PMVT is characterized by QRS complexes that vary in shape and amplitude from beat to beat and appear to twist from upright to negative or negative to upright and back, resembling a spindle. The ventricular rate is 150 to 300 beats/min and is typically 200 to 250 beats/min.

OBJ: Describe the ECG characteristics, possible causes, signs and symptoms, and initial emergency care for PMVT.

31. D. When a delay or interruption in impulse conduction from the atria to the ventricles occurs as a result of a transient or permanent anatomic or functional impairment, the resulting dysrhythmia is called an *AV block*. A BBB is a disruption in impulse conduction from the bundle of His through either the right or left bundle branch to the Purkinje fibers. With SA block, which is also called *sinus exit block*, the pacemaker cells within the SA node initiate an impulse but it is blocked as it exits the SA node. With sinus arrest, the pacemaker cells of the SA node fail to initiate an electrical impulse for one or more beats, resulting in absent PQRST complexes on the ECG.

OBJ: Describe the ECG characteristics, possible causes, signs and symptoms, and emergency management for first-degree AV block.

32. B. The rSR′ pattern is characteristic of RBBB. The rSR′ pattern is sometimes referred to as an "M" or "rabbit ear" pattern.

OBJ: Describe the appearance of RBBB and LBBB as seen in lead V_1.

33. B. A first-degree AV block is present when there is a 1:1 relationship between P waves and QRS complexes and the PR interval is constant and more than 0.20 second in duration (prolonged).

OBJ: Describe the ECG characteristics, possible causes, signs and symptoms, and emergency management for first-degree AV block.

34. D. Second-degree AV blocks are types of *incomplete* blocks because at least some of the impulses from the SA node are conducted to the ventricles. With third-degree AV block, there is a *complete* block in conduction of impulses between the atria and the ventricles.

OBJ: Describe the ECG characteristics, possible causes, signs and symptoms, and emergency management for third-degree AV block.

35. B. Second-degree 2:1 AV block is characterized by P waves that are normal in size and shape, but every other P wave is not followed by a QRS. The atrial rate is twice the ventricular rate. Because there are no two PQRST cycles in a row from which to compare PR intervals, 2:1 AV block cannot be conclusively classified as type I or type II. To determine the type of block with certainty, it is necessary to continue close ECG monitoring of the patient until the conduction ratio of P waves to QRS complexes changes to 3:2, 4:3, and so on, which would enable PR interval comparison. With second-degree AV block in the form of 2:1 AV block, the level of the block can be located within the AV node or within the His-Purkinje system.

OBJ: Describe 2:1 AV block and advanced second-degree AV block.

36. B. The terms *advanced* or *high-grade second-degree AV block* may be used to describe three or more consecutive P waves that are not conducted. For example, with 3:1 AV block, every third P wave is conducted (i.e., followed by a QRS complex); with 4:1 AV block, every fourth P wave is conducted.

OBJ: Describe 2:1 AV block and advanced second-degree AV block.

37. A. When the presence of BBB is suspected, an examination of V_1 can reveal whether the block affects the right or the left bundle branch.

OBJ: Describe the appearance of RBBB and LBBB as seen in lead V_1.

38. D. *Capture* refers to the successful conduction of an artificial pacemaker's impulse through the myocardium, resulting in depolarization. A pacemaker spike is a vertical line on the ECG that indicates the pacemaker has discharged. Sensitivity is the extent to which an artificial pacemaker recognizes intrinsic cardiac electrical activity. Inhibition is a pacemaker response in which the output pulse is suppressed when an intrinsic event is sensed.

OBJ: Discuss the terms *triggering, inhibition, pacing, capture, electrical capture, mechanical capture,* and *sensitivity*.

39. B. The 12-lead ECG provides a 2.5-second view of each lead because it is assumed that 2.5 seconds is long enough to capture at least one representative complex. However, a 2.5-second view is not long enough to properly assess rate and rhythm, so at least one continuous rhythm strip is usually included at the bottom of the tracing.

OBJ: Describe a systematic method for analyzing a 12-lead ECG.

40. C. Although a right ventricular infarction may occur by itself, it is more commonly associated with an inferior MI, and it should be suspected when ECG changes suggesting an inferior infarction are seen.

OBJ: Recognize the changes on the ECG that may reflect evidence of myocardial ischemia, injury, or infarction.

41. B. *Poor R-wave progression* is a phrase used to describe R waves that decrease in size from V_1 to V_4. This is often seen in an anteroseptal infarction but may be a normal variant in young people, particularly in young women. Other causes of poor R-wave progression include LBBB, left ventricular hypertrophy, and severe chronic obstructive pulmonary disease (particularly emphysema).

OBJ: Distinguish patterns of normal and abnormal R-wave progression.

42. The right atrium receives deoxygenated blood from the superior vena cava (which carries blood from the head and upper extremities), the inferior vena cava (which carries blood from the lower body), and the coronary sinus (which receives blood from the intracardiac circulation).

OBJ: Identify and describe the chambers of the heart and the vessels that enter or leave each.

43. A beat originating from the AV junction that appears later than the next expected sinus beat is called a <u>junctional escape beat</u>.
OBJ: Describe the ECG characteristics and possible causes for junctional escape beats.

44. A rapid, wide-QRS rhythm associated with pulselessness, shock, or heart failure should be presumed to be <u>ventricular tachycardia</u>.
OBJ: Describe the ECG characteristics, possible causes, signs and symptoms, and initial emergency care for monomorphic VT.

45. PACs associated with a wide QRS complex are called <u>aberrantly conducted</u> PACs, indicating conduction through the ventricles is abnormal.
OBJ: Describe the ECG characteristics, possible causes, signs and symptoms, and initial emergency care for PACs.

46. <u>Diastole</u> is the period of relaxation during which a heart chamber is filling.
OBJ: Identify and discuss each phase of the cardiac cycle.

47. The thick, muscular middle layer of the heart wall that contains the atrial and ventricular muscle fibers necessary for contraction is the <u>myocardium</u>.
OBJ: Identify the three cardiac muscle layers.

48. Delivery of an electrical current timed for delivery during the QRS complex is called <u>synchronized cardioversion</u>.
OBJ: Discuss the indications and procedure for synchronized cardioversion.

49. Sometimes, when a PAC occurs very prematurely and close to the T wave of the preceding beat, only a P wave may be seen with no QRS after it (appearing as a pause). This type of PAC is termed a <u>nonconducted</u> (or *blocked*) *PAC*.
OBJ: Describe the ECG characteristics, possible causes, signs and symptoms, and initial emergency care for PACs.

50. If the AV junction paces the heart, the electrical impulse must travel in a <u>backward</u> (retrograde) direction to activate the atria.
OBJ: Describe the location, the function, and, when appropriate, the intrinsic rate of the following structures: the SA node, the AV bundle, and the Purkinje fibers.

51. A demand pacemaker is also known as a <u>synchronous</u> or <u>noncompetitive</u> pacemaker.
OBJ: Explain the differences between single-chamber and dual-chamber pacemakers and between fixed-rate and demand pacemakers.

52. The axes of leads I, II, and III form an equilateral triangle with the heart at the center (Einthoven's triangle). If the augmented limb leads are added to this configuration and the axes of the six leads move in a way in which they bisect each other, the result is the <u>hexaxial reference system</u>.
OBJ: Explain the term *electrical axis* and its significance.

53.

Leads	Heart Surface Viewed
II, III, aVF	<u>Inferior</u>
V_1, V_2	<u>Septal</u>
V_3, V_4	<u>Anterior</u>
I, aVL, V_5, V_6	<u>Lateral</u>

OBJ: Relate the cardiac surfaces or areas represented by the ECG leads.

54. The pathway of blood flow through the normal heart and lungs to the systemic circulation:

1	Right atrium	9	Left ventricle
8	Mitral valve	5	Pulmonary arteries
11	Aorta	2	Tricuspid valve
3	Right ventricle	6	Pulmonary veins
4	Pulmonic valve	10	Aortic valve
7	Left atrium	12	Systemic circulation

OBJ: Beginning with the right atrium, describe blood flow through the normal heart and lungs to the systemic circulation.

55.
1. Assess regularity (atrial and ventricular)
2. Assess rate (atrial and ventricular)
3. Identify and examine waveforms
4. Assess intervals (e.g., PR, QRS, QT) and examine ST segments
5. Interpret the rhythm and assess its clinical significance

OBJ: Describe a systematic approach to the analysis and interpretation of cardiac dysrhythmias.

56. A dual-chamber pacemaker stimulates the right atrium and right ventricle sequentially (stimulating first the atrium and then the ventricle), mimicking normal cardiac physiology and thus preserving the atrial contribution to ventricular filling (atrial kick).
OBJ: Explain the differences between single-chamber and dual-chamber pacemakers and between fixed-rate and demand pacemakers.

57. ECG monitoring may be used to (1) monitor a patient's heart rate; (2) evaluate the effects of disease or injury on heart function; (3) evaluate pacemaker function; (4) evaluate the response to medications (e.g., antiarrhythmics); (5) obtain a baseline recording before, during, and after a medical procedure; and (6) evaluate for signs of myocardial ischemia, injury, and infarction.
OBJ: Explain the purpose of ECG monitoring.

58. An abnormal (i.e., pathologic) Q wave is more than 0.04 second in duration or more than one third the height of the following R wave in that lead. MI is one possible cause of abnormal Q waves.
OBJ: Define and describe the significance of each of the following as they relate to cardiac electrical activity: P wave, QRS complex, T wave, U wave, PR segment, TP segment, ST segment, PR interval, QRS duration, and QT interval.

59. A sinus rhythm has a rate of 60 to 100 beats/min. A sinus tachycardia has a rate of 101 to 180 beats/min.

OBJ: Describe the ECG characteristics, possible causes, signs and symptoms, and emergency management of sinus tachycardia.

60. Artifact may be caused by loose electrodes, broken wires or ECG cables, muscle tremor, patient movement, external chest compressions, or 60-cycle interference.

OBJ: Define the term *artifact* and explain methods that may be used to minimize its occurrence.

61. Coarse VF is 3 mm or more in amplitude. Fine VF is less than 3 mm in amplitude.

OBJ: Describe the ECG characteristics, possible causes, signs and symptoms, and initial emergency care for VF.

62. The AV junction may assume responsibility for pacing the heart under any of the following circumstances:
   1. The SA node fails to discharge (such as sinus arrest).
   2. An impulse from the SA node is generated but blocked as it exits the SA node (e.g., SA block).
   3. The rate of discharge of the SA node is slower than that of the AV junction (e.g., a sinus bradycardia or the slower phase of a sinus arrhythmia).
   4. An impulse from the SA node is generated and is conducted through the atria but is not conducted to the ventricles (e.g., an AV block).

OBJ: Describe the location, the function, and, when appropriate, the intrinsic rate of the following structures: the SA node, the AV bundle, and the Purkinje fibers.

63. Because the atria do not contract effectively and expel all of the blood within them, blood may pool within them and form clots. A clot may dislodge on its own or because of conversion to a sinus rhythm. A stroke can result if a clot moves from the atria and lodges in an artery in the brain.

OBJ: Describe the ECG characteristics, possible causes, signs and symptoms, and initial emergency care for AFib.

64. On the ECG, the ST segment represents early ventricular repolarization, and the T wave represents ventricular repolarization.

OBJ: Define and describe the significance of each of the following as they relate to cardiac electrical activity: P wave, QRS complex, T wave, U wave, PR segment, TP segment, ST segment, PR interval, QRS duration, and QT interval.

65.

ECG Finding	AVNRT	Atrial Flutter	Atrial Fibrillation
Rhythm	**Ventricular rhythm is usually very regular**	**Atrial rhythm is regular; ventricular rhythm is regular or irregular**	**Ventricular rhythm is usually irregularly irregular**
Rate (beats/min)	**150 to 250**	**Atrial rate is typically 240 to 300; ventricular rate variable—determined by AV blockade**	**Atrial rate is 300 to 600; ventricular rate is variable**
P waves (lead II)	**P waves often hidden in QRS complex**	**No identifiable P waves; saw-tooth flutter waves present**	**No identifiable P waves; fibrillatory waves present; erratic, wavy baseline**
PR interval	**If P waves are seen, the PRI will usually measure 0.12 to 0.20 sec**	**Not measurable**	**Not measurable**
QRS duration	**0.11 sec or less unless abnormally conducted**	**0.11 sec or less unless abnormally conducted**	**0.11 sec or less unless abnormally conducted**

OBJ: Describe the ECG characteristics, possible causes, signs and symptoms, and initial emergency care for AVNRT, atrial flutter, and AFib.

66. During pacing, the cardiac monitor is observed for electrical capture, usually evidenced by a wide QRS and broad T wave. In some patients, electrical capture is less obvious, indicated only as a change in the shape of the QRS. Mechanical capture is evaluated by assessing the patient's right upper extremity or right femoral pulses.

OBJ: Discuss the terms *triggering, inhibition, pacing, capture, electrical capture, mechanical capture,* and *sensitivity.*

67. The four primary characteristics of cardiac cells are listed below:
   1. Automaticity
   2. Excitability (i.e., irritability)
   3. Conductivity
   4. Contractility

OBJ: Describe the primary characteristics of cardiac cells.

68. The term *anatomically contiguous leads* refers to leads that "see" the same area of the heart. Two leads are contiguous if they look at the same or adjacent areas of the heart or if they are numerically consecutive *chest* leads.

OBJ: Relate the cardiac surfaces or areas represented by the ECG leads.

69.

Ventricular rhythm	Second-Degree AV Block Type II	2:1 AV Block
Ventricular rhythm	**Irregular**	**Regular**
PR interval	**Constant**	**Constant**
QRS width	**Narrow or wide**	**Narrow or wide**

OBJ: Describe 2:1 AV block and advanced second-degree AV block.

70.

ECG Finding	Idioventricular Rhythm	Accelerated Idioventricular Rhythm	Monomorphic Ventricular Tachycardia
Rhythm	**Essentially regular**	**Essentially regular**	**Usually regular**
Rate (beats/min)	**20 to 40**	**41 to 100; some experts consider the rate 41 to 120**	**101 to 250; some experts consider the rate 121 to 250**
P waves (lead II)	**Usually absent**	**Usually absent**	**Usually absent**
PR interval	**None**	**None**	**None**
QRS duration	**0.12 sec or greater**	**0.12 sec or greater**	**0.12 sec or greater**

OBJ: Describe the ECG characteristics, possible causes, signs and symptoms, and initial emergency care for an idioventricular rhythm, accelerated idioventricular rhythm, and monomorphic VT.

Posttest Rhythm Strip Answers

Note: Because of the distortion of ECGs that can occur during printing, a range of acceptable measurements is provided in the rhythm strip answers throughout this textbook.

71. Fig. 10.1
Rhythm: Regular
Rate: 88 beats/min
P waves: Inverted before each QRS; 1:1 relationship
PR interval: 0.12 to 0.14 second
QRS duration: 0.06 second
QT interval: 0.44 to 0.48 second
Interpretation: Accelerated junctional rhythm at 88 beats/min

72. Fig. 10.2
Rhythm: Irregular
Rate: 80 beats/min
P waves: Upright before each QRS; an early P wave distorts the T wave of beat 3
PR interval: 0.12 to 0.14 second
QRS duration: 0.06 to 0.08 second
QT interval: 0.36 second
Interpretation: Sinus rhythm at 80 beats/min with a nonconducted PAC and ST-segment depression

73. Fig. 10.3
Rhythm: Ventricular irregular; atrial regular
Rate: Ventricular about 70 beats/min; atrial 107 beats/min
P waves: Upright; more Ps than QRSs
PR interval: Lengthening
QRS duration: 0.08 second
QT interval: 0.32 second
Interpretation: Second-degree AV block type 1 at 70 beats/min

74. Fig. 10.4
Rhythm: Irregular
Rate: 90 beats/min
P waves: Upright before most QRS complexes; none visible for 3 early beats
PR interval: 0.16 second (sinus beats)
QRS duration: 0.06 second (sinus beats)
QT interval: 0.32 second (sinus beats)
Interpretation: Sinus rhythm at 90 beats/min with ventricular trigeminy

75. Fig. 10.5
Rhythm: Irregular
Rate: 70 beats/min
P waves: None visible; fibrillatory waves present
PR interval: None
QRS duration: 0.08 second (atrial beats)
QT interval: Unable to determine
Interpretation: AFib at 70 beats/min with a ventricular complex

76. Fig. 10.6
Rhythm: Regular
Rate: 88 beats/min
P waves: Upright before each QRS; 1:1 relationship
PR interval: 0.16 second
QRS duration: 0.06 to 0.08 second
QT interval: 0.32 to 0.36 second
Interpretation: Sinus rhythm at 88 beats/min; artifact is present

77. Fig. 10.7
Rhythm: Irregular
Rate: 30 beats/min (junctional beats) to 56 beats/min (sinus beats)
P waves: None with junctional beats; upright with sinus beats

PR interval: None with junctional beats; 0.18 second with sinus beats

QRS duration: 0.04 second (junctional beats); 0.08 second (sinus beats)

QT interval: 0.36 second

Interpretation: Junctional bradycardia at 30 beats/min to sinus bradycardia at 56 beats/min

78. **Fig. 10.8**

Rhythm: Regular

Rate: 65 beats/min

P waves: Upright before each QRS, some are notched; 1:1 relationship

PR interval: 0.16 second

QRS duration: 0.08 second

QT interval: 0.32 to 0.36 second

Interpretation: Sinus rhythm at 65 beats/min with ST-segment elevation (STE)

79. **Fig. 10.9**

Rhythm: Irregular

Rate: About 440 beats/min

P waves: None

PR interval: None

QRS duration: 0.12 to 0.14 second

QT interval: None

Interpretation: PMVT at about 440 beats/min

80. **Fig. 10.10**

Rhythm: Atrial and ventricular rhythms are essentially regular

Rate: Ventricular 45 beats/min; atrial 107 beats/min

P waves: Upright; more Ps than QRSs

PR interval: None

QRS duration: 0.14 to 0.16 second

QT interval: 0.40 to 0.44 second

Interpretation: Third-degree AV block at 45 beats/min with a wide QRS

81. **Fig. 10.11**

Rhythm: Regular

Rate: 83 beats/min

P waves: Inverted before each QRS; artifact is present

PR interval: 0.12 second

QRS duration: 0.08 second

QT interval: 0.36 second

Interpretation: Accelerated junctional rhythm at 83 beats/min with deeply inverted T waves

82. **Fig. 10.12**

Rhythm: Irregular

Rate: About 110 beats/min; 54 beats/min (sinus beats)

P waves: Sinus P waves; none with ventricular beats

PR interval: 0.12 second (sinus beats)

QRS duration: 0.06 to 0.08 second (sinus beats)

QT interval: 0.28 second (sinus beats)

Interpretation: Sinus bradycardia at 54 beats/min with ventricular bigeminy; rate about 110 beats/min if ventricular beats counted in the rate

83. **Fig. 10.13**

Rhythm: Regular

Rate: 150 beats/min

P waves: Flutter waves visible

PR interval: None

QRS duration: 0.08 second

QT interval: Unable to determine

Interpretation: Atrial flutter with a rapid ventricular response of 150 beats/min

84. **Fig. 10.14**

Rhythm: Regular

Rate: 180 beats/min

P waves: None visible

PR interval: Unable to determine

QRS duration: 0.06 second

QT interval: 0.20 to 0.24 second

Interpretation: AVNRT at 180 beats/min

85. **Fig. 10.15**

Rhythm: Regular

Rate: Ventricular 42 beats/min; atrial 71 beats/min

P waves: Upright; more Ps than QRSs

PR interval: None

QRS duration: 0.12 second

QT interval: 0.48 second

Interpretation: Third-degree AV block at 42 beats/min with a wide QRS, a prolonged QT interval, and STE

86. **Fig. 10.16**

Atrial paced activity? No

Ventricular paced activity? Yes

Pacemaker malfunction? No

Interpretation: Ventricular paced rhythm with 100% capture at 65 pulses/min

87. **Fig. 10.17**

Rhythm: Irregular

Rate: 100 beats/min

P waves: Upright before each QRS; the P wave of beat 7 is early and distorts the T wave of the preceding beat

PR interval: 0.16 second (sinus beats)

QRS duration: 0.04 to 0.06 second (sinus beats)

QT interval: 0.28 to 0.30 second (sinus beats)

Interpretation: Sinus rhythm at 100 beats/min with a PAC; beat 7 is the PAC

88. **Fig. 10.18**

Rhythm: Irregular

Rate: 140 beats/min

P waves: None consistently visible

PR interval: None

QRS duration: 0.06 to 0.10 second

QT interval: 0.28 to 0.32 second

Interpretation: AFib with a ventricular response of 140 beats/min; ST-segment depression in lead II

89. **Fig. 10.19**

Atrial paced activity? Yes

Ventricular paced activity? Yes

Pacemaker malfunction? No

Interpretation: Dual-chamber paced rhythm with 100% capture at 71 pulses/min

90. **Fig. 10.20**

Rhythm: Irregular

Rate: 60 beats/min

P waves: Upright before each QRS; a PQRST complex is missing

PR interval: 0.16 second

QRS duration: 0.06 to 0.08 second

QT interval: 0.32 to 0.36 second

Interpretation: Sinus rhythm at 60 beats/min with an episode of SA block

91. **Fig. 10.21**

Rhythm: Irregular

Rate: 110 beats/min

P waves: Upright before most QRSs; inverted with beats 8 and 10

PR interval: 0.12 to 0.16 second (sinus beats)

QRS duration: 0.06 to 0.08 second (sinus beats)

QT interval: 0.24 to 0.28 second (sinus beats)

Interpretation: Sinus tachycardia at 110 beats/min with two PJCs

92. **Fig. 10.22**

Rhythm: Regular

Rate: 69 beats/min

P waves: Upright; 1:1 relationship

PR interval: 0.36 second

QRS duration: 0.10 to 0.11 second

QT interval: 0.40 to 0.44 second

Interpretation: Sinus rhythm at 69 beats/min with first-degree AV block and STE

93. **Fig. 10.23**

Rhythm: Ventricular irregular; atrial regular

Rate: Ventricular 60 beats/min; atrial 100 beats/min

P waves: Upright; more Ps than QRSs

PR interval: Lengthening

QRS duration: 0.04 second

QT interval: 0.28 second

Interpretation: Second-degree AV block type I at 60 beats/min with STE; although the complexes on the right side of the rhythm strip show 2:1 conduction, comparison of the PR intervals of beats 1 and 2 enable a diagnosis of second-degree type I AV block

94. **Fig. 10.24**

Atrial paced activity? Yes

Ventricular paced activity? Yes

Pacemaker malfunction? No

Interpretation: Dual-chamber paced rhythm with 100% capture at 70 pulses/min

95. **Fig. 10.25**

Rhythm: Regular

Rate: 73 beats/min

P waves: None visible

PR interval: None

QRS duration: 0.12 to 0.14 second

QT interval: 0.32 second

Interpretation: Accelerated idioventricular rhythm at 73 beats/min

96. **Fig. 10.26**

Rhythm: Irregular

Rate: 90 beats/min

P waves: No identifiable P waves; fibrillatory waves present

PR interval: None

QRS duration: 0.06 to 0.08 second

QT interval: Unable to determine; no consistently identifiable T waves

Interpretation: AFib at 90 beats/min

97. **Fig. 10.27**

Rhythm: Irregular

Rate: 60 beats/min

P waves: Upright before most QRSs; none visible with beat 4

PR interval: 0.16 to 0.18 second

QRS duration: 0.08 second

QT interval: 0.44 second

Interpretation: Sinus rhythm at 60 beats/min with an episode of sinus arrest and a junctional escape beat

98. **Fig. 10.28**

Rhythm: Irregular

Rate: 60 beats/min

P waves: Upright before each QRS

PR interval: 0.20 to 0.22 second

QRS duration: 0.06 to 0.08 second

QT interval: 0.36 to 0.38 second

Interpretation: Sinus arrhythmia with first-degree AV block at 60 beats/min; artifact is present

99. **Fig. 10.29**

Rhythm: Irregular

Rate: 80 beats/min

P waves: Upright before each QRS; some are smooth and rounded, others are pointed

PR interval: 0.16 to 0.20 second

QRS duration: 0.08 second

QT interval: 0.36 second

Interpretation: Sinus rhythm at 80 beats/min with PACs (beats 3 and 5 are PACs)

100. **Fig. 10.30**

Rhythm: Irregular

Rate: 120 beats/min

P waves: Upright with sinus beats; none with ventricular beats

PR interval: 0.18 second (sinus beats)

QRS duration: 0.06 second (sinus beats)
QT interval: 0.28 second (sinus beats)
Interpretation: Sinus tachycardia at 120 beats/min with two uniform PVCs

101. **Fig. 10.31**
Rhythm: Regular
Rate: 130 beats/min
P waves: Upright; 1:1 relationship
PR interval: 0.16 second
QRS duration: 0.06 to 0.08 second
QT interval: 0.28 second
Interpretation: Sinus tachycardia at 130 beats/min with ST-segment depression; artifact is present

102. **Fig. 10.32**
Rhythm: Regular
Rate: 55 beats/min
P waves: Flutter waves present
PR interval: None
QRS duration: 0.08 second
QT interval: Unable to determine
Interpretation: Atrial flutter at 55 beats/min

103. **Fig. 10.33**
Rhythm: Regular
Rate: 69 beats/min
P waves: Upright and peaked; 1:1 relationship
PR interval: 0.16 second
QRS duration: 0.08 second
QT interval: 0.32 second
Interpretation: Sinus rhythm at 69 beats/min with ST-segment depression and inverted T waves

104. **Fig. 10.34**
Rhythm: Regular
Rate: 225 beats/min
P waves: None visible
PR interval: None
QRS duration: 0.06 second
QT interval: Unable to determine
Interpretation: AVNRT at 225 beats/min with ST-segment depression

105. **Fig. 10.35**
Atrial paced activity? No
Ventricular paced activity? Yes
Pacemaker malfunction? No
Interpretation: Ventricular paced rhythm with a PVC, a paced beat, nonsustained monomorphic VT, and a paced beat; paced interval 71 pulses/min

106. **Fig. 10.36**
Rhythm: Irregular
Rate: 70 beats/min
P waves: Vary in size and shape
PR interval: Varies
QRS duration: 0.08 to 0.12 second
QT interval: 0.40 to 0.44 second

Interpretation: Underlying rhythm is sinus but pacemaker site varies; ventricular rate 70 beats/min; patient with known WPW pattern; note the delta waves

107. **Fig. 10.37**
Rhythm: Irregular
Rate: 50 beats/min
P waves: Upright; none visible before the QRS with beat 3, but an inverted P wave appears after it
PR interval: 0.24 second
QRS duration: 0.08 second
QT interval: 0.32 to 0.36 second
Interpretation: Sinus rhythm at 50 beats/min with a first-degree AV block, an episode of sinus arrest, a junctional escape beat, and ST-segment depression

108. **Fig. 10.38**
Rhythm: Ventricular absent; atrial regular
Rate: Ventricular none; atrial 40 beats/min
P waves: Upright
PR interval: None
QRS duration: None
QT interval: None
Interpretation: P-wave asystole

109. **Fig. 10.39**
Rhythm: None
Rate: None
P waves: None
PR interval: None
QRS duration: None
QT interval: None
Interpretation: Ventricular fibrillation

110. **Fig. 10.40**
Atrial paced activity? Yes
Ventricular paced activity? Yes
Pacemaker malfunction? Yes—failure to capture and failure to sense
Interpretation: Dual-chamber pacemaker with failure to capture (seventh spike) and failure to sense (eighth spike) at 71 pulses/min

111. **Fig. 10.41**
Rhythm: Ventricular essentially regular; atrial essentially regular
Rate: Ventricular 37 beats/min; atrial 100 beats/min
P waves: Upright; more Ps than QRSs
PR interval: None
QRS duration: 0.08 to 0.10 second
QT interval: Unable to determine because T waves are not clearly visible
Interpretation: Third-degree AV block at 37 beats/min

112. **Fig. 10.42**
Rhythm: Regular
Rate: 39 beats/min
P waves: None visible

PR interval: None
QRS duration: 0.18 second
QT interval: 0.32 second
Interpretation: Idioventricular rhythm at 39 beats/min

113. **Fig. 10.43**
Rhythm: Ventricular regular; atrial regular
Rate: Ventricular 36 beats/min; atrial 108 beats/min
P waves: Upright; more Ps than QRSs; 3:1 relationship
PR interval: 0.16 second
QRS duration: 0.08 to 0.10 second
QT interval: Unable to determine
Interpretation: Advanced second-degree AV block with 3:1 conduction at 36 beats/min

114. **Fig. 10.44**
Rhythm: Irregular
Rate: 120 beats/min
P waves: Vary in size, shape, and direction
PR interval: Varies
QRS duration: 0.08 to 0.10 second
QT interval: 0.24 to 0.28 second
Interpretation: Multifocal atrial tachycardia at 120 beats/min

115. **Fig. 10.45**
Rhythm: Irregular
Rate: 50 beats/min
P waves: Upright; the P wave of beat 3 is early
PR interval: 0.16 second
QRS duration: 0.08 second
QT interval: 0.40 to 0.44 second
Interpretation: Sinus rhythm at 50 beats/min with a PAC

116. **Fig. 10.46**
Rhythm: Irregular
Rate: 100 beats/min (sinus beats); 136 beats/min (ventricular beats)
P waves: Low amplitude but upright with sinus beats
PR interval: 0.16 to 0.20 second (sinus beats)
QRS duration: 0.08 second (sinus beats); 0.12 second (ventricular beats)
QT interval: 0.34 second (sinus beats)
Interpretation: Sinus rhythm at 100 beats/min with a run of monomorphic VT at 136 beats/min

117. **Fig. 10.47**
Rhythm: Irregular
Rate: 68 beats/min (sinus beats); 75 beats/min (junctional beats)
P waves: Upright with sinus beats; inverted with junctional beats
PR interval: 0.16 second (sinus beats)
QRS duration: 0.08 second
QT interval: 0.28 to 0.32 second
Interpretation: Sinus rhythm at 68 beats/min to an accelerated junctional rhythm at 75 beats/min

118. **Fig. 10.48**
Rhythm: Irregular
Rate: 50 beats/min (top strip)
P waves: Vary in size, shape, and direction
PR interval: Varies
QRS duration: 0.06 to 0.08 second
QT interval: 0.40 to 0.44 second
Interpretation: Wandering atrial pacemaker at 50 beats/min

119. **Fig. 10.49**
Rhythm: Ventricular irregular; atrial regular
Rate: Ventricular 50 beats/min; atrial 167 beats/min
P waves: Upright and notched; more Ps than QRSs
PR interval: 0.26 second; the PR intervals before and after the nonconducted P waves are constant
QRS duration: 0.12 to 0.14 second
QT interval: Unable to determine
Interpretation: Second-degree AV block type II at 60 beats/min with ST-segment depression

120. **Fig. 10.50**
Rhythm: Regular
Rate: 150 beats/min
P waves: One P wave appears after each QRS
PR interval: None
QRS duration: 0.06 second
QT interval: 0.20 second
Interpretation: Junctional tachycardia at 150 beats/min

121. **Fig. 10.51**
Rhythm: Irregular
Rate: 83 beats/min (sinus beats)
P waves: Flutter waves initially present; sinus P waves present for last 3 beats
PR interval: 0.20 second (sinus beats)
QRS duration: 0.08 to 0.10 second (sinus beats)
QT interval: 0.36 to 0.40 second (sinus beats)
Interpretation: Atrial flutter with a period of asystole to sinus rhythm at 83 beats/min

122. **Fig. 10.52**
Rhythm: Regular
Rate: 45 beats/min
P waves: Low amplitude but upright
PR interval: 0.20 to 0.24 second
QRS duration: 0.10 to 0.12 second
QT interval: 0.36 to 0.40 second
Interpretation: Sinus bradycardia at 45 beats/min with first-degree AV block and horizontal ST segments; artifact is present

123. **Fig. 10.53**
Rhythm: Irregular
Rate: 110 beats/min
P waves: Upright; the P wave of beat 5 is early and inverted
PR interval: 0.16 second (sinus beats)
QRS duration: 0.06 second (sinus beats)
QT interval: Unable to determine
Interpretation: Sinus tachycardia at 110 beats/min with a PJC (beat 5 is the PJC)

124. Fig. 10.54
Rhythm: Ventricular regular; atrial regular
Rate: Ventricular 40 beats/min; atrial 79 beats/min
P waves: Upright; more Ps than QRSs
PR interval: 0.28 second
QRS duration: 0.06 to 0.08 second
QT interval: 0.48 second (prolonged)
Interpretation: 2:1 AV block at 40 beats/min with a prolonged QT interval

125. Fig. 10.55
Rhythm: Irregular
Rate: 30 beats/min (junctional beats)
P waves: Upright (sinus beats); none with junctional beats
PR interval: 0.16 second (sinus beats); none (junctional beats)
QRS duration: 0.06 to 0.08 second
QT interval: 0.36 to 0.38 second
Interpretation: Sinus beat, two junctional beats, sinus beat; ST-segment depression; artifact is present

126. Fig. 10.56
Rhythm: Irregular
Rate: 80 beats/min
P waves: Upright; the P wave of beat 3 is early and distorts the previous T wave
PR interval: 0.16 second
QRS duration: 0.06 second
QT interval: Unable to determine
Interpretation: Sinus rhythm at 80 beats/min with a PAC and STE

127. Fig. 10.57
Rhythm: Regular
Rate: 79 beats/min
P waves: None visible
PR interval: None
QRS duration: 0.06 second
QT interval: 0.36 to 0.38 second
Interpretation: Accelerated junctional rhythm at 79 beats/min

128. Fig. 10.58
Rhythm: Irregular
Rate: 40 beats/min
P waves: Upright; some are notched
PR interval: 0.20 second
QRS duration: 0.08 second
QT interval: 0.44 second
Interpretation: Sinus bradycardia at 40 beats/min with an episode of sinus arrest

129. Fig. 10.59
Rhythm: Irregular
Rate: 90 beats/min
P waves: Fibrillatory waves are present
PR interval: None
QRS duration: 0.08 to 0.10 second
QT interval: Unable to determine
Interpretation: AFib at 90 beats/min

130. Fig. 10.60
Rhythm: Irregular
Rate: 56 beats/min (sinus beats)
P waves: Upright with sinus beats; none with ventricular beats
PR interval: 0.16 second (sinus beats)
QRS duration: 0.06 second (sinus beats)
QT interval: Unable to determine
Interpretation: Sinus bradycardia at 56 beats/min with multiform ventricular bigeminy, a run of VT, and ST-segment depression

131. Fig. 10.61
Rhythm: Irregular
Rate: 130 beats/min
P waves: Vary in size, shape, and direction
PR interval: Varies
QRS duration: 0.08 second
QT interval: Varies
Interpretation: Multifocal atrial tachycardia at 130 beats/min

132. Fig. 10.62
Rhythm: Irregular
Rate: 50 beats/min
P waves: Upright; more Ps than QRSs
PR interval: Lengthens (visible in last three beats)
QRS duration: 0.08 to 0.10 second
QT interval: 0.40 to 0.44 second
Interpretation: Second-degree AV block type I at 50 beats/min with ST-segment depression; note the presence of 2:1 AV block at the start of the rhythm strip

133. Fig. 10.63
Rhythm: Ventricular regular; atrial regular
Rate: Ventricular 34 beats/min; atrial 68 beats/min
P waves: Upright; more Ps than QRSs; 2:1 relationship
PR interval: 0.14 to 0.16 second
QRS duration: 0.10 second
QT interval: 0.52 second (prolonged)
Interpretation: 2:1 AV block at 34 beats/min with ST-segment depression, a prolonged QT interval, and tall T waves

134. Fig. 10.64
Rhythm: Irregular
Rate: 60 beats/min
P waves: Upright; early P wave after beat 3; no P wave with beat 4
PR interval: 0.22 to 0.24 second
QRS duration: 0.08 second (sinus beats)
QT interval: 0.36 to 0.40 second
Interpretation: Sinus rhythm at 60 beats/min with a first-degree AV block, a nonconducted PAC, and a ventricular escape beat

135. Fig. 10.65
Rhythm: Irregular
Rate: 50 beats/min
P waves: Upright before each QRS; a PQRST complex is missing
PR interval: 0.16 second
QRS duration: 0.08 second
QT interval: 0.32 to 0.36 second
Interpretation: Sinus bradycardia at 50 beats/min with an episode of SA block

136. Fig. 10.66
Rhythm: Irregular
Rate: About 330 beats/min
P waves: None
PR interval: None
QRS duration: Varies
QT interval: Unable to determine
Interpretation: PMVT at about 330 beats/min

137. Fig. 10.67
Rhythm: Regular
Rate: Ventricular 90 beats/min; atrial 180 beats/min
P waves: Upright before each QRS; others are hidden in the T waves; 2:1 relationship
PR interval: 0.16 second
QRS duration: 0.06 second
QT interval: 0.24 to 0.28 second
Interpretation: Atrial tachycardia at 90 beats/min with 2:1 block and STE

138. Fig. 10.68
Rhythm: Regular
Rate: 88 beats/min
P waves: Upright
PR interval: 0.16 to 0.20 second
QRS duration: 0.10 to 0.12 second (notched)
QT interval: 0.32 second
Interpretation: Sinus rhythm at 88 beats/min with an incomplete BBB

139. Fig. 10.69
Rhythm: Regular
Rate: 60 beats/min
P waves: None visible
PR interval: None
QRS duration: 0.12 to 0.14 second
QT interval: 0.28 to 0.32 second
Interpretation: Accelerated idioventricular rhythm at 60 beats/min with tall T waves; artifact is present

140. Fig. 10.70
Rhythm: Ventricular irregular; atrial regular
Rate: Ventricular 30 beats/min; atrial 79 beats/min
P waves: Upright; more Ps than QRSs
PR interval: 0.14 second
QRS duration: 0.16 second
QT interval: 0.40 to 0.42 second
Interpretation: Advanced second-degree AV block at 30 beats/min with a wide QRS and STE

141. Fig. 10.71
Rhythm: Regular
Rate: 115 beats/min
P waves: Upright; 1:1 relationship
PR interval: 0.16 second
QRS duration: 0.08 second
QT interval: 0.28 second
Interpretation: Sinus tachycardia at 115 beats/min with STE in V_4; artifact is present

142. Fig. 10.72
Rhythm: Irregular
Rate: 60 beats/min
P waves: Upright (sinus beats); inverted after the QRS in beat 5
PR interval: 0.14 second (sinus beats)
QRS duration: 0.06 second
QT interval: 0.40 to 0.44 second
Interpretation: Sinus rhythm at 60 beats/min with a PJC

143. Fig. 10.73
Rhythm: Regular
Rate: 45 beats/min
P waves: None visible
PR interval: None
QRS duration: 0.08 to 0.11 second
QT interval: 0.48 to 0.52 second (prolonged)
Interpretation: Junctional rhythm at 45 beats/min with STE and a prolonged QT interval

144. Fig. 10.74
Rhythm: Irregular
Rate: 40 beats/min
P waves: Upright (sinus beats); none with beat 2
PR interval: 0.36 second (sinus beats)
QRS duration: 0.06 second (sinus beats)
QT interval: 0.36 to 0.38 second
Interpretation: Sinus bradycardia at 40 beats/min with first-degree AV block and a PJC

145. Fig. 10.75
Rhythm: Irregular
Rate: 71 beats/min (sinus beats)
P waves: Upright before each QRS; one early P wave distorts the T wave of beat 4 (most clearly seen in lead MCL_1)
PR interval: 0.20 second (lead II)
QRS duration: 0.12 second (lead II)
QT interval: 0.40 to 0.44 second (lead II)
Interpretation: Sinus rhythm at 71 beats/min with a wide QRS and a nonconducted PAC

Index

Note: Pages followed by "*f*" refer to figures.